Pediatric Surgery, Flowcharts and Clinical Algorithms

Edited by Sameh Shehata

Published in London, United Kingdom

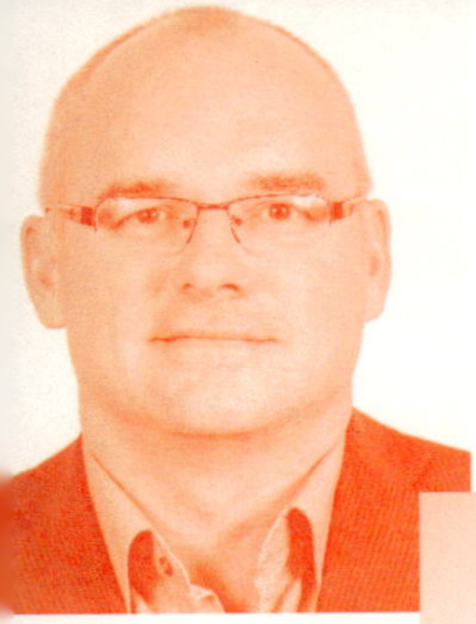
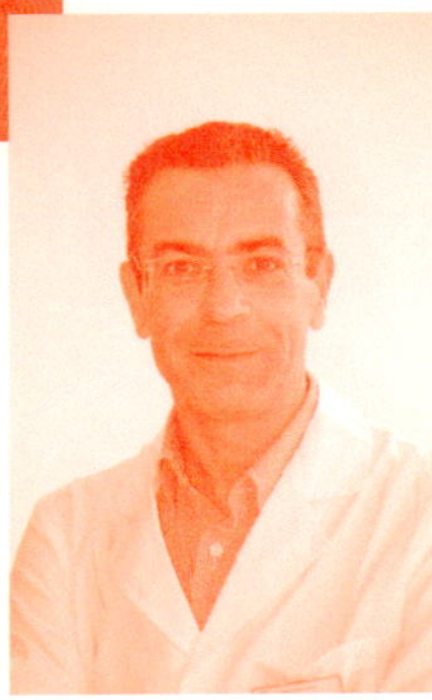
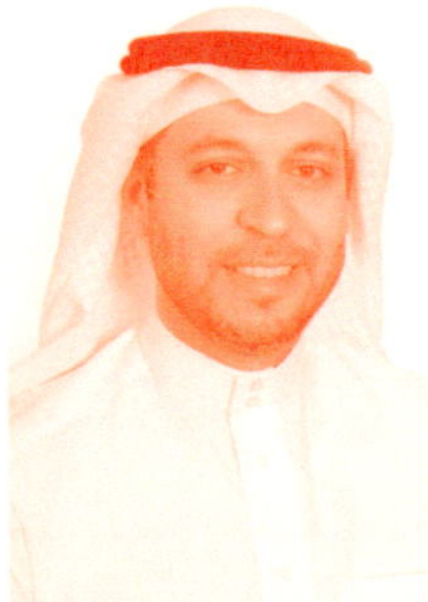
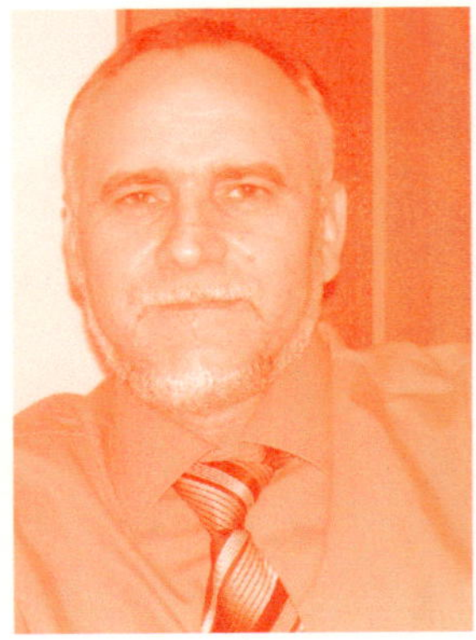
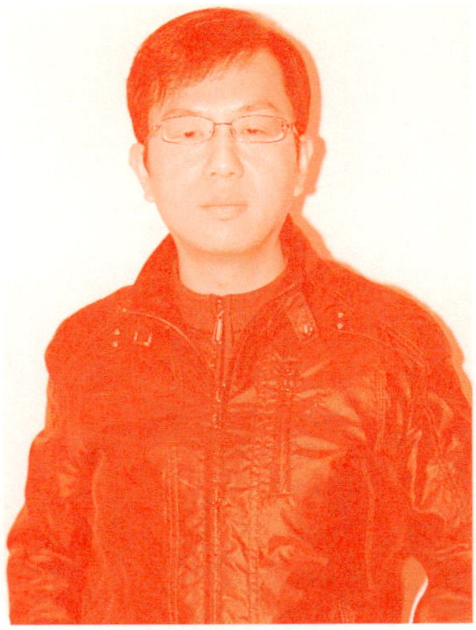
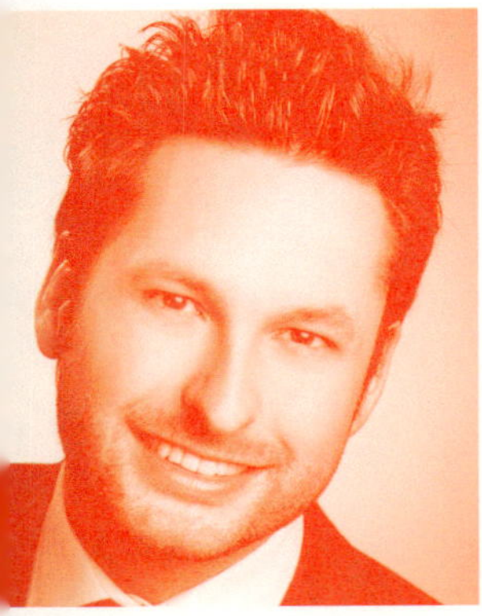
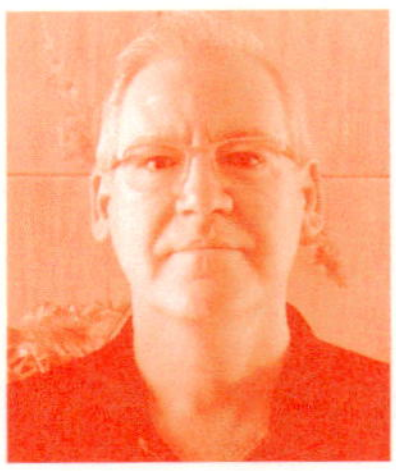

IntechOpen

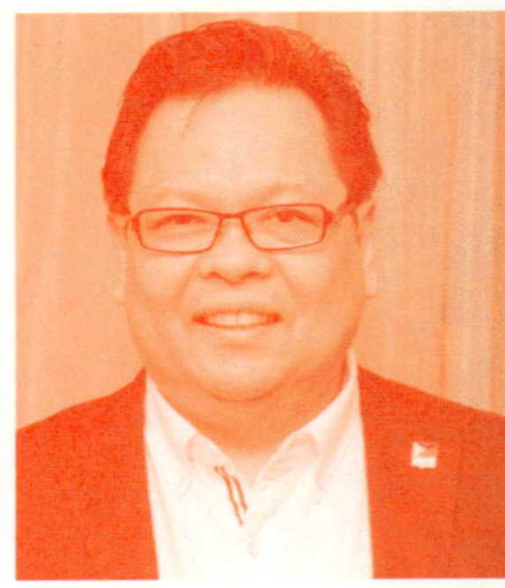
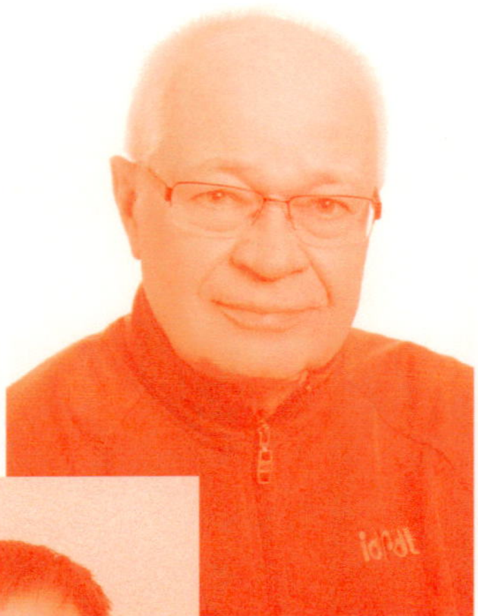
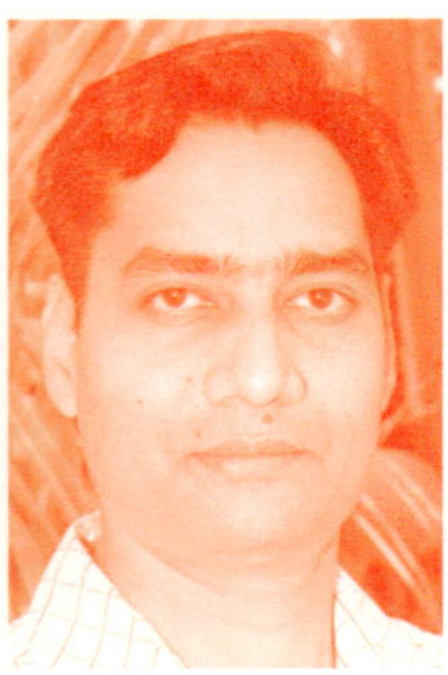
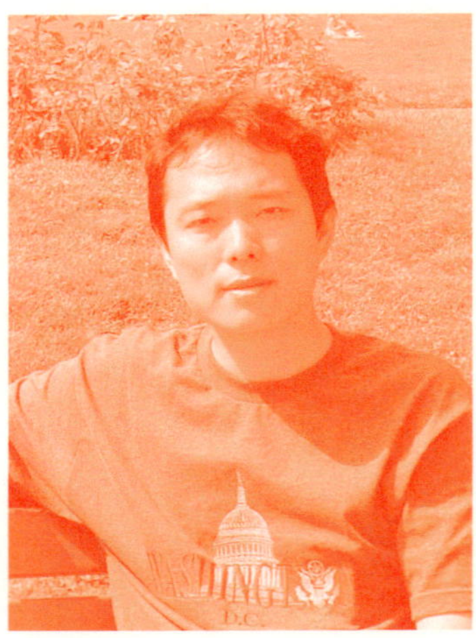
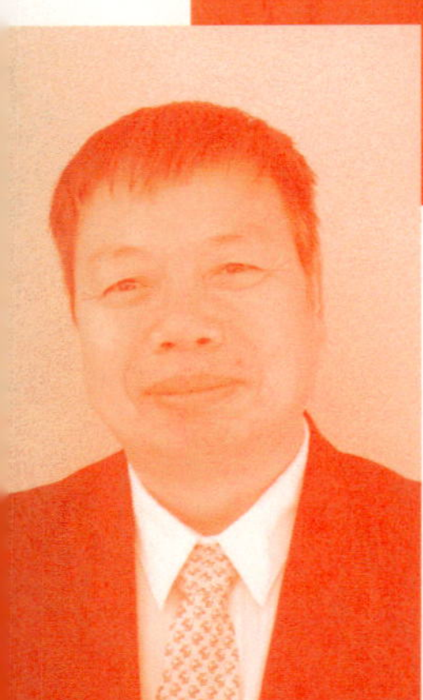
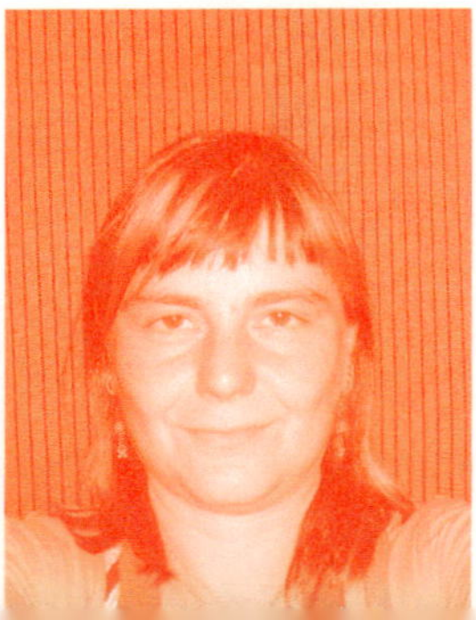

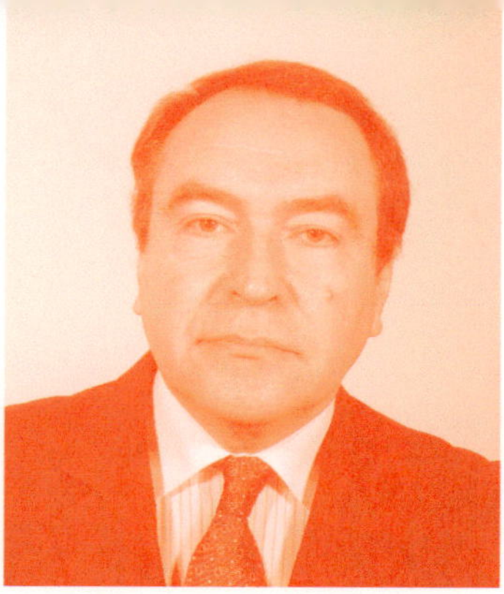
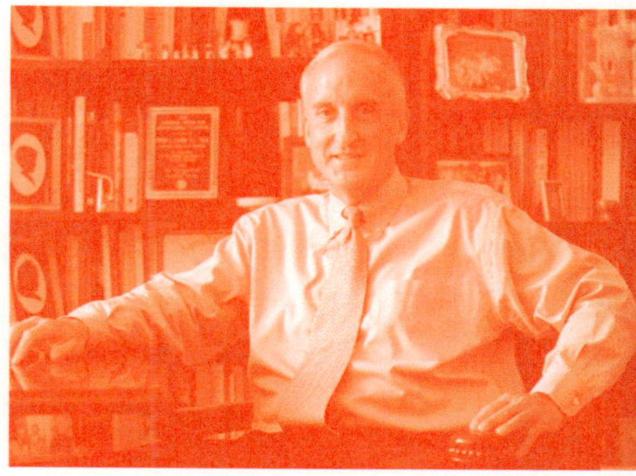
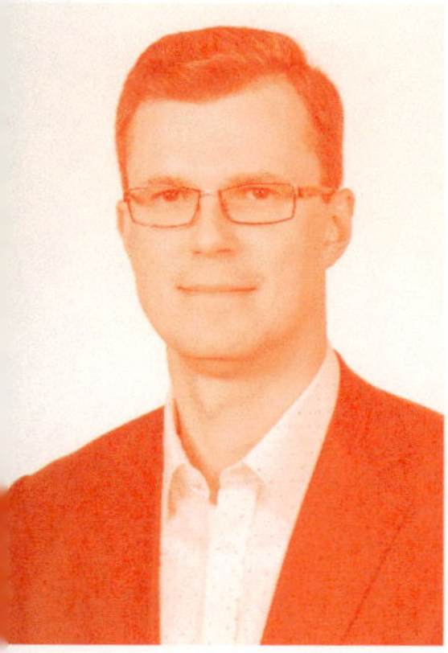
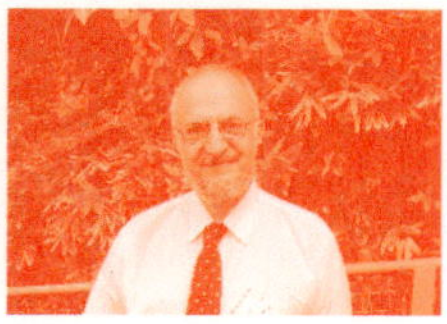
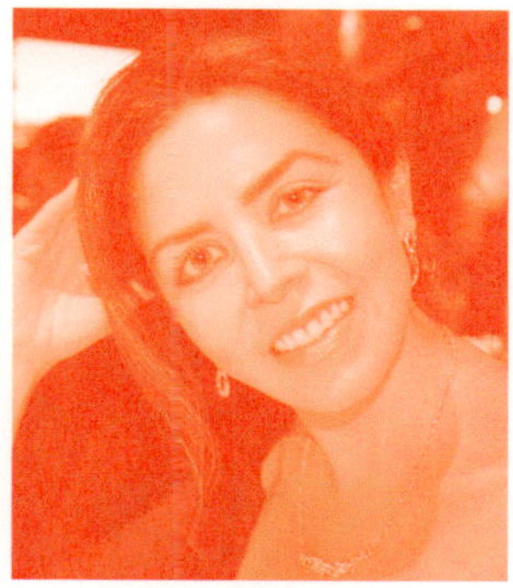

Supporting open minds since 2005

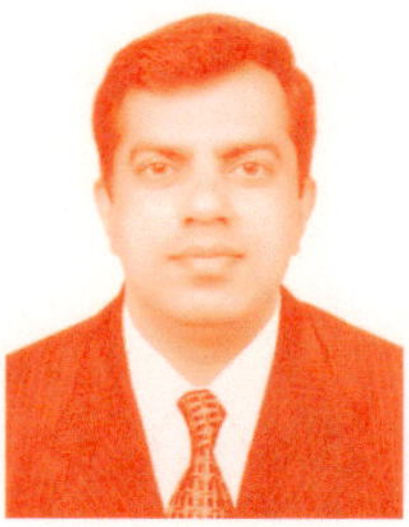
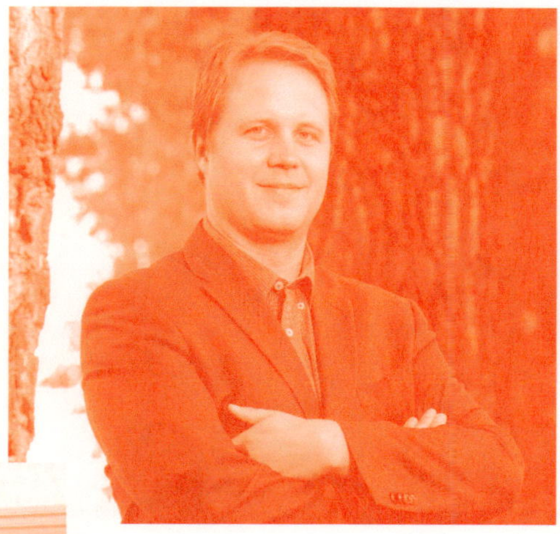
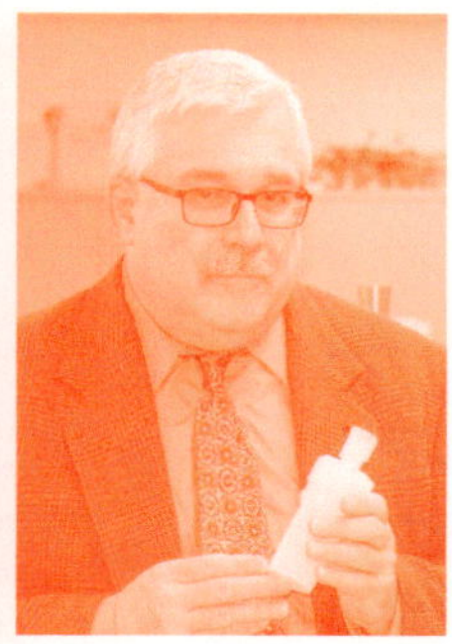
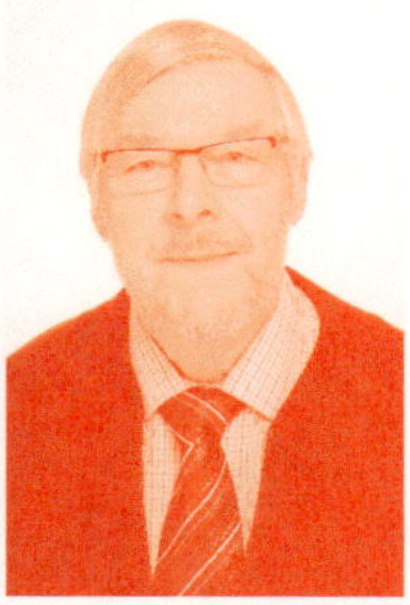
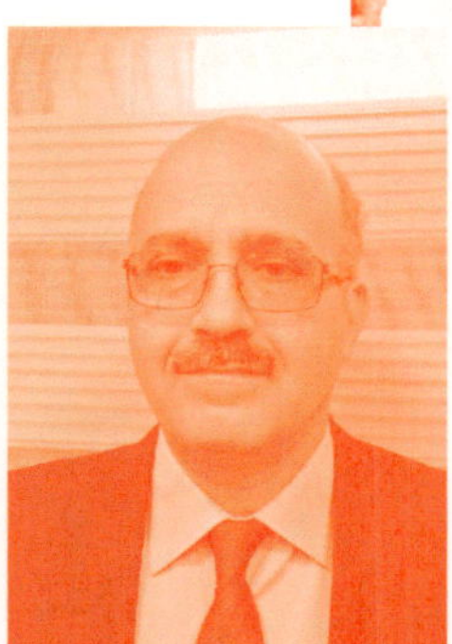
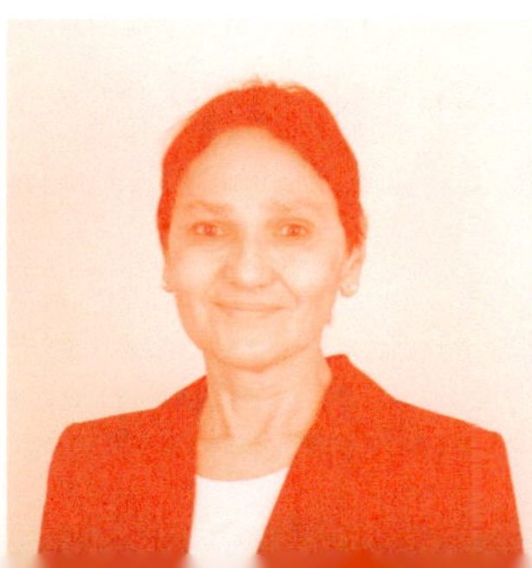
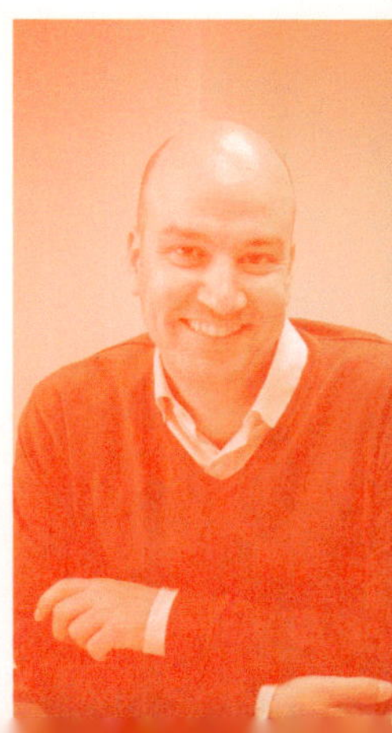

Pediatric Surgery, Flowcharts and Clinical Algorithms
http://dx.doi.org/10.5772/intechopen.78837
Edited by Sameh Shehata

Contributors
Omogiade Udefiagbon, Owolabi Oni, Hasan Özkan Gezer, Alaa Obeida, Aly Shalaby, Samuel Osei-Nketiah, Willam Appeadu-Mensah, Ahmed Abdelghffar Helal, Ameen Alsaggaf, Yazeed Owiwi, Syed Salahuddin, Enaam Raboei, Mazen Zaidan, Alaa Ghallab, Rita Verma, Archana Kota

First published in London, United Kingdom, 2019 by IntechOpen
IntechOpen is the global imprint of INTECHOPEN LIMITED, registered in England and Wales, registration number: 11086078, 7th floor, 10 Lower Thames Street, London, EC3R 6AF, United Kingdom
Printed in Croatia

British Library Cataloguing-in-Publication Data
A catalogue record for this book is available from the British Library

Additional hard and PDF copies can be obtained from orders@intechopen.com

Pediatric Surgery, Flowcharts and Clinical Algorithms
Edited by Sameh Shehata
p. cm.
Print ISBN 978-1-78923-995-9
Online ISBN 978-1-78923-996-6
eBook (PDF) ISBN 978-1-83962-856-6

For EU product safety concerns:
IN TECH d.o.o., Prolaz Marije Krucifikse Kozulić 3, 51000 Rijeka, Croatia, info@intechopen.com or visit our website at intechopen.com.

Meet the editor

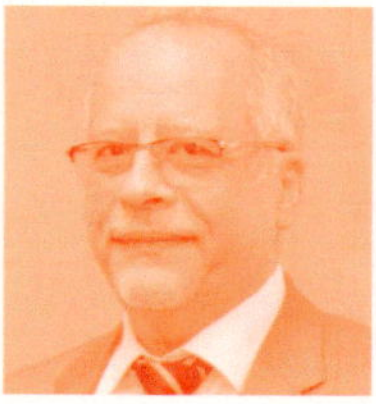

Prof Sameh Shehata is a professor and past chairman of the Pediatric Surgery Department, Faculty of Medicine, University of Alexandria, Egypt. He is the president-elect of the World Federation of Associations of Pediatric Surgery (WOFAPS) and the current president of the International Pediatric Endosurgery Group's (IPEG) Middle East chapter.

Dr. Shehata is the innovator of the laparoscopic traction technique for intra-abdominal testis, known as the "Shehata technique," which is widely practiced now in many centers worldwide.

Dr. Shehata is on the editorial boards of many national and international pediatric surgery journals, including *JPS*, *Medicine*, *Annals of Pediatric Surgery*, and the *International Journal of Urology*.

He has shared as a speaker, keynote speaker, moderator, and panelist at more than 250 national and international meetings.

Contents

Preface

Pediatric Surgery, Flowcharts and Clinical Algorithms is for readers interested in pediatric surgery. It provides updated information about some common topics together with suggested algorithms to assist the clinical management of different disease presentations.

The section on fetal surgery includes a chapter by Dr. Ahmed Abdelghaffar Helal that covers the most common anomalies encountered in fetal screening and possible fetal interventions as well as their success rates and the possible risks to the fetus and the mother.

The section on gastrointestinal disorders includes three chapters. "Gastrointestinal Surgical Disorders in Neonates" by Dr. Rita Verma covers the common gastrointestinal disorders in pediatric surgery, suggested diagnostic approaches, and updated management protocols together with prognosis.

"Oesophageal Atresia: Drowning a Child in His/Her Own Saliva" by Dr. Samuel Osei-Nketiah, and Dr. William Appeadu-Mensahm is a comprehensive review of esophageal atresia starting with a detailed description of the embryology, anatomy and physiology of the esophagus, and ending with antenatal and post-natal diagnosis and resuscitative management.

The chapter also describes different classifications systems and prognostic indicators as well as the surgical strategy for long-gap esophageal atresia, including early and late postoperative complications.

"Meconium Ileus" by Dr. Omogiade Ernest Udefiagbon covers the salient features of meconium ileus including an interesting algorithm to assist in decision making whether using operative or non-operative management.

The hepatobiliary section includes a chapter on "Choledochus Cysts" by Dr. Hasan Özkan Gezer that covers the history and etiology of these malformations and the different classification systems used over time. It discusses investigatory workup as well as the different management options for the different types of cysts, including open and laparoscopic approaches with discussion of the possible postoperative complications.

The section on abdominal wall defects includes a chapter on "Gastroschisis" by Dr. Alaa Obeida and Dr. Aly Shalaby. It covers the important aspects of gastroschisis including etiology and antenatal detection with special emphasis on gastroschisis in low- to middle-income countries. The chapter includes an important section on intraoperative decision making in some of the difficult comorbidities

The section on minimally invasive surgery includes a chapter about "Single-Port Laparoscopic Surgery" by Dr. Enaam Raboei, which is about the tips and tricks of single-incision laparoscopic surgery, clearly showing the advantages and disadvantages of the technique, and some practical examples and personal experience for its application in common pediatric surgical procedures.

The chapter authors have made a great effort to bring the most updated information about these conditions to the pediatric surgeon to facilitate decision making and achieve best results and prognosis.

Sameh Shehata
Alexandria University,
Alexandria, Egypt

Section 1

Fetal Surgery

Chapter 1

Principles of Fetal Surgery

Ahmed Abdelghaffar Helal

Abstract

Fetal therapy (in utero therapy) is a type of special therapy which aims to prevent or correct congenital anomalies in fetus, and prevents their severe consequences on later fetal development. It includes the use of in utero human fetal stem cell transplantation, fetal gene therapy and gene-editing technology as a new treatment for fetal genetic disorders. It started with open fetal surgery and then significantly advancing with innovations, toward minimally invasive fetal procedures, which are undoubtedly the future of fetal surgery, with the goal of providing the best possible fetal outcome, while minimizing the morbidity and mortality to the mother. The goal of fetal treatments is to decrease both fetal and maternal risks and prevent premature rupture of membranes. Fetal ultrasound and MRI are crucial for successful fetal interventions. Moreover, multidisciplinary fetal teams, including fetal surgeon, ultrasonographer, perinatologist, and anesthesiologist, are essential for optimum care to both mother and fetus. Finally, any new modality of fetal therapy must be thoroughly evaluated in animal models before clinical practice. In this chapter, we discuss the basic principles of fetal surgery, milestones of fetal surgery, specific fetal anomalies that are amenable for fetal surgery, successful fetal surgery criteria and future of fetal surgery.

Keywords: fetal therapy, in utero therapy, fetal team, minimally invasive fetal procedures

1. Introduction

Fetal surgery or in utero therapy tries to prevents or corrects multiple congenital anomalies in the fetus to prevent their severe consequences on later fetal development. It started with open fetal surgery then innovations toward minimally invasive procedures have occurred. In this chapter, we discuss the basic principles of fetal surgery, the general history of its development, important specific conditions and procedures used to treat them, and the future of the field.

2. Key points

- The goal of fetal treatments is to decrease both fetal and maternal risk and prevent premature rupture of membranes.

- Real-time ultrasound and fetal MRI is crucial to the implementation and success of fetal procedures.

IntechOpen

- Multidisciplinary fetal teams, including a fetal surgeon, ultrasonographer, perinatologist, and anesthesiologist, are critical to the delivery of optimum care.

3. History and general principles of fetal surgery

In 1963 first fetal intervention was performed (**Table 1**), the first fetal transfusion was reported by Liley. He used Tuohy needle (size 16-G) into the fetal peritoneal space. He injected a contrast material into the amniotic cavity to localize the fetal abdomen and the swallowed contrast opacify the fetal bowel. In the 1970s, endoscopy was used for direct visualization of the fetus, and the first fetal blood sampling or biopsy tissue was reported, however because of the limited technical skill, the therapeutic uses were not applicable [1, 2]. After that, with more use of ultrasound as non-invasive diagnostic tool, the use of diagnostic fetoscopy was replaced with percutaneous needle-based techniques under ultrasound guidance. In the 1980s open fetal surgery was started (direct exposure of the fetus by maternal laparotomy and hysterostomy), then open fetal surgery was replaced with a less invasive fetoscopy, where video camera was inserted inside the uterus under ultrasound guides. At first, fetoscopy was performed in amniotic fluid medium, using a single port to enter the uterine cavity and with a side way working channel. However, amniotic fluid medium poses many limitations for many fetal surgeries especially that require dissection and suture. Low quality images in the fluid medium, and any bleeding will prevent an adequate imaging, and it can end the procedure. Moreover, the "fluctuation" of the fetus during the intervention prevent maintenance of the ideal accessible position. In 2010 Kohl et al. use low insufflation pressure carbon dioxide of amniotic cavity which was left with some amount of amniotic fluid [3–6].

First fetal intervention	1963
Direct visualization of the fetus	1970
Start of open fetal surgery	1982
Thoraco-amniotic fetal shunt placement	1987
Treatment of twin–twin transfusion syndrome by laser ablation	1990
Closure of fetal myelomeningocele using fetoscopy	1997
Treatment of fetal congenital diaphragmatic hernia by tracheal clipping (Fetendo technique)	1997
Excision of fetal amniotic band using fetoscopy	1997
Treatment of fetal congenital diaphragmatic hernia by fetoscopic balloon tracheal occlusion technique	2001

Table 1.
Time scales for important fetal surgeries.

4. Milestones in development of fetal surgery

Criteria for fetal surgery are summarized in **Table 2**.

4.1 Ethical considerations

The ethical issues in the field of fetal surgery are complex because the medical intervention is always invasive, often experimental, involves at least two patients the mother and fetus, and the success rate is difficult to measure. On the

I.	Prompt diagnosis of the pathology and associated anomalies.
II.	Pathophysiology of the disease is documented, and overall prognosis is promising
III.	No curative postnatal treatment.
IV.	Animal models prove feasibility of the in utero technique, preventing serious effects of the pathology.
V.	Fetal therapy performed in specialized multi-disciplinary fetal care centers within clear procedure with local ethics committee approval and signed informed maternal or parent consent.

Table 2.
Successful fetal surgery criteria.

other hand, strong evidence on the benefits of fetal surgery are not present, with many centers considered fetal surgery as an experimental technique to correct fetal anomalies. Controlled randomized studies to evaluate the effects of fetal surgeries on both mother and fetus are still needed. More often, doctors attempt fetal surgery in clinical settings without reporting post-operative outcomes in medical journals. The overall goal of fetal interventions is clear: to improve the health of fetus by intervening before birth to correct or treat prenatally diagnosed abnormalities. Mother and fetus that undergo these interventions must have the same protection afforded to other study participants, with detailed explanation of both short and long-term risks and benefits of these interventions on both the mother and the fetus. Therefore, diagnostic or therapeutic fetal intervention, cannot be performed without mother explicit informed consent (**Table 2**) [7–10].

4.2 Surgical techniques and procedures

4.2.1 Surgical team

In fetal surgery, there are complex diseases and two patients, so careful planning and open communication before, during, and after surgery between the members of the multidisciplinary care team are essential. The team must include pediatric surgery, obstetrics, pediatric anesthesia, obstetric anesthesia, cardiology, radiology, otolaryngology, neonatology, neonatal nursing, and operative room nursing [11, 12].

During any fetal procedures, the use of ultrasound will guide the pediatric surgeon and/or obstetrician and allow for monitor the fetus during surgery. The surgeon should actively communicate with the anesthesia team, as well as nursing and scrub staff, throughout the procedure. Also, the presence of knowledgeable technical support staff familial with the specialized equipment and instrument is essential [13, 14].

4.2.2 Surgical approach

Currently, fetal surgery can be classified into three broader areas; open fetal surgery, minimally invasive fetal surgery and EXIT procedures. Each procedure is subdivided into several subdivisions, in an attempt to treat a wide number of severe pathologies that would compromise the fetus. During minimally invasive fetal surgeries a small skin incision on the mother's abdomen was done. The location of the placenta, as well as the intrauterine pathology will guide the site of the planned incision. 1–2 mm instruments were used to access the fetus are to minimize maternal morbidity. Also, curved instruments may be used to avoid injury to anteriorly placed placenta. During fetal access, any present fluid (ascites, pleural effusions, cystic structures, or the bladder) are aspirated or shunted into the amniotic space. During fetal cardiac valvuloplasty and radiofrequency ablation for treatment of complicated twin gestation, needle-based access is very helpful [15–20].

4.3 Fetoscopic procedures

Usually all patients submitted for a fetoscopic procedure are often pre-medicated with a tocolytic agent. Local or regional anesthesia are usually used. The surgery can be performed in the surgical theater, labor or delivery unit, or in the ultrasound department (depends on gestational age of the fetus). The used instruments, particularly, endoscopes have undergone numerous evolution, based on prototypes developed in animal models. Fetoscopes diameters are between 1.0 and 2.0 mm. Sharp trocars have been developed to accommodate the wide range of diameters used for different operations. Operative fetoscopy is a sonoendoscopic enterprise that has evolved so that the surgical team can see the ultrasound and fetoscopic images simultaneously. Basically, the ultrasound is used to identify an appropriate entry point to direct the trocar into the amniotic cavity, avoiding the placenta and the fetus as well as maternal organs, such as the bowel and bladder. However, some operators have documented the safety, in their hands, of a transplacental approach. Despite this experience, most operators still attempt to avoid the placenta. Nowadays, fetoscopic technique is indicated when direct visualization of the fetus (more than ultrasonography) is needed, as in treatment of cases of twin to twin transfusion syndrome, posterior urethral valves, constricting amniotic bands, and tracheal balloon occlusion for treatment of congenital diaphragmatic hernia. Fetoscopic procedures are performed using 1.2- to 3.0-mm endoscopes. Pictured is a 3 mm 0° endoscope, adjustable length, with a 1-mm working channel (**Figure 1**) [21–29].

4.4 EXIT procedures

EXIT procedures principles is to perform controlled delivery to allow for fetal intervention and establishment of airway prior to cord clamping/cutting. Indications of EXIT procedures includes severe airway obstruction or likelihood of cardiopulmonary insufficiency at birth. Cervical masses, congenital lung malformations (CLM), congenital high airway obstruction (CHAOS), pulmonary agenesis, transition to ECMO. It performed under general anesthesia (fetal anesthesia, uterine relaxation), with maintenance of placental circulation and dorsal supine leftward tilt. Steps includes; Pfannenstiel incision, then customized hysterotomy based on placental location, partial delivery of fetus, and placement of

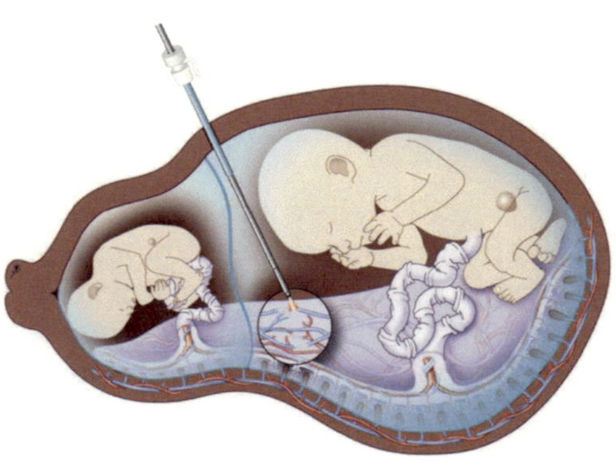

Figure 1.
Fetoscopic laser ablation of abnormal chorionic vessels for TTTS.

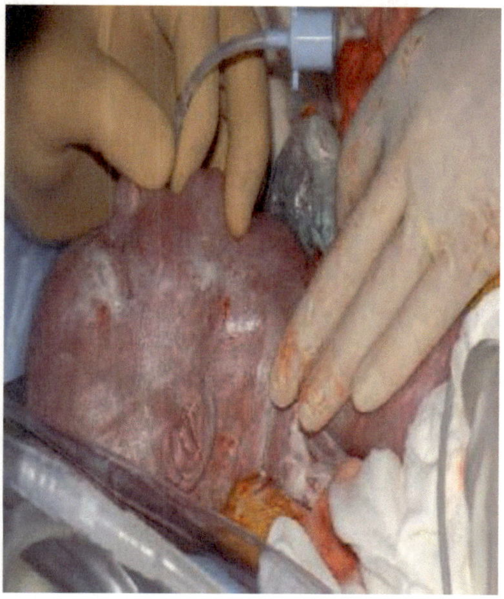

Figure 2.
Successful oro-tracheal intubation during the EXIT procedure.

monitors, fetal airway establishment during surgical intervention then delivery was completed with, transition of the baby to postnatal care, and finally completion of cesarean section (**Figure 2**) [30, 31].

4.4.1 Anesthetic care

Before anesthesia, all physiological changes associated with pregnancy must be considered. The effects of pregnancy on mother pulmonary and cardiovascular function must be considered. Adequate precautions should be taken to prevent hypoxemia and aspiration. The magnesium sulfate used in tocolysis may decreases capillary oncotic pressure and increases capillary permeability with increased risk of pulmonary edema. Aorto-caval compression must be prevented by using left uterine displacement. The doses of anesthetic drugs must be adjusted. Maternal local anesthesia can be effectively used for most needle-based and single port fetoscopic procedures. When multiple ports or caesarian section could be necessary, regional anesthesia; epidural or combined spinal epidural can be added. On the other hand, fetal anesthesia is indicated only for endoscopic procedures performed directly on the fetus. All fetal anesthetic drugs are typically administered through intramuscular route and consists of opiates and non-depolarizing muscle relaxants. Atropine is usually given to avoid fetal bradycardia. For placental or cord procedures with no direct fetal contact, the risk–benefit of fetal anesthesia should be weighed [32–35].

5. Drawbacks of fetal surgery

The drawbacks of fetal surgery, includes bleeding, amniotic fluid leak, chorioamnionic separation, chorioamnionitis, premature rupture of membranes, preterm labor, preterm birth, and fetal loss. Premature rupture of membranes, preterm labor is the most common complication of minimally invasive fetal surgery, with high morbidity, including oligohydramnios, chorioamnionitis, and preterm delivery. However, accurate analysis of the frequency of these complications are difficult due to variations in both the assessment of the complication as well as reporting methods. Factors increasing the risk during minimally invasive fetal procedures include the number of ports and the diameter of the used instruments. A systematic review of 1376 minimally invasive fetal procedures for lower urinary tract obstruction, and twin reversed arterial perfusion reported that increased diameter of the instrument and increased number of ports are major predictors of iatrogenic premature rupture of membranes [36–38].

Following open fetal procedure, risk of hysterotomy scar weakness may interrupt both current and future labor. Some cases of uterine scar rupture after open fetal procedure was reported, starting from the second trimester, may be caused only by the uterine distension (with no uterine contractions) which form significant risk to both mother and fetus. Moreover, maternal counseling about the risk of delivery complications must be considered. On the other hand, minimally invasive fetal procedures do not preclude vaginal delivery. However, long-term follow-up of subsequent pregnancies after these procedures is not available, beside the complications of repeat caesarian section, significant advantage of minimally invasive fetal procedures should be considered [39, 40].

6. Certain problems amenable for fetal surgery

Some important indications for fetal interventions are summarized in **Table 3**.

6.1 Twin gestations

6.1.1 Twin–twin transfusion syndrome (TTTS)

Monochorionic (shared) placenta with A-V, V-V, A-A connections and unbalanced flow between two twins

- Donor – low flow, oligohydramnios, high output heart failure, brain ischemia, small

- Recipient – fluid overload, polyhydramnios, congestive heart failure, hydrops fetalis, large

Prognosis: 80–90% mortality for both if untreated.

Fetal Surgery

- High-volume amnioreduction historically (survival of at least one twin 60%)

- Fetoscopic laser ablation of vascular connections

  Offered to Stage II or greater
  Selective A-V or nonselective

76% single survivor, 36% dual survivors.

The donor twin usually develops hypovolemia, leading to oliguria and oligohydramnios from reduced renal perfusion, and the recipient twin suffers the consequences of hypervolemia, including polyuria and polyhydramnios. Both twins are at risk for significant morbidity [41, 42].

Basic principles for TTTS interventions are to prevent preterm delivery caused by polyhydramnios, through removing the excess amniotic fluid surrounding

Fetal surgery	Why to interfere?
I-Surgery on the fetus	
Congenital diaphragmatic hernia	Avoidance of pulmonary hypoplasia and pulmonary hypertension
Sacrococcygeal teratoma	Stop of steal phenomenon, avoid cardiac failure and polyhydramnios
Thoracic space-occupying lesions	Avoid pulmonary hypoplasia and cardiac failure
Lower urinary tract obstruction	Avoid renal failure and pulmonary hypoplasia
Cardiac malformations	Avoid hypoplasia or progressing damage to developing heart
Myelomeningocele	Repair of exposed spinal nerves, stop cerebrospinal fluid leakage, prevent hydrocephaly and hindbrain herniation
II- Placenta, cord or membranes surgery	
Complicated monochorionic pregnancies:	Arrest of feto-fetal transfusion and its consequences
Twin–twin transfusion syndrome (TTTS)	Avoid preterm delivery
Twin-reversed-arterial-perfusion sequence (TRAP) and other discordant anomalies	Avoid damage to co-twin
Twin-anemia polycythaemia sequence	In some conditions (TTTS/TRAP) reversal of cardiac failure and polyhydramnios
III- Selective intra-uterine growth restriction	
Amniotic band syndrome	Avoid deformities and functional loss
Chorioangioma	Avoid of cardiac failure, hydrops fetoplacental and polyhydramnios

Table 3.
Some important indications for fetal surgery.

the recipient twin, with improved fetal circulation by decreasing pressure on the chorionic plate. In 1990, fetoscopic laser was used to coagulate the crossing superficial blood vessels separating the 2 fetal circulations and destroying the inter-twin vessels that cause discordant twin–twin transfusion. Nowadays, laser ablation is the preferred treatment for TTTS between 16 and 26 weeks of gestation. The procedure is performed through a single uterine access site using a fetoscope and thin laser (**Table 4**) [43–45].

6.1.2 Twin reversed arterial perfusion

One normal twin acts as a "pump" for a cardiac, a cephalic twin via A-A anastomoses

I	Presence of Poly and oligohydramnios
II	Stage I plus non-visualized bladder in donor twin
III	Stage II plus seriously abnormal Doppler (umbilical artery absent or reversed end-diastolic velocity, ductus venosus reversed flow, pulsatile umbilical venous flow)
IV	Stage III plus evidence of hydrops in either twin
V	Fetal death

Table 4.
Staging of TTTS.

Normal twin much like donor twin in TTTS with R/O high output heart failure, hydrops fetalis, 50% mortality

Fetal Surgery

- Open hysterotomy/delivery
- Fetoscopic ligation
- Bipolar cautery/harmonic scalpel division
- Thermal/laser coagulation
- RFA of acardiac/acephalic cord insertion

6.1.3 Selective fetal reduction

In addition to TTTS, other serious problem that can affect monochorionic twin pregnancies, includes severe intrauterine growth restriction, structural anomalies, twin anemia polycythemia sequence, and TRAP sequence, or a cardiac twinning. In some complicated monochorionic pregnancies, elective fetal reduction is recommended especially for high risk of hemodynamic compromise or intrauterine fetal death, aimed to prevent neurologic injury or demise to the co-twin. Fetal intra-cardiac potassium chloride injection is contraindicated in these pregnancies, because of risk of transmission between twins and selective termination must be performed with interruption of blood flow to the fetus. This interruption usually performed through ligation of the umbilical cord, fetoscopic laser coagulation, ultrasound-guided and bipolar cord coagulation. Selective fetal reduction was seriously indicated in complicated twin pregnancies what is TRAP sequence. In TRAP sequence, one twin is incompatible with life due to absent or rudimentary heart, as well as absence of other vital structures, as head (anencephaly). This twin usually has no placental blood supply, and it receives its blood supply directly through vascular connections from the second normal twin (acts as pump twin). Therefore, the normal twin will rapidly develop high-output heart failure, with more than 50% mortality rate. Selective fetal reduction aims to stop blood flow to incompatible with life twin, and save the life of normal (pump) twin. In the largest review from 12 fetal centers from the North American Fetal Therapy Network registry data, identified 98 patients who underwent percutaneous radio frequency ablation of a cardiac twin. In this series, the overall survival of the normal (pump) twin to 30 days was 80% [46–50].

6.2 Lower urinary tract obstruction (LUTO)

LUTO can be caused by stenosis of the urethral meatus, valves, urethral atresia, ectopic insertion of a ureter or peri-vesical tumors. Bladder shunts are effective for urine diversion, restoring amniotic fluid and thereby preventing pulmonary hypoplasia. Whether shunting effectively salvages renal function is uncertain. For that, prior accurate assessment of renal function is required. The actual anatomical cause of LUTO proved to be an important predictor. Posterior urethral valves do much better in the long run, while babies with urethral atresias or the Prune Belly phenotype do less well. At the moment, the two commonly used techniques, are percutaneous vesico-amniotic shunting, under ultrasound guide, where double pigtail stent is inserted, usually combined with amnio-infusion. The second procedure is fetal cystoscopy, where fetoscope is inserted into the fetal bladder, to diagnose the source of obstruction and to ablate PUV. The commonly used methods to ablate the valve, includes guide wires, hydro-ablation and laser-ablation. The first open clinical fetal surgical intervention for a case of lower urinary tract obstruction (LUTO), not eligible for shunt placement. Instead, fetal ureterostomies were successfully created. There were no maternal complications, but unfortunately the fetus never produced any urine. On the other hand, main complications of shunting include; failure to insert the catheter, occlusion of the catheter, dislocation, and sometimes fistula formation. In order to conclude and evaluate the results of in-utero VAS, and its long-term outcomes, randomized, controlled trial, "Percutaneous vesico-amniotic shunting versus conservative management for fetal Lower Urinary Tract Obstruction" (PLUTO), was performed in the United Kingdom, Ireland, and the Netherlands from 2006 to 2012. The study performed on 31 cases (16 submitted to VAS, 15 undergo conservative treatment). Study reported that fetal cystoscopy, although it is more invasive than VAS, it has the advantage of confirming the diagnosis of PUV, and more accurate in selection of patients who will benefit from valve ablation. In other multi-centric retrospective study includes 50 cases submitted to fetal cystoscopies for treatment of LUTO, 30 fetuses were diagnosed with PUV and were treated with laser-ablation. Other 13 fetuses were diagnosed with urethral atresia, 5 fetus diagnosed with urethral stenosis, and 2 fetuses diagnosed with trisomy 18 (not treated). The results of the 54 fetuses with normal karyotype were, 32.4 weeks mean delivery gestational age, and 34.8% overall 2 years' survival. For PUV patients treated with laser-ablation, 53.6% 2 years' survival. Although 20% (6 of the 30) developed recurrence of LUTO symptoms, and further fetal procedure was performed in 10% (3 patients). Postnatal ablation of PUV was needed in 10 of the 17 survivors. Normal renal function at 2 years of age, was achieved in 75% of infants with PUV (12 of the 16), which considered more promising than the 29% reported in the PLUTO trial with VAS. Reports up to date indicate that, minimally invasive fetal procedure (in selected cases of LUTO), can improve the survival when compared to expectant treatment. However, studies of long term renal function are less encouraging [51–56].

6.3 Intrauterine myelo-meningocele (IMM)

IMM, or Spina bifida, is defined as failure of complete closure of the neural tube with exposure of the spinal canal structures. Lumbar or cervical vertebral levels are the most commonly affected sites, however IMM can occur anywhere along the spine. Neurologic deficits with motor and somato-sensory abnormalities are the most feared complications. In addition, bowel and bladder function may be affected due to injury of autonomic nervous system. Moreover, mostly all patients with IMM will develop Arnold-Chiari II malformation affecting hindbrain, with non-communicating hydrocephalus, which requires ventriculo-peritoneal shunting. Although mortality of IMM was low in the perinatal period, its long-term neurologic morbidity may be fatal, and up to 30% of patients may die before adulthood [57–60].

6.3.1 IMM repair

At the moment, the compared outcomes of pre-natal versus post-natal repair of IMM showed that; although prenatal surgery has an increased risk of preterm delivery, pre-natal repair had significantly better outcomes than the post-natal repair. Pre-natal repair for IMM decrease the risk of death and subsequent needs for shunting (nearly at age of 12 months). Also, pre-natal repair improves scores of mental and motor function (at 30 months). However, pre-natal repair was associated with an increased risk of preterm delivery and uterine dehiscence at labor. Therefore, the potential benefits of pre-natal repair must be balanced against the risks of prematurity and maternal morbidity [61–65]. In a retrospective review of 54 children evaluated for lower extremity neuro-motor function and short-term ambulatory function following fetal myelomeningocele closure, they concluded that fetal myelomeningocele repair results in better than predicted lower extremity neuro-motor function at birth and short-term ambulatory status. However, these children continue to demonstrate movement incoordination which is characteristic for children with Spina-bifida. In retrospective study evaluated the incidence and clinical implications of the development of cutaneously derived intradural inclusion cysts (ICs) following fetal myelomeningocele closure through parental questionnaire. They concluded that intradural ICs can develop following fetal myelomeningocele repair. ICs long-term complications in these children may include deterioration of bladder function, and loss of lower-extremity function after fetal myelomeningocele closure. Koh et al. 2006 compared urodynamic findings in patients who underwent pre-natal closure of IMM with those of patients who underwent post-natal closure. All pre-natally treated patients had lower lumbo-sacral lesions on neurological examination. In comparison, 39% of post-natally treated patients showed lack of sphincter activity at newborn examination, with similar findings noted at 1-year evaluation. Regarding bladder function, all pre-natally treated patients showed detrusor over-activity, compared to 38% of post-natally treated patients, up to 1-year evaluation. They concluded that fetal closure of IMM is associated with a higher incidence of complete denervation of the external urethral sphincter and detrusor over-activity compared to post-natal repair. Open fetal IMM closure has been extensively studied and its benefits to the fetus have been proven. Minimally invasive fetoscopic repair is technically difficult, with high risk of membrane separation and premature rupture of membrane, and its benefits to the fetus have not been proved. Therefore, minimally invasive IMM repair still needs further more studies to confirm its validity for clinical applications [66–70].

6.4 Congenital diaphragmatic hernia (CDH)

One in 2500 live infant births may be affected with CDH. It consists of abnormal defect in the fetal diaphragm, resulting in herniation of all or part of abdominal viscera into the thoracic cavity (according to the defect size). Pulmonary hypoplasia and pulmonary hypertension, usually present as a result of abnormal development of the lungs and pulmonary vasculature, this may cause persistent fetal circulation and respiratory failure with increased mortality rate. Despite great improvement in its diagnosis and treatment, infant mortality from isolated CDH still about 20–30%. Poor prognostic indicators by ultrasonography include low lung-to-head ratio, liver herniation into the thoracic cavity, and low total lung volume detected by fetal MRI. Initial experimental studies using sheep models demonstrated that prenatal repair of the diaphragmatic hernia could reverse the pulmonary hypoplasia caused by a surgically created CDH. The first clinical experience in humans likewise involved open fetal surgery. High fetal mortality rate is associated with this approach, because of umbilical vein kinking during reduction of the herniated liver into the fetal abdomen. Therefore, all recent studies consider that minimally invasive methods, taking the upper hand for treatment of CDH, as it stimulates lung growth in utero, while open fetal repair of the diaphragmatic defect was abandoned from the clinical use. Preliminary experimental studies in fetal lambs were promising, demonstrating that fetal tracheal occlusion improved fetal lung growth and reducing the severity of pulmonary hypoplasia. In cases of severe CDH, postnatal mortality appears to be significantly lower with in utero surgical intervention. Studies of fetal endoscopic tracheal occlusion (FETO) performed in cases of severe CDH have demonstrated a significantly higher survival rate compared with control fetuses that did not undergo

FETO. Severe PAH occurred in 47% of fetuses that underwent FETO, but in 89% of patients in the prenatal expectant management group (**Figure 3**) [58, 71, 72].

So, fetal surgeons prefer minimally invasive procedures to avoid large hysterotomy and adequately visualize and access the fetal trachea. In 1997 the first fetal endoscopic (Fetendo) tracheal clipping, was done in human fetus, where maternal laparotomy was done, then 4 trocars was inserted through uterus to access and clip the fetal trachea. For the fear of serious complications of tracheal damage and vocal cord paralysis during clipping, fetoscopic balloon tracheal occlusion technique was introduced, in which no fetal neck dissection and only single uterine port was needed. Fetal endoscopic tracheal occlusion (FETO) is usually performed between 26 and 30 weeks of gestation., A trocar is placed through the maternal abdomen into the amniotic cavity guided by ultrasound, and fetoscope is inserted through the fetal mouth, then advanced into the fetal trachea. Once the carina has been retched, the balloon is inflating with physiologic solution and left just above the carina. The correct position is then checked by ultrasound imaging. In some studies, the tracheal balloon was removed at the time of delivery through ex utero intrapartum therapy. However, balloon removal before birth not only allows for the possibility of vaginal birth, but also was shown to increase pneumocyte cells differentiation type II, with increasing surfactant production. Currently, tracheal occlusion can be reversed in utero, by performing second fetoscopic procedure (typically at 34 weeks of gestation) [73, 74]. A multicenter European series including 210 cases of FETO with severe CDH (liver up and lung-to-head ratio ≤ 1) they reported 48.0% rate of survival to discharge, with 47.1% incidence of premature rupture of membrane. Up to date meta-analysis comparing survival outcome between FETO and a contemporary control group, reported that FETO improves survival compared with standard perinatal care in fetuses with isolated CDH and severe pulmonary hypoplasia (lung-to-head ratio ≤ 1). 46.3% of fetuses (Fifty-one of 110) who had undergone FETO survived to discharge, compared with 5.9% (6 of 101) in the control group, giving the FETO group more significant survival chance. However, the true benefits of FETO are difficult to determine because the severity of CDH was not measured uniformly and there was great variability in the postnatal care of these infants. International, randomized controlled studies to evaluate the role of intrauterine fetal surgery in CDH cases with moderate and severe pulmonary hypoplasia is still needed [75].

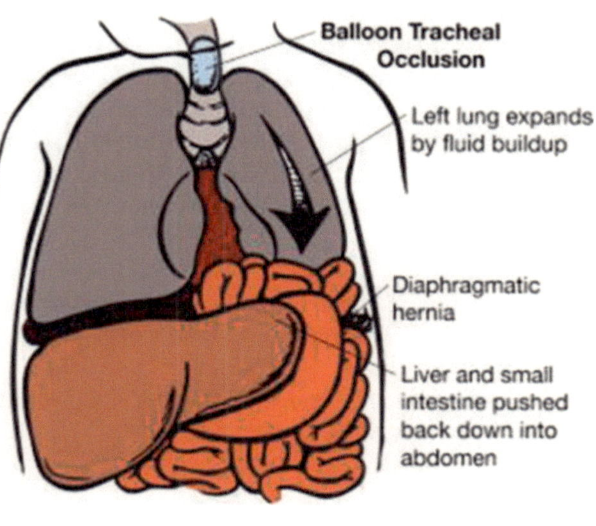

Figure 3.
Tracheal occlusion in fetus with congenital diaphragmatic hernia (CDH) to increases lung volume, decreases herniation of abdominal viscera, and improves postnatal lung function.

6.5 Amniotic band syndrome (ABS)

Amniotic band syndrome can lead to fetal death from umbilical cord strangulation and/or congenital limb deformity or loss, presumed to result from ischemia caused by constriction bands that interfere with vascular perfusion. There is increasing experience with intrauterine release of congenital constrictions and evidence is mounting that this therapy may help save/restore some limb function and morphology. The location of the bands and timing of fetal damage will affect the presentation, severity, and outcome of the condition. For example, pseudosyndactyly or limb amputation can be the results of constriction bands at the extremities, whereas more midline bands can result in craniofacial, thoracic, or abdominal defects, and may be fatal. The etiology of this syndrome is unknown, and theories range from a genetic basis or early disruption of the germinal disc to traumatic disruption of the membranes later in fetal development. Fetoscopic release of amniotic bands using minimally invasive surgery, can help in preservation of life and or limb saving in cases of ABS. The present acceptable functional outcome in 50% of cases is promising, although, clear selection criteria are needed to justify the risk of this in-utero invasive procedure, through increased experience and larger studies on this type of therapy for ABS (**Figure 4**).

In cases of extremity involvement by amniotic band syndrome, the band must be released using fetoscope to save the normal development of the limb and allow for normal limb function. Ultrasound imaging can easily diagnose the problem, showing; distal limb edema and interrupted blood flow by Doppler, with or without visualization of the constricting band. Although, the available reports include small case series, its results suggest that fetuses must have distal arterial limb flow detected by Doppler in order to benefit from intervention. Moreover, data from recent studies reported that fetuses with single limb involvement tend to do better than those with multiple involved limbs. Surprising, the incidence of PROM with this procedure seem to be higher than for other fetoscopic procedures, (reported rates up to 78%). Although, small number of cases were reported in all available studies, and considering the learning curve in this studies, it could also be related to inherent membrane problems in these fetuses [76, 77].

6.6 Sacrococcygeal teratoma (SCT)

Although the mortality rate is 5% for SCT diagnosed in the newborn, the mortality rate is about 50% for fetal SCT. Rupture of the tumor, or hemorrhage inside, or high output heart failure, and premature labor, form the main causes of fetal loss. Every attempt at interventions, to prevent this high prenatal mortality are the target of study of several fetal centers. Resection of the tumor (in utero) should be consider for treatment of pre-mature patients with early signs of heart failure or placentomegaly.

- Removal of the external part of the tumor is usually preferred, followed by later removal of its pelvic extension.

- Alternatively, radio-frequency, or thermal ablation can be used to occlude supplying arteries to the tumor.

It is important to note the related morbidity of all mentioned procedures, like risk of preterm delivery, beside procedure failure rate. The related morbidity can be reduced with minimally invasive procedures, however, the fear from decreased efficacy in local control, still a significant problem. Moreover, these less invasive

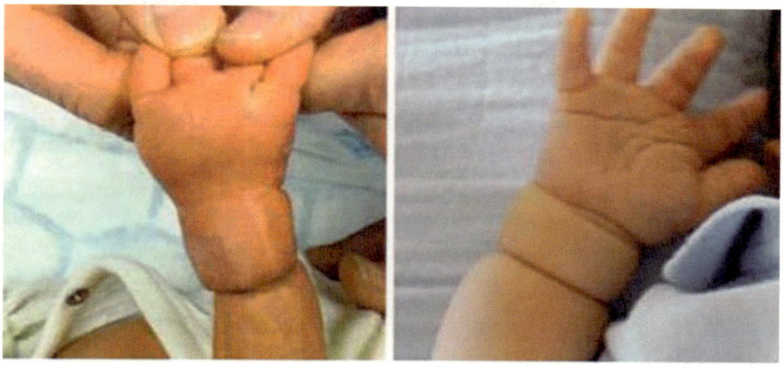

Figure 4.
Some amniotic bands may constrict fetal limbs, and may be serious to cause limb amputation.

procedures should be used as early as possible, preferably before early signs of heart failure, to prevent IUFD. Certainly the best option is complete tumor resection, if possible. A systematic review on 34 cases of SCT from 1980 to 2013, using minimally invasive fetal procedures, they reported 44% (14/32) overall survival with 29.7 ± 4.0 weeks, as mean gestational delivery age. They considered heart failure as a bad prognostic indicator, (30% survival rate (6/20)). Another review compares two minimally invasive procedures, direct tumor control, and vascular occlusion of the tumor feeding vessels. Study included 33 cases, 11 cases submitted to vascular occlusion (group A) and 22 submitted to direct tumor control (group B). They reported 63.6% (7/11) survival in vascular ablation (group A) compared to 40.9% (9/22) in direct tumor control (group B). They claimed that reduction of the tumor blood supply slowly appears safer than rapid tumor necrosis which may lead to hemorrhage inside the tumor. Regarding outcomes of fetuses with large SCTs and fetal hydrops before viability, due to rarity of the tumor the available small case series suggest that fetal intervention does confer a survival advantage. However, randomized trials are needed to make a valuable conclusion, also long-term outcomes data are needed. Because these procedures are associated with significant risks, so to get the best benefit these patients must be performed only in specialized centers, and must be limited to cases presented with both high-output heart failure and fetal hydrops [78].

6.7 Cystic pulmonary airway malformations (CPAM)

Most prenatally detected lung lesions are cystic pulmonary airway malformations (CPAM), broncho-pulmonar sequestrations or so called 'hybrid' lesions, containing features of both. The outcome of most lesions are favorable even without pre-natal intervention, despite often impressive appearance at mid-gestation. During pregnancy many lesions may regress, or disappear completely. Therefore, non-operative treatment (watchful waiting) is preferred by most fetal surgeons. Surprisingly, pressure effect or hemo-dynamic changes may cause sudden physiologic derangements, which may end with progressive heart failure and intrauterine demise. Therefore, pre-natal intervention may be warranted to improve outcome. Pre-natal interventions for fetal lung lesions aim to alleviate the pressure effect of the mass by partial or complete removal of the lesion. Many surgical and non-surgical options have been reported.

- In macrocystic lesions, needle thoraco-centesis or thoraco-amniotic shunt drainage under ultrasound guided may be used for decompression.

- In microcystic lesions, cysts are too small for drainage. In these cases, open fetal surgery has been performed.

- When a systemic feeding vessel is found, percutaneous laser coagulation or injection of a sclerosing agent can be successful.

Routine ultrasound used as screening method for detection of congenital lung lesions and require referral to a specialist center. Other co-existing problems of the fetus should be carefully evaluated to determine, the magnitude of related complications, delivery place, time and type, and if intra-uterine intervention is needed. Minimally invasive intra-uterine fetal intervention for severe lesions can greatly improve the prognosis of these fetuses. In a large study of thoraco-amniotic shunt placement for congenital lung mass or pleural effusion, performed on 75 fetuses at Children's Hospital of Philadelphia, they showed 55% decrease in congenital cystic adenomatoid malformation volume and 27% of cases showed complete drainage of pleural effusion (73% showed partial drainage of effusions) with hydrops resolution in 83% of fetuses (43/53), which was greatly correlated with survival. Survival to delivery was 93% (70/75), median gestational age was 36 weeks, with 68% (51/75) long-term survival rate. Fifty-six percent of fetuses were delivered at an average of 10 weeks after shunt placement. Duration of stay in the neonatal intensive care unit of 21 days, with for greater than 24 hours. This series affirms the survival benefit risk patients, but underscores the risks inherent to in utero intensive neonatal therapy required [79, 80].

7. Future of fetal surgery

Minimally invasive treatment is undoubtedly the future of fetal surgery, with the goal of providing the best possible outcome for the fetus, while minimizing the morbidity or mortality to the mother. So the concept of treating two patients at the same time is the challenging goal. To this end, significant efforts are being made toward safest methods for fetal intervention, particularly premature rupture of membranes. Currently a collaboration between University of California San Francisco, the University of California Berkeley, and Caltech is focusing on the development of a biocompatible adhesive (methyldihydroxyphenylalanine-based polymers) to preseal amniotic membranes before fetal surgery to prevent PPROM. This formula is currently under development and called "Amnioseal" which can be delivered just below the uterus to preseal the fetal membrane before amniotic access. At the moment, prenatal stem cell transplantation and gene therapy is under extensive research to treat a wide range of genetic conditions, and to extend the current application of fetal surgical intervention for only correction of structural fetal anomalies. The in utero stem cell transplantation will prevent the process of abnormal immune development before the fetus cellular differentiations. Two types of fetal stem cell therapy are currently under investigations for potential clinical use the in utero hematopoietic stem cell transplantation and mesenchymal stem cell transplantation. Many recent clinical trials of in utero hematopoietic stem cell transplantation reported that it has had a limited success in recipients without underlying immunodeficiency, however, some experimental data in a large animal model of intrauterine hematopoietic stem cell transplantation have demonstrated clinically relevant levels of chimerism, may be supporting its role for inherited hematologic disorders. On the other hand, the use of in utero human fetal mesenchymal stem cell transplantation has been reported for osteogenesis imperfect, although the preliminary results are promising, it temporally results. Finally, the studies of fetal gene therapy and gene-editing technology as a new treatment lines for fetal genetic disorders, are significantly advancing in the field of fetal therapy. However, the safety and long-term effect of these new types of treatment must be thoroughly evaluated in animal models before its applications in clinical practice.

Author details

Ahmed Abdelghaffar Helal
Pediatric Surgery Department, Faculty of Medicine, Al-Azhar University, Cairo, Egypt

*Address all correspondence to: helalhmada@azhar.edu.eg

References

[1] Adzick NS. Fetal surgery for spina bifida: Past, present, future. Seminars in Pediatric Surgery. 2013;**22**:10-17

[2] Adzick NS, Thom EA, Spong CY, et al. A randomized trial of prenatal versus postnatal repair of myelomeningocele. The New England Journal of Medicine. 2011;**364**:993e1004

[3] American College of Obstetricians and Gynecologists. Committee on ethics; American Academy of Pediatrics, committee on bioethics. Committee opinion no. 501: Maternalefetal intervention and fetal care centers. Obstetrics and Gynecology. 2011;**118**(Pt 1):405e10

[4] Bamforth JS. Amniotic band sequence: Streeter's hypothesis reexamined. American Journal of Medical Genetics. 1992;**44**:280-287

[5] Biffl WL, Spain DA, Rietsma AM, et al. Responsible development and application of surgical innovations: A position statement of the Society of University Surgeons. Journal of the American College of Surgeons. 2008;**206**:1204e9

[6] Chan JK, Gotherstrom C. Prenatal transplantation of mesenchymal stem cells to treat osteogenesis imperfecta. Frontiers in Pharmacology. 2014;**5**:223

[7] Chervenak FA, McCullough LB. An ethically justified framework for clinical investigation to benefit pregnant and fetal patients. The American Journal of Bioethics. 2011;**11**:39e49

[8] Chervenak FA, McCullough LB. The Professional Responsibility Model of Perinatal Ethics. Berlin: Walter de Gruyter; 2014

[9] Cignini P, Giorlandino C, Padula F, et al. Epidemiology and risk factors of amniotic band syndrome, or ADAM sequence. Journal of Prenatal Medicine. 2012;**6**:59-63

[10] Deprest JA, Flake AW, Gratacos E, et al. The making of fetal surgery. Prenatal Diagnosis. 2010;**30**:653-667

[11] Ehrenberg-Buchner S, Stapf AM, Berman DR, et al. Fetal lung lesions: Can we start to breathe easier? American Journal of Obstetrics and Gynecology. 2013;**208**:151.e1-151.e7

[12] Graves EC, Harrison RM, Padilla EB. Minimally invasive fetal surgery. Clinics in Perinatology. 2017;**44**(4):729-751

[13] Harrison MR, Adzick NS, Bullard KM, et al. Correction of congenital diaphragmatic hernia in utero VII: A prospective trial. Journal of Pediatric Surgery. 1997;**32**:1637-1642

[14] Harrison MR, Adzick NS, Flake AW, et al. Correction of congenital diaphragmatic hernia in utero: VI. Hard-earned lessons. Journal of Pediatric Surgery. 1993;**28**:1411-1417

[15] Jani J, Cannie M, Done E, et al. Relationship between lung area at ultrasound examination and lung volume assessment with magnetic resonance imaging in isolated congenital diaphragmatic hernia. Ultrasound in Obstetrics & Gynecology. 2007b;**30**:855-860

[16] Jani J, Nicolaides KH, Gratacos E, et al. Fetal lung-to-head ratio in the prediction of survival in severe left-sided diaphragmatic hernia treated by fetal endoscopic tracheal occlusion (FETO). American Journal of Obstetrics and Gynecology. 2006b;**195**:1646-1650

[17] Jani J, Nicolaides KH, Keller RL, et al. Observed to expected lung

area to head circumference ratio in the prediction of survival in fetuses with isolated diaphragmatic hernia. Ultrasound in Obstetrics & Gynecology. 2007a;**30**:67-71

[18] Jani JC, Nicolaides KH, Gratacos E, et al. Severe diaphragmatic hernia treated by fetal endoscopic tracheal occlusion. Ultrasound in Obstetrics & Gynecology. 2009;**34**:304-310

[19] Javid P, Jaksic T, Skarsgard E, Lee S. Survival rate in congenital diaphragmatic hernia: The experience of the Canadian neonatal network. Journal of Pediatric Surgery. 2004;**39**:657-660

[20] Johnson MP, Corsi P, Badfield W, et al. Sequential urinalysis improves evaluation of fetal renal function in obstructive uropathy. American Journal of Obstetrics and Gynecology. 1995;**173**:59-65

[21] Johnson MP, on behalf of NAFTNet. The north American fetal therapy network (NAFTNet): A new approach to collaborative research in fetal diagnosis and therapy. Seminars in Fetal & Neonatal Medicine. 2009;**15**:52-57

[22] Keller BA, Hirose S, Farmer DL. Fetal therapy. In: Milunsky A, editor. Genetic Disorders and the Fetus: Diagnosis, Prevention, and Treatment. 7th ed. Hoboken (NJ): John Wiley & Sons, Inc.; 2016. pp. 989-1011

[23] Kunisaki S, Barnewolt C, Estroff J, et al. Ex utero intrapartum treatment with extracorporeal membrane oxygenation for severe congenital diaphragmatic hernia. Journal of Pediatric Surgery. 2007;**42**:98-106

[24] Kunisaki SM, Fuchs JR, Kaviani A, et al. Diaphragmatic repair through fetal tissue engineering: A comparison between mesenchymal amniocyte- and myoblast-based constructs. Journal of Pediatric Surgery. 2006;**41**:34-39

[25] Lam YH, Tang MHY, Shek TWH. Thermocoagulation of fetal sacrococcygeal teratoma. Prenatal Diagnosis. 2002;**22**:99-101

[26] Lee H, Wagner AJ, Sy E, et al. Efficacy of radiofrequency ablation for twin-reversed arterial perfusion sequence. American Journal of Obstetrics and Gynecology. 2007;**196**:459.e1-459.e4

[27] Lenclen R, Ciarlo G, Paupe A, et al. Neurodevelopmental outcome at 2 years in children born preterm treated by amnioreduction or fetoscopic laser surgery for twin-to-twin transfusion syndrome: Comparison with dichorionic twins. American Journal of Obstetrics and Gynecology. 2009;**201**:291.e1-291.e5

[28] Lewi L, Jani J, Blickstein I, et al. The outcome of monochorionic diamniotic twin gestations in the era of invasive fetal therapy: A prospective cohort study. American Journal of Obstetrics and Gynecology. 2008;**199**:514.e1-514.e8

[29] Lewi L, Jani J, Cannie M, et al. Intertwin anastomoses in monochorionic placentas after fetoscopic laser coagulation for severe twin-to-twin transfusion syndrome: Is there more than meets the eye? American Journal of Obstetrics and Gynecology. 2006;**194**:790-795

[30] Liechty K. Ex utero intrapartum therapy. Seminars in Fetal & Neonatal Medicine. 2010;**15**:34-39

[31] Liechty KW, Crombleholme TM, Flake AW, et al. Intrapartum airway management for giant fetal neck masses: The EXIT procedure (ex utero intrapartum treatment). American Journal of Obstetrics and Gynecology. 1997;**177**:870-874

[32] Liggins GC, Howie RN. A controlled trial of antepartum glucocorticoid treatment for prevention of the respiratory distress syndrome in

premature infants. Pediatrics. 1972;**50**:515-525

[33] Liley AW. Intrauterine transfusion of fetus in haemolytic disease. British Medical Journal. 1963;**2**:1107-1109

[34] Louw JH, Barnard CN. Congenital intestinal atresia; observations on its origin. Lancet. 1955;**269**:1065-1067

[35] Luks FI, Deprest JA, Vandenberghe K, et al. Fetoscopy-guided fetal endoscopy in a sheep model. Journal of the American College of Surgeons. 1994;**178**(6):609-612

[36] Luks FI, Deprest JA. Endoscopic fetal surgery: A new alternative? European Journal of Obstetrics, Gynecology, and Reproductive Biology. 1993;**52**:1-3

[37] Luks FI, Gilchrist BF, Jackson BT, Piasecki GJ. Endoscopic tracheal obstruction with an expanding device in a fetal lamb model:Preliminary considerations. Fetal Diagnosis and Therapy. 1996b;**11**:67-71

[38] Luks FI, Peers KH, Deprest JA, et al. The effect of open and endoscopic fetal surgery on uteroplacental oxygen delivery in the sheep. Journal of Pediatric Surgery. 1996a;**31**:310-314

[39] Luks FI, Wild YK, Piasecki GJ, De Paepe ME. Short-term tracheal occlusion corrects pulmonary vascular anomalies in the fetal lamb with diaphragmatic hernia. Surgery. 2000;**128**:266-272

[40] MacKenzie TC, David AL, Flake AW, et al. Consensus statement from the first international conference for in utero stem cell transplantation and gene therapy. Frontiers in Pharmacology. 2015;**6**:15

[41] MacKenzie TC. Fetal surgical conditions and the unraveling of maternal-fetal tolerance. Journal of Pediatric Surgery. 2016;**51**:197-199

[42] Makin EC, Hyett J, Ade-Ajayi N, et al. Outcome of antenatally diagnosed sacrococcygeal teratomas: Single-center experience (1993-2004). Journal of Pediatric Surgery. 2006;**41**:388-393

[43] Mallik AS, Fichter MA, Rieder S, et al. Fetoscopic closure of punctured fetal membranes with a cellular human amnion plugs in a rabbit model. Obstetrics and Gynecology. 2007;**110**:1121-1129

[44] Mann S, Johnson MP, Wilson RD. Fetal thoracic and bladder shunts. Seminars in Fetal & Neonatal Medicine. 2010;**15**:28-33

[45] Manning FA, Harrison MR, Rodeck C. Catheter shunts for fetal hydronephrosis and hydrocephalus. Report of the international Fetal surgery registry. The New England Journal of Medicine. 1986;**315**:336-340

[46] McClain LE, Flake AW. In utero stem cell transplantation and gene therapy: Recent progress and the potential for clinical application. Best Practice & Research. Clinical Obstetrics & Gynaecology. 2016;**31**:88-98

[47] McCurdy CM, Childers JM, Seeds JW. Ligation of the umbilical cord of an acardiac–acephalus twin with an endoscopic intrauterine technique. Obstetrics and Gynecology. 1993;**82**:708-711

[48] McHugh K, Afaq A, Broderick N, et al. Tracheomegaly: A complication of fetal endoscopic tracheal occlusion in the treatment of congenital diaphragmatic hernia. Pediatric Radiology. 2010;**40**:674-680

[49] Mettauer NL, Pierce CM, Cassidy JV, et al. One year survival in congenital diaphragmatic hernia, 1995-2006. Archives of Disease in Childhood. 2009;**94**:407

[50] Meuli M, Meuli-Simmen C, Yingling CD, et al. In utero repair of

experimental myelomeningocele saves neurological function at birth. Journal of Pediatric Surgery. 1996;**31**:397-402

[51] Moise K. The history of fetal therapy. American Journal of Perinatology. 2014;**31**:557e66

[52] Senat MV, Deprest J, Boulvain M, et al. A randomized trial of endoscopic laser surgery versus serial amnioreduction for severe twin-to-twin transfusion syndrome at midgestation. The New England Journal of Medicine. 2004;**351**:136-144

[53] Peranteau WH, Adzick NS, Boelig MM, et al. Thoracoamniotic shunts for the management of fetal lung lesions and pleural effusions: A single-institution review and predictors of survival in 75 cases. Journal of Pediatric Surgery. 2015;**50**:301-305

[54] Peranteau WH, Boelig MM, Khalek N, et al. Effect of single and multiple courses of maternal betamethasone on prenatal congenital lung lesion growth and fetal survival. Journal of Pediatric Surgery. 2016;**51**:28-32

[55] Roelofs LA, Eggink AJ, Hulsbergen-van de Kaa CA, et al. Fetal abdominal wall repair with a collagen biomatrix in an experimental sheep model for gastroschisis. Tissue Engineering. Part A. 2008a;**14**:2033-2040

[56] Roelofs LA, Eggink AJ, Hulsbergen-van de Kaa CA, et al. Fetal bladder wall regeneration with a collagen biomatrix and histological evaluation of bladder exstrophy in a fetal sheep model. Fetal Diagnosis and Therapy. 2008b;**24**:7-14

[57] Rosenkrantz JG, Simon RC, Carlisle JH. Fetal surgery in the pig with a review of other mammalian fetal techniques. Journal of Pediatric Surgery. 1968;**3**:392-397

[58] Roybal JL, Santore MT, Flake AW. Stem cell and genetic therapies for the fetus. Seminars in Fetal & Neonatal Medicine. 2010;**15**:46-51

[59] Ruano R, Aubry MC, Barthe B, et al. Quantitative analysis of pulmonary vasculature by 3D-power Doppler ultrasonography in isolated congenital diaphragmatic hernia. American Journal of Obstetrics and Gynecology. 2006;**195**:1720-1728

[60] Ruano R, Duarte S, Bunduki V, et al. Fetal cystoscopy for severe lower urinary tract obstruction—Initial experience of a single Centre. Prenatal Diagnosis. 2010;**30**:30-39

[61] Ruano R, Sananes N, Sangi-Haghpeykar H, et al. Fetal intervention for severe lower urinary tract obstruction: A multicenter case-control study comparing fetal cystoscopy with vesicoamniotic shunting. Ultrasound in Obstetrics & Gynecology. 2015;**45**:452-458

[62] Rychik J, Tian Z, Bebbington M, et al. The twin-twin transfusion syndrome: Spectrum of cardiovascular abnormality and development of a cardiovascular score to assess severity of disease. American Journal of Obstetrics and Gynecology. 2007;**197**:392.e1-392.e8

[63] Sala P, Prefumo F, Pastorino D, Buffi D, Gaggero CR, Foppiano M, et al. Fetal surgery: An overview. Obstetrical & Gynecological Survey. 2014;**69**:218e28

[64] Sartoris J, Varnholt V, Dahlheim D, Schaible T. CDH in Mannheim—Algorithm and results. Monatschr Kinderheilkd. 2006;**153**:717

[65] Sokol J, Shimizu Bohn D, et al. Fetal pulmonary artery diameter measurements as a predictor of morbidity in antenatally diagnosed congenital diaphragmatic hernia: A prospective study. American Journal of Obstetrics and Gynecology. 2006;**195**:470-477

[66] Sroka M, Swiatokowska-Freund M, Golebiewski A, et al. Fetal surgery: Future or way leading to nowhere. First experiences. Przeglad Pediatryczny. 2007;**37**:7-9

[67] Stege G, Fenton A, Jaffray B. Nihilism in the 1990s. The true mortality of CDH. Pediatrics. 2003;**112**:532-535

[68] Stirnemann JJ, Nasr B, Quarello E, et al. A definition of selectivity in laser coagulation of chorionic plate anastomoses in twin-to-twin transfusion syndrome and its relationship to perinatal outcome. American Journal of Obstetrics and Gynecology. 2008;**198**:62.e1-62.e6

[69] Sviggum HP, Kodali BS. Maternal anesthesia for fetal surgery. Clinics in Perinatology. 2013;**40**:413-427

[70] Tsao K, Hawgood S, Vu L, et al. Resolution of hydrops fetalis in congenital cystic adenomatoid malformation after prenatal steroid therapy. Journal of Pediatric Surgery. 2003;**38**:508-510

[71] van der Wildt B, Luks FI, Steegers EA, et al. Absence of electrical uterine activity after endoscopic access for fetal surgery in the rhesus monkey. European Journal of Obstetrics, Gynecology, and Reproductive Biology. 1995;**58**:213-214

[72] Van Mieghem T, Klaritsch P, Dońe E, et al. Assessment of fetal cardiac function before and after therapy for twin-to-twin transfusion syndrome. American Journal of Obstetrics and Gynecology. 2009;**200**:400.e1-400.e7

[73] Van Peborgh P, Rambaud C, Ville Y. Effect of laser coagulation on placental vessels: Histological aspects. Fetal Diagnosis and Therapy. 1997;**12**:32-35

[74] Ville Y, Hyett J, Hecher K, Nicolaides K. Preliminary experience with endoscopic laser surgery for severe twin–twin transfusion syndrome. The New England Journal of Medicine. 1995;**332**:224-227

[75] Ville Y, Hyett JA, Vandenbussche F, Nicolaides KH. Endoscopic laser coagulation of umbilical cord vessels in twin reversed arterial perfusion sequence. Ultrasound in Obstetrics & Gynecology. 1994;**4**:396-398

[76] Ville Y. Twin-to-twin transfusion syndrome: Time to forget the Quintero staging system? Ultrasound in Obstetrics & Gynecology. 2007;**30**:924-927

[77] Welsh A, Agarwal S, Kumar S, et al. Fetal cystoscopy in the management of fetal obstructive uropathy: Experience in a single European Centre. Prenatal Diagnosis. 2003;**23**:1033-1041

[78] Westerburg B, Feldstein V, Sandberg P, et al. Sonographic prognostic factors in fetuses with sacrococcygeal teratoma. Journal of Pediatric Surgery. 2000;**35**:322-326

[79] Clewell WH, Johnson ML, Meier PR, Newkirk JB, Zide SL, Hendee RW, et al. The New England Journal of Medicine. 1982;**306**:1320-1325

[80] Kohl T, Herin R, Heep A, et al. Percutaneous fetoscopic patch coverage of spina bifida aperta in the human—Early clinical experience and potential. Fetal Diagnosis and Therapy. 2006;**21**:185-193

Section 2

Gastrointestinal Disorders

Chapter 2

Necrotizing Enterocolitis

Rita Prasad Verma and Archana Kota

Abstract

Necrotizing enterocolitis (NEC) is the commonest inflammatory gastrointestinal disorder of newborn infants, occurring primarily in premature neonates. Presenting as a medical and surgical emergency, it is associated with significant morbidity and mortality. NEC is characterized by acute intestinal inflammation and necrosis with intramural dissection of gas, pathognomically appearing as pneumatosis intestinalis on radiography. The incidence and mortality, with an inverse relationship to maturation, range between 3–11% and 17–20% respectively. Mortality may be up to 50% in extremely premature infants who require surgery for intestinal perforation or gangrene. The exact etiopathogenesis is unknown. Over 90% of infants are premature and more than 98% are enterally fed. NEC presents with feeding intolerance and abdominal distension, which may rapidly progress to cardiorespiratory decompensation and death in severe cases. Intestinal dysbiosis and its functional and immunological immaturity are proposed to play roles in the pathogenesis. While exact triggers are undetermined, the disease is marked by an anomalous immunological response of enterocytes to inflammation, invoking cytokines and chemokines. NEC is treated with bowel rest, antibiotics, cardiorespiratory support, parenteral nutrition, and blood products transfusion. Approximately 30% of cases require surgery and a significant number of survivors suffer from neurological deficits, intestinal dysfunction, and post surgical short bowel syndrome.

Keywords: necrotizing enterocolitis, preterm infants, pneumatosis intestinalis, intestinal gangrene, intestinal perforation, intestinal dysbiosis, short bowel syndrome, feeding intolerance, heme positive stools, abdominal distension, cardiovascular decompensation

1. Introduction

Necrotizing enterocolitis (NEC) is an acquired, multifactorial and devastating gastrointestinal disease associated with high morbidity and mortality in preterm neonates. With an incidence of about 7% in infants with BW < 1500 g and mortality up to 30%, NEC presents as a medical and surgical emergency [1, 2]. It is characterized by ischemia, necrosis, and inflammation of bowel wall with invasion by gas-forming organisms and intramural dissection of gas, characteristically appearing as pneumatosis intestinalis in radiological and pathological studies. While exact etiology is undetermined, the pathogenesis is believed to be an anomalous innate immune response to an altered, less diverse intestinal microbiota by the highly immunoreactive enterocytes of premature infants, leading to inflammation and tissue necrosis [3, 4]. The clinical presentation can be severe with cardiorespiratory collapse, shock, and disseminated intravascular coagulopathy (DIC), escalating to multisystem failure and death [2]. About one third of the cases require surgical intervention due to intestinal perforation and gangrene [5]. NEC is the commonest gastrointestinal (GI) disorder of preterm newborn infants, although term infants can be affected. NEC is associated with significant adverse outcomes, and approximately half of the survivors suffer from abnormal neurodevelopment independent of maturational status at birth. It is one of the most important causes of intestinal failure in children. Despite substantial advances in its diagnosis, prevention, and management strategies, the incidence has not changed, especially in very low birth weight neonates, and the morbidity and mortality associated with necrotizing enterocolitis continue to be high.

2. Epidemiology

NEC constitutes about 2–5% of all NICU admissions. The incidence reported in 2012 by the Canadian Neonatal Network (CNN) in infants less than 33 weeks of gestational age (GA) was 5.1% [1]. In the United States the incidence is estimated to be 1–3 per 1000 live births [2, 6], while its prevalence is 0.3–2.4 per 1000 live births. There is considerable variability in incidence among different geographical locations and neonatal intensive care units [6–8]. Henry and Moss noted an overall incidence of 3–7% in 2005 [5]. A review by the National Institute of Child Health and Human Development (NICHD) Neonatal Research Network data from 1998 to 2001 reported a 7% incidence of NEC among very low birth weight infants [9], while a more recent report from the network in 2010 documented an incidence of 11–15% in neonates < 1500 g or < 32 weeks at birth [10]. The incidence was found to be relatively unchanged at approximately 7% in infants weighing <1500 g in another report published in 2011 [11]. Ninety percent of the infants are preterm and the rest term or late preterm. Incidence and mortality are inversely related to GA and birth weight (BW). Mortality in preterm infants from NEC may be up to 30–50%, and 27% of infants require surgical intervention with an overall case fatality rate of 15% [5, 11, 12]. The mortality rate is higher in surgical NEC and African American males [13]. Forty-six percent of survivors suffer from abnormal neurodevelopment, and 12% of all cases of GI failure in children are due to NEC [14]. The risk and mortality associated with NEC were stratified according to BW and GA in a cohort of extremely premature infants in who the overall incidence was estimated to be 7.5% (**Tables 1** and 2) [2].

Despite the variability in incidence among studies with rates ranging between 3 and 15% in VLBW infants, a relative stability in the incidence over time has been noted. Survival in NEC has not changed in the past five decades, the average mortality being 20–30% and up to 50% in infants requiring surgical management [10]. The proportion of neonates with NEC requiring surgical intervention has

Birth weight (grams)	Risk of NEC(%)	Mortality with NEC (%)
501-750	12	42
751-1000	9	29
1001-1250	6	21
1251-1500	3	16

Table 1.
Risk and mortality associated with NEC based on birth weight.

Gestational Age (in weeks)	Risk of NEC (percent %)
22	11
23	16
24	11
25	9
26	10
27	8
28	8

Table 2.
Risk of NEC based on gestational age.

also remained stable at approximately 30% [15]. The reasons for such observations are the decreasing gestational age limit for neonatal viability and increased survival of extremely premature infants with advances in neonatal care. Practice implementations, such as standardizing enteral feeding guidelines, exclusive feedings of own mother's milk, using donor breast milk when mother's milk is not available, minimizing duration of empiric antibiotics after birth, and avoiding packed red blood cells (PRBC) transfusions as well as antacid use in preterm infants, are associated with a decrease in incidence of NEC in very low birth weight infants [16].

3. Etiology and risk factors

The exact etiology of NEC is undetermined and multiple risk factors have been forwarded. NEC occurs in a stereotypic relation at chronological age of onset to the gestational age at birth, the younger the gestation, the later the onset; and requires that the infant be fed [1, 11]. In one study the median age at onset in infants with a GA of less than 26 weeks was 23 days compared to a median age of 11 days for more mature infants with a GA of greater than 31 weeks [17]. Prematurity is the single greatest risk factor with almost 90% patients being premature. Enteral feeding is the second most common feature with over 98% of cases having a history of feeding. However, rate of advancement unless excessive, trophic, and early versus late and colostrum feeding are not conclusively proven to have any effect on the occurrence of NEC [18]. Other suggested risk factors are the 5 min Apgar score < 7, outborn status, body temperature 0f 36°C at 1 h of age, cesarean section, use of indomethacin with or without dexamethasone, sepsis, use of inotropes, severe metabolic acidosis, patent ductus arteriosus (PDA), gastroschisis, severe anemia, polycythemia, packed red blood cell (PRBC) transfusion, use of H2 antagonist, exposure to empirical antimicrobials, and black and Hispanic ethnicity [19]. Approximately 10% of cases occur in term and late preterm infants. Risk factors for NEC in term infants are nonhuman milk feeding; preexisting illnesses, such as congenital heart disease; primary gastrointestinal disorders; sepsis; polycythemia; respiratory disease; hypotension; neonatal abstinence; fetal growth restriction; and perinatal hypoxia [20]. Despite the fact that no predilection for sex, race, or ethnicity has been conclusively established, a higher incidence is observed in male African American infants than in any other single demographic. This could be related to the higher incidence of prematurity in this ethnic group than in the general US population. Hypoxic ischemic injury is no longer considered a major predisposing factor in the development of NEC except in term babies [21].

4. Pathology

NEC primarily affects the ileum and colon, the commonest location being ileocecal area [22]. The entire gastrointestinal tract may be involved in severe cases. On gross examination, the bowel loops are distended with areas of hemorrhage, congestion, necrosis, and pneumatosis (**Figure 1**). On microscopic examination, signs of inflammation, mucosal edema, bacterial invasion, submucosal and intramural gas bubbles, and ischemic transmural necrosis are seen. Intestinal perforation may happen when the entire thickness of bowel is involved leading to pneumoperitoneum, peritonitis, and portal venous gas (**Figure 2**). Microscopically, the predominant feature is coagulation necrosis, suggesting an ischemic origin of NEC. The aggregated inflammatory cells are both acute and chronic, such as neutrophils, lymphocytes, and macrophages representing an appropriate response to pathogenic bacterial invasion and tissue necrosis. Epithelial regeneration, granulation tissue formation and fibrosis may be seen suggesting reparative histological process [23]. Common pathogens isolated in NEC are Enterobacteriaceae including *Escherichia*, *Salmonella*, *Enterobacter*, and *Klebsiella* (68%); staphylococcal species (26%); clostridium species (4%); viruses including rota, echo, corona, and toro (11%); and candida (1%). No organism is isolated in 3% of cases.

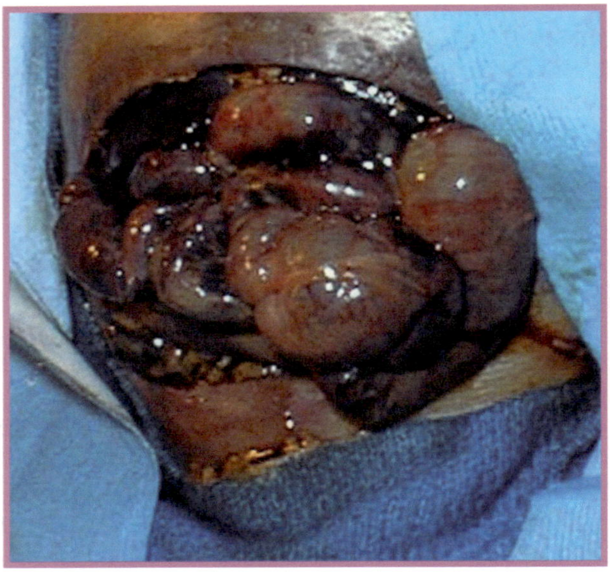

Figure 1.
Macroscopic appearance of necrotizing enterocolitis showing necrotic bowel loops. [Courtesy of Renu Sharma, MD, Professor of Pediatrics, University of Florida at Jacksonville, USA].

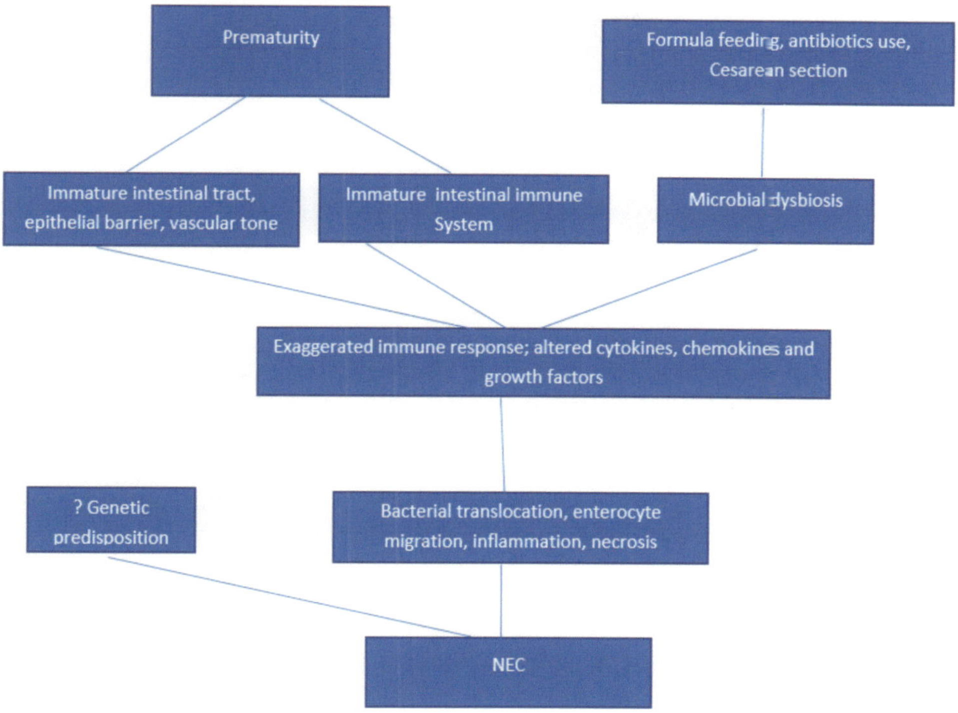

Figure 2.
Schematic presentation of pathogenesis of NEC.

5. Pathogenesis

The pathogenesis of NEC is complex, multifactorial, and incompletely defined. The disorder is believed to be a composite result of intestinal immaturity, aberrant immunological response, and gut microbial dysbiosis [3, 4, 23, 24]. It almost never occurs when the intestinal immune system is mature and intact, even when other risk factors are present. Experimental NEC does not occur in sterile environment. Research support the hypothesis that NEC in the preterm infant results from a multifactorial process that requires the concurrent presence of an immature intestinal tract and immune system leading to increased susceptibility, factors causing disruption of the normal intestinal bacterial microbiome with growth of potentially pathogenic bacteria, and an exaggerated inflammatory host response with the release of cytokines and chemokines (**Figure 2**). A genetically determined predisposition to necrotizing enterocolitis has been also proposed implying the contribution of genetic polymorphisms in the pro-inflammatory cytokines associated with NEC [25]. The combination of compromised intestinal epithelial barrier; underdeveloped and anomalous immune defense; abnormal mesenteric vascular development, tone, and flow; and altered luminal microbiota shaped by formula feedings, antibiotic exposure, and cesarean delivery presumably leads to intestinal inflammation and gangrene. NEC is triggered when several risk factors heighten neonatal intestinal inflammation and an irreversible borderline is surpassed.

5.1 Intestinal immaturity, dysbiosis, and barrier dysfunction

Immaturity of neonatal intestinal mucosal barrier and mucosal immune system is characterized by decreased mucus coat, altered mucus protein, reduced Ig A, and abnormal epithelial membrane and tight junctions [4, 26, 27]. Preterm intestinal mucosa is highly immunoreactive, and fetal human enterocytes have been shown to evoke excessive immunological and inflammatory response compared to adults. An imbalance between epithelial cell injury and repair leads to a gut barrier failure and a consequent cycle of bacterial invasion, immune activation, uncontrolled inflammation, and gut necrosis (**Figure 2**).

5.2 Feeding and immature GI function

Premature GIT is relatively deficient in digestive functions and peristaltic motility in addition to immune responses [28]. Dysfunctional gastric emptying and increased gastric pH add to gut barrier disruption and epithelial permeability [4, 29–31]. Aggressive feeding with peristaltic dysmotility leads to stasis of intraluminal contents and intestinal dilatation, which may further impair epithelial barrier (EB). These, in concurrence with microbial dysbiosis, result in abnormal signal transduction across the EB with consequent inflammation, apoptosis, and necrosis. The balance between the pro-inflammatory and anti-inflammatory signaling is affected with an inappropriate response to pathogenic microorganisms.

5.3 Role of cytokines and chemokines

NEC is associated with increased expression of inflammatory cytokines, such as tumor necrosis factor (TNF), interleukin (IL)-1β, IL-6, IL-8/CXC-motif ligand 8 (CXCL8), IL 10 monocyte chemoattractant protein-1/CC-motif ligand (CCL)-2, macrophage inflammatory protein-1β/CCL3, and C-reactive protein in plasma and affected tissues [32]. These cytokines can disrupt the epithelial barrier and augment intestinal injury. Serum levels of cytokines/chemokines are elevated in NEC, and increased TLR4 and abnormal IkB/NFkB suggest excessive abnormal immunological response [33–35]. Lower blood TGF-β and interleukin (IL)-2 and higher IL-8 levels are found in ELBW infants with NEC. A developmental immaturity is noted in IkB expression, the molecule that inhibits cytokines activation via NFkB in NEC. Recently the role of toll-like receptor 4 (TLR4) signaling in the pathogenesis of NEC has been highlighted. Hypoxia, infection, and prematurity accentuate the expression of TLR4 in the intestinal mucosa. TLR4 is subsequently activated by enteric bacteria, triggering an inflammatory cascade which results in increased gut mucosal injury and reduced epithelial repair. Activation of cytoplasmic innate immune receptors, NOD2 and TLR9 leads to inhibition of TLR4, with restoration of the intestinal epithelial barrier and reduction in severity of NEC in experimental models. Other factors implicated in pathogenesis of NEC are platelet-activating factor, nitric oxide, reactive oxygen species, and transforming growth factors. However, despite success in animal model systems, no significant improvement in treatment and outcomes of NEC has been achieved due to an incomplete understanding of the developing immune system in premature infants and inability to replicate them in animal models [32].

6. Clinical presentation

NEC presents acutely with feeding intolerance, heme-positive stools, abdominal distension, gastric residuals, and vomiting in a previously stable and feeding preterm infant. Commonly associated nonspecific symptoms are temperature instability, apnea, bradycardia, oxygen desaturation, and lethargy. There may be abdominal wall erythema, abdominal tenderness, and decreased or absent bowel sounds (**Figure 3**). As the disease process advances, cardiorespiratory

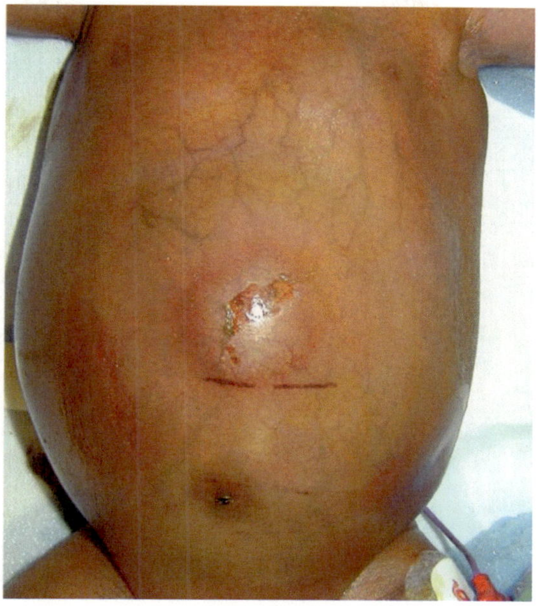

Figure 3.
Abdominal distension, erythema and skin ulceration in a case of necrotizing enterocolitis. [Courtesy of Renu Sharma, MD, Professor of Pediatrics, University of Florida at Jacksonville, USA].

decompensation, septic shock, and multi-organ failure may supervene. The diagnosis is confirmed by the presence of pneumatosis intestinalis in abdominal X-ray which is pathognomonic of NEC (**Figure 4**). The course may be mild to moderate with recovery with antibiotics, GI rest, and correction of biochemical and hematological anomalies, or fulminant with early signs of severe systemic

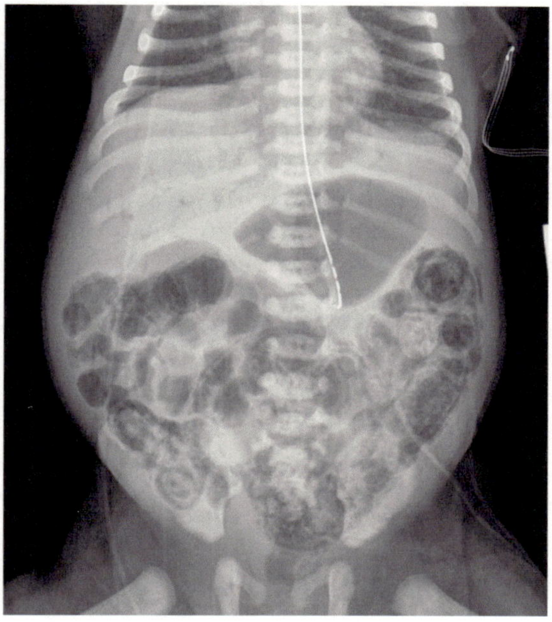

Figure 4.
Extensive pneumatosis with branching linear lucencies in the liver, consistent with portal venous gas. [Courtesy of Dr. Renu Aggarwal, Attending Neonatologist, NYU Winthrop Hospital, Mineola, NY, USA].

	STAGE	SYSTEMICSIGNS	ABDOMINALSIGNS	RADIOGRAPHIC SIGNS
IA	Suspected	Temperature instability, apnea, bradycardia, lethargy	Gastric residuals, abdominal distension, emesis, guaiac-positive stool	Normal or intestinal dilation; mild ileus
IB	Suspected	Same as IA	Gross bloody stool	Same as IA
IIA	Definite, mildly ill	Same as IA	IA, IB plus decreased or absent bowel sounds with/without abdominal tenderness	Intestinal dilation, ileus, pneumatosis intestinalis
IIB	Definite, moderately ill	IIA plus mild metabolic acidosis and mild thrombocytopenia	IIA plus abdominal tenderness plus absent bowel sounds with/without abdominal cellulitis, or right lower quadrant mass, absent bowel sounds	IIA plus abdominal tenderness plus absent bowel sounds with/without abdominal cellulitis, or right lower quadrant mass, absent bowel sounds
IIIA	Advanced, severely ill, intact bowel	IIB plus hypotension, bradycardia, severe apnea, combined respiratory and metabolic acidosis, DIC, neutropenia, anuria	IIB plus signs of peritonitis, marked abdominal tenderness, distension, and abdominal wall erythema	IIB plus definite ascites
IIIB	Advanced, severely ill, perforated bowel	Same as IIIA	Same as IIIA	IIB plus pneumoperitoneum

Adapted from: .Neu J. Necrotizing enterocolitis: the search for a unifying pathogenic theory leading to prevention. Pediatr Clin North Am. 1996;43(2):409–43:

Table 3.
Modified Bell's staging criteria for necrotizing enterocolitis in neonates [33].

inflammatory response and poor response to correction of metabolic and hematological derangements, such as severe metabolic acidosis, hyponatremia, hyperglycemia, thrombocytopenia, DIC, anemia, and neutropenia, eventually progressing to death.

Age of onset varies in an inverse relationship with GA at birth, and the average post menstrual gestational age of NEC is estimated to be 31–32 weeks. In a cohort of preterm infants under 33 weeks gestational age, NEC presented at a mean of 7 days in more mature infants, while it was delayed to 32 days in lower birth weight and gestational age neonates [1]. The average age of onset has been reported to be 20.2 days for babies born at less than 30 weeks' estimated gestational age, 13.8 days for babies born at 31–33 weeks, and 5.4 days for babies born after 34 weeks of gestation. Term infants develop necrotizing enterocolitis much earlier, with the average age of onset within the first week or within the first 1–2 days of life [36].

To classify the severity of NEC based on clinical findings, a staging criterion was proposed by Bell in 1978 which was later modified (**Table 3**) [37]. In about one third of cases, NEC is suspected but not confirmed (stage I), and symptoms resolve gradually with treatment. In 25–40% of cases, the progression of NEC is fulminant with signs of peritonitis and sepsis and the rapid development of DIC and shock (stage III). About 30% of the cases may develop intestinal perforation, peritonitis, and other complications necessitating surgical intervention. Mean LOS is 62 days in surgical and 36 days in medical NEC cases [15]. Surgical NEC cases incur higher hospital costs.

7. Laboratory and radiological investigations

In all cases of NEC, CBC with diff, blood culture, C-reactive protein, serum electrolytes, pH, lactate, acid-base indicators, arterial blood gases, and pertinent radiography should be done. The characteristic anomalies are metabolic or mixed acidosis, high C-reactive protein (CRP), hyponatremia, hyperglycemia, thrombocytopenia, neutropenia, or leukocytosis with high I/T ratio. CSF studies are suggested, and peritoneal fluid analysis for bacteria and fecal material should be done if paracentesis abdominis is performed for therapeutic or diagnostic purposes. Presentation of NEC is similar to, or may be associated with sepsis, and the differentiation is confirmed by the presence of pneumatosis intestinalis (PI) on radiography (**Figure 5**). Apart from PI other radiological features of NEC are ileus, bowel wall thickness, and bowel perforation with peritoneal air. Bowel wall thickening, with or without echogenicity, indicates increasing inflammation, swelling, and perfusion of the area. Bowel loops may be separated by the presence of peritoneal fluid and give an impression of thickening. Thin bowel wall with a central echogenic focus and a hypoechoic rim, called pseudo-kidney sign, if present, may indicate necrotic bowel and imminent perforation. Ultrasound detection of small air bubbles in the bowel wall as in pneumatosis intestinalis can be spatially differentiated from air bubbles in stool that can sometimes be misdiagnosed as pneumatosis on radiographs. Ultrasonography also can detect intermittent gas bubbles in the liver parenchyma and portal venous system that are not detected on radiography. Ultrasound is more sensitive in detecting peritoneal fluid collections. Doppler ultrasound is dynamic and permits real-time visualization of bowel wall thickness, peristalsis, and perfusion. It is more sensitive than abdominal radiography in detecting bowel necrosis [15]. Evidence of free peritoneal air and ascites indicate intestinal perforation. Contrast enemas are not recommended if NEC is suspected, as it may result in bowel perforation with extravasation of contrast material into the peritoneum. Near-infrared spectroscopy (NIRS) is a new, noninvasive method of estimating local tissue hemoglobin oxygen saturation by measuring the difference between oxyhemoglobin and deoxyhemoglobin and may have utility in diagnosing intestinal ischemia in NEC. Fortune et al. demonstrated cerebro-splanchnic oxygenation ratio < 0.75 to have a positive predictive value of 0.75 for intestinal ischemia, whereas, if above 0.75, intestinal ischemia is excluded with a negative predictive value of 0.96 [38].

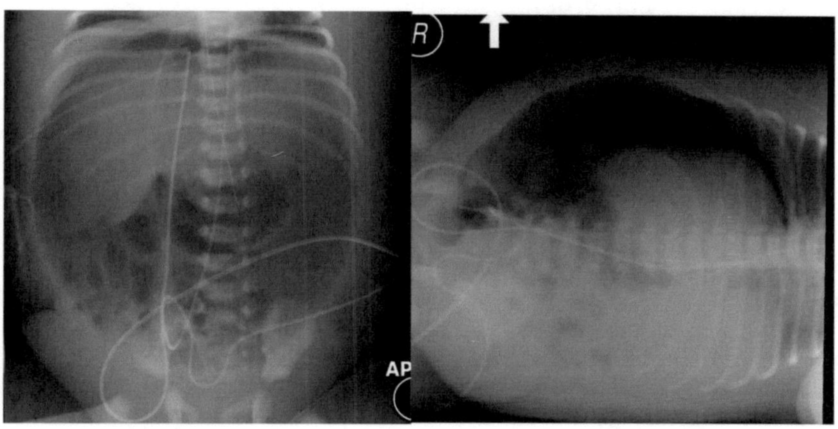

Figure 5.
On left: massive pneumoperitoneum with visualization of falciform ligament, massive lucency involving the entire abdomen, visualization of the liver margin. On right: left lateral decubitus radiograph demonstrating massive lucency with visualization of the liver margin and bowel. [Courtesy of Dr. Renu Aggarwal, Attending Neonatologist, NYU Winthrop Hospital, Mineola, NY, USA].

7.1 Differentiating medical and surgical NEC: use of biomarkers

Pneumoperitoneum is not a very reliable clinical feature for surgical NEC and is observed in less than half of all infants with intestinal perforation or necrosis [15, 39]. Clinical deterioration despite maximal medical therapy is considered a relative indication for surgical intervention. Research has been done to identify a dependable predictor for intestinal necrosis. The most commonly used biochemical markers for bowel necrosis among pediatric surgeons are platelet count (99%), C-reactive protein (CRP) concentration (90%), white blood cell count (83%), lactate levels (43%), fecal calprotectin 10%, and interleukin (IL)-6 or interleukin-8 10% [40]. Fecal calprotectin is a marker of intestinal inflammation and can differentiate between local Bell stage II and systemic Bell III NEC with 76% sensitivity and 92% specificity [41]. Fecal levels of another protein, S100A12, are noted to be higher in infants with suspected NEC who subsequently develop bowel perforation. Unremitting and relentlessly high CRP levels despite treatment may indicate advanced stage of NEC and bowel necrosis. IL-8 levels have been shown to be significantly elevated in patients developing surgical NEC compared to medically managed NEC [42]. The levels can also discriminate NEC totalis from focal and multifocal diseases and predict 60-day mortality [43]. Maximum concentration of CRP and duration of CRP elevation are increased in infants who developed intestinal strictures following NEC, while the negative predictive value of CRP levels <10 mg/dL for stricture development is 100% [44]. Intestinal fatty acid-binding protein (I-FABP), a marker of intestinal injury and progression to severe NEC, is located in mature enterocytes of small intestinal villi and is released into the blood stream after cell disruption and subsequently excreted into the urine. At onset of symptoms, I-FABP concentrations have been shown to be significantly higher in infants who later developed surgical NEC [45]. Other biomarkers being investigated for surgical NEC are serum amyloid A protein, liver fatty acid-binding protein, urine peptides, and heart rate characteristic index.

8. Differential diagnosis

Blood stream infection can present like NEC and must be ruled out. Sepsis and other conditions that can cause feeding intolerance, rectal bleeding, abdominal distension, gastric retention of feed, or intestinal perforation can be differentiated from NEC by the absence of radiologic evidence of pneumatosis intestinalis and the characteristic combination of rectal bleeding presenting as heme-positive or grossly bloody stools, abdominal distention, bilious vomiting, and gastric aspirates as seen in NEC. Spontaneous intestinal perforation is characterized by a single noninflammatory perforation that is typically located at the terminal ileum or colon. It occurs primarily in infants with birth weight <1000 g and is differentiated from NEC by the presence of less severe systemic signs and absence of pneumatosis intestinalis. Infectious enteritis may present with frequent, occasionally bloody stools with abdominal distension but no pneumatosis. Congenital anomalies of GIT, such as Hirschsprung disease, small bowel atresia, meconium ileus, and acquired conditions like volvulus and intussusception, present with intestinal obstruction and at times secondary enterocolitis. Abdominal radiography differentiates these conditions from NEC. Anal fissures can result in rectal bleeding and can be detected on pertinent thorough physical examination. Milk protein allergy-induced enterocolitis may present with heme-positive stools and other GI symptoms similar to NEC in preterm infants but no pneumatosis. Such patients respond to dietary modification by switching the formula to extensively hydrolyzed or amino acid-based ones and may have eosinophilia along with thrombocytosis.

9. Management

The basic principles of management of NEC are bowel decompression and rest, antibiotics coverage, cardiorespiratory support, fluid resuscitation, provision of blood products, and surgical intervention if indicated. The management strategies according to Bell's staging are outlined in **Table 4**. Surgical consultation is obtained in all stages of NEC including stage 1. Total parenteral nutrition (TPN) should be provided during the period that the infant is nil by mouth.

9.1 Medical management

The principles are as follows: (1) bowel decompression and rest, (2) parenteral hydration and nutrition, (3) respiratory and cardiovascular support, (4) antibiotic therapy, (5) general supportive care, (6) fluid resuscitation, and (7) serial close laboratory monitoring and radiologic surveillance. The focus is on limiting the progression of the disease. Intermittent or continuous nasogastric suction is done for bowel decompression, TPN is provided to ensure nutrition, and fluid is replaced to correct third space losses. Adequate cardiorespiratory support is of paramount value, and hematologic anomalies, such as DIC, anemia, and thrombocytopenia, are promptly corrected. Metabolic abnormalities, such as metabolic acidosis, hyponatremia, and hyper- or hypoglycemia, are appropriately treated. Even though an infectious agent has not been identified or attributed to NEC, antibiotics are routinely used in its treatment. Observational data reveal that 20–30% cases of NEC have bacteremia, and pathogenic bacteria are recovered from pathologic specimens and peritoneal fluid. Epidemic outbreaks of NEC are common, and the clinical picture improves with antibiotics. The efficacy of antibiotic agents is documented in experimental animal models for NEC. The commonly used empiric broad-spectrum antibiotic combinations are as follows: ampicillin gentamicin (or amikacin), ampicillin, gentamicin (or amikacin) and clindamycin or ampicillin, cefotaxime, and metronidazole. Ceftazidime is an alternative choice for cefotaxime. Other antibiotic combinations are tazobactam and gentamicin (or amikacin); vancomycin, piperacillin-tazobactam, and gentamicin; and meropenem and vancomycin if methicillin-resistant staphylococcus or ampicillin-resistant enterococcus infections are suspected. Amikacin may be used in centers with significant gentamicin resistance. Metronidazole or clindamycin is added to cover anaerobic bacteria, especially in cases where infant is fed orally before NEC supervenes.

Evaluation of progression of the disease is important in order to take appropriate and timely steps to avoid further damage to the bowel. Serial laboratory monitoring is routinely performed. At diagnosis stool for guaiac test, complete blood and differential neutrophil counts, blood culture, CSF study if indicated, C-reactive protein, platelet count, serum electrolytes, pH, creatinine, blood urea nitrogen, and acid-base studies are obtained and monitored q 12 or 24 h or more frequently

NEC Bell's stage	Treatment
1a and 1b	Antibiotics × 3 days, NPO
2a	NPO, antibiotics × 7–10 days
2b	NPO, antibiotics × 14 days
3a	As in 2b plus, fluid resuscitation, inotropic and ventilator support, blood products
3b	As in 3a plus surgery

Table 4.
Management principles of NEC [65].

if needed. In addition, arterial blood gas values are measured and repeated every 4–6–12 h as per the severity of respiratory decompensation. Serial lactate levels are helpful in monitoring progression of the necrotic process and assessing systemic status. Worsening or persistent metabolic acidosis and persistent hyperglycemia or thrombocytopenia are poor prognostic signs. Improvement in metabolic acidosis is a positive prognostic sign but may be misleading if blood circulation to the necrotic bowel is completely severed and the generated lactic acid cannot enter the circulation. Blood in stools is not predictive of resolution or outcome. Radiographic monitoring is done with abdominal radiograph performed in supine position during the initial phase of illness. A lateral decubitus view is simultaneously obtained with the infant's left side down to visualize the presence of free air over the liver. It should be repeated q 6–12 h as per the severity and progression of the disease and when improvement is obtained less frequently. In the initial stages q 4–6 h may be appropriate and advisable. Supine cross-table lateral view may be done to visualize layering of free air under umbilical area if patient is too sick to move or put in a decubitus position (**Figure 2**). Radiography is discontinued when pneumatosis resolves and bowel gas pattern normalizes.

9.2 Surgical management

The only definite indication for surgery is intestinal perforation. Other relative indications, which are highly suggestive of bowel perforation or necrosis, are abdominal mass, fixed dilated bowel loop, positive paracentesis, and severe metabolic acidosis that is unresponsive to treatment (**Figures** 5 and **6**) [46]. Signs that indicate peritonitis or bowel necrosis are unremitting clinical deterioration, worsening or unrelenting metabolic acidosis, and DIC or thrombocytopenia. Signs of ascites and intestinal obstruction may be present. Perforation can occur without evidence of free air on the radiograph as the timing of study may not coincide with the occurrence of perforation and the free air may get absorbed. Likewise, pneumatosis may not be always caught on serial X-rays. Under such conditions other signs and clinical judgment should be used to assess the severity and need for surgery. As clinical parameters may not be reliable to assess progression to surgical from medical NEC, abnormalities in biochemical markers, such as platelet count, CRP, WBC count, blood lactate, fecal calprotectin, and serum IL-6 and IL-8 may be used. Surgical procedures performed in cases of NEC are exploratory laparotomy with resection of the affected intestinal region or primary peritoneal drainage (PPD). PPD is preferred as the initial procedure in ELBW infants and is performed in the NICU at bedside with analgesia and local anesthesia. Laparotomy is done in an operating room under general anesthesia and may require a second surgical procedure for reanastomosis.

In primary peritoneal drainage abdomen is prepped with iodine solution, and local anesthesia is administered. Small transverse incision is made at McBurney's point and abdominal wall layers bluntly dissected to enter the peritoneal cavity. A rush of air and the presence of meconium are generally encountered. Cultures are obtained, and then peritoneal cavity is copiously irrigated with warm saline solution. Following this Penrose drain is gently threaded into the abdomen and secured. The drain site is observed over the subsequent days. When there is no intestinal or meconium drainage, the drain is backed out daily until removed. After the return of bowel function, a trial of feeding can be started, or the patency of the gastrointestinal tract may be determined with a contrast study. In laparotomy the procedure includes resection of the affected bowel segment and placement of a proximal enterostomy (usually an ileostomy) and distal mucous fistula. Primary reanastomosis, if required, usually is performed 8–12 weeks after the initial procedure, depending

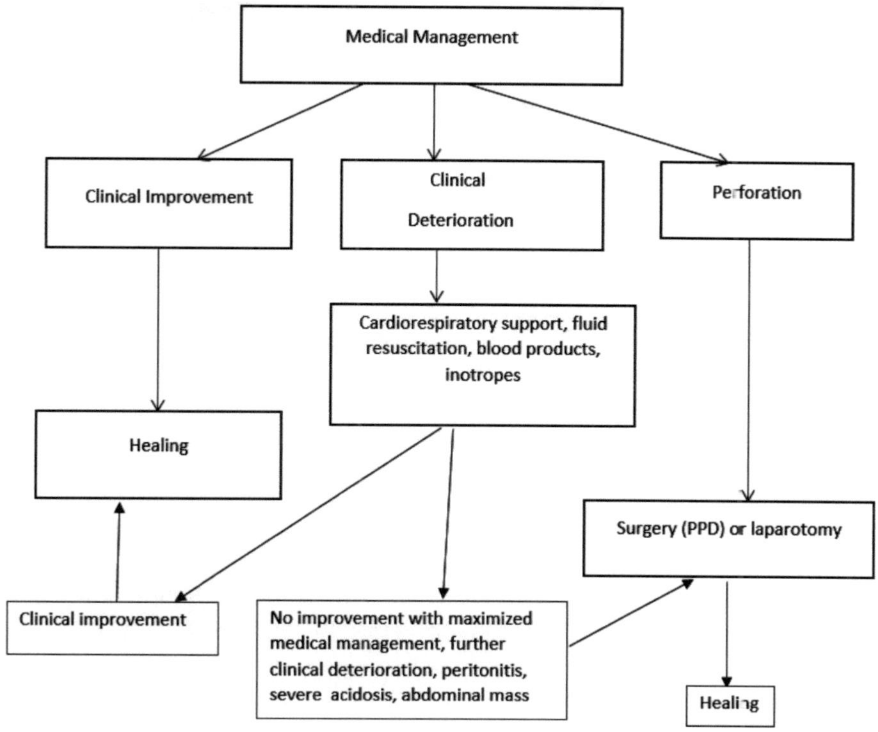

Figure 6.
Flow chart outlining management principles in NEC.

upon the infant's clinical condition. A contrast enema usually is performed before the reanastomosis to detect intestinal strictures. If NEC affects only a short segment of bowel, and the resection is limited, some surgeons perform a primary anastomosis. Complications associated with ileostomies are fluid and electrolyte abnormalities, delayed resumption of oral feedings, poor growth, and stenosis of the enterostomy site. An alternative approach is placement of an intestinal patch and peritoneal drain instead of resection and enterostomy. Preservation of ileocecal valve is a favorable prognostic sign. When a substantial length of bowel is affected, resection is restricted to segments of definite necrosis or perforation to avoid the risk of short bowel syndrome. If the potential viability of some segments is uncertain, one approach is to place peritoneal drains and plan a second operation in 2–3 days to reexamine the bowel and excise necrotic segments.

Recently, standard and fluorescein laparoscopy has been used in cases of NEC when there is no evidence of perforation, but clinical deterioration with maximum support continues, and a diagnosis for the presence and extent of bowel necrosis needs to be made in order to decide against, or in favor of, surgical exploration and its type [47]. Laparoscopy can also identify infants who do not need surgical intervention as it can visualize the viability and perfusion status of the bowel. According to a Cochrane review by Smith and Thyoka, which included eight reports and 44 patients, laparoscopy was able to diagnose NEC in 91% of the cases and exclude in 9% [48]. Moreover, additional surgical intervention was avoided in eight (18%) infants. Among those who did not require surgery, NEC was excluded in four (9%), while two (5%) had no perforation or intestinal gangrene, and two (5%) had NEC totalis which contraindicated surgery. Thirty-six infants out of 44 required surgery following laparoscopy, which included placement of a peritoneal drain (9) or a stoma (20) and intestinal resection and anastomosis (7). Perforation was detected in 25 out of 44 (57%) infants and was missed in one case which subsequently required laparotomy. Six (14%) infants died due to NEC totalis and two of ongoing and recurrent NEC following recovery from the acute episode of each. The authors concluded that laparoscopy is a useful procedure in the management of NEC, with one-fifth of patients not requiring further surgery. However, due to the lack of enough evidence about its utility and benefits, the procedure is generally not undertaken in the routine management of NEC.

9.3 Comparison of laparotomy and PPD

There are limited data about the superiority of one procedure over other. In a multicenter controlled study, 117 infants who were <34 weeks of gestation with perforated NEC were randomized to PPD or laparotomy. No differences were noted in mortality (34.5 versus 35.5%), TPN dependence on postoperative day 90 (47.2 versus 40%), and length of hospital stay (126 ± 58 versus 116 ± 56 days) [49]. A subgroup analysis of cases with extensive pneumatosis intestinalis, GA less than 25 weeks, and serum pH less than 7.30 at presentation showed no significant advantage of one procedure over the other. In another randomized multicenter trial of 69 extremely low birth weight (ELBW) infants with NEC or SIP, no difference in the survival rates was noted between the two interventions, while 74% treated with PPD subsequently required laparotomy [50]. A cohort study from the NICHD neonatal research group reported no difference in mortality rate, and 24% treated with PPD required subsequent laparotomy. Blakely et al. reported that PPD is more likely to result in a composite outcome of death or neurodevelopmental impairment at 18–22 months postmenstrual age [51]. However in their study, PPD was performed in infants who were more premature (gestational age 24.7 versus 25.7 weeks), were more likely to be hypotensive, required higher respiratory support, and were more likely to have a pre-operative diagnosis of SIP. Most of these studies are compromised by a lack pf power.

9.4 Post-surgery intestinal failure and short bowel syndrome

About 9% of NEC cases result in short bowel syndrome (SBS) with incidence inversely related to GA and almost 42% in intestinal failure and SBS [52, 53]. Such infants suffer from significant malabsorption and are at risk for sepsis, cholestasis, and liver failure due to prolonged parenteral nutrition (PN). It is suggested that infants with residual small bowel length ≤ 10% of expected small bowel length may develop SBS. The cumulative probability of weaning from PN by 24 months is 96% in infants with >50 cm of residual small bowel compared to 38% in those who have <50 cm of residual small bowel. Those with ≥41 cm of residual bowel are significantly more likely to achieve enteral autonomy than those with less than 41 cm [53]. In general, those with post-resection length of remaining bowel less than 25% of the normal small bowel length have higher chances of developing SBS. The length of remaining bowel, however, is not the sole or best predictor of SBS. Infants at risk of SBS are as follows: parenteral antibiotics or mechanical ventilation on the day of onset of NEC, birth weight less than 750 g, enteral nutrition before the diagnosis of NEC, percentage of bowel resected, and placement and duration of a diverting jejunostomy. The intestines continue to grow after resection and contribute to the process of attaining enteral autonomy.

9.5 Surgical procedures for short bowel syndrome

In a NICHD cohort, 95% of cases of SBS were due to NEC with an overall incidence of 0.7% of infants <1500 g at birth [52]. Approximately 42% of cases of NEC in infants <1500 g of BW who undergo surgery develop intestinal failure and SBS, risk factors being lower birth weight, antibiotics use, positive pressure ventilation on the day of NEC, feeding, and lower post-resection length of remaining bowel [53]. Intestinal tailoring and lengthening procedure, also called "autologous intestinal reconstruction surgery" are performed in conditions where likelihood of weaning from PN is low despite rigorous intestinal rehabilitation measures. The criteria for surgery, tentative and not well supported by studies, include dilated small intestine, failure to attain intestinal autonomy, and absence of liver failure and GI dysmotility. The procedures aim at surgical lengthening of the bowel to increase the absorptive area and tapering or plicating the dilated bowel to improve motility. There is not enough literature on the subject to assess its clinical advantage. Bianchi procedure is a longitudinal intestinal lengthening and tailoring procedure (LILT) and may be successful in improving absorption and nutritional status but requires multiple anastomoses. Complications of this procedure include fistula formation, anastomotic stenosis, or leakage and sepsis [54]. The 6-year survival rate is 45%, and survivors have residual bowel length greater than 40 cm and no liver disease. The Bianchi procedure is not recommended in neonates with liver disease or intestine length less than 50 cm. The serial transverse enteroplasty procedure (STEP) is a substitute for LILT which increases the girth of bowel. It has a simpler technique that does not need bowel anastomoses, and the tapering can be performed on dilated bowel. STEP increases intestinal length, improves intestinal absorptive capacity, and may decrease the risk of D-lactic acidosis due to bacterial overgrowth. STEP is more favored over other techniques as the weaning from parenteral nutrition is faster and the need for later transplants lesser. There is no difference in early complications, growth rates, or survival between the two procedures, and nearly half of patients operated achieve enteral autonomy, with the median time to wean from parenteral nutrition (PN) being 21 months postoperatively. Patients whose bowel re-dilates after a lengthening procedure have worse overall outcomes. Complications of STEP include gastrointestinal bleeding, staple line leak, hematoma, abscess formation, stricture, pleural effusion, obstruction, a need for transplantation, and even death. In a recent publication, the rate of independence from PN post-STEP was reported as 58% with parenteral calories decreasing from 71 to 36% within 1 month and to 12% after 1 year. The total increase in intestinal length achieved was about 49% [54].

Small bowel transplantation (SBT) may be considered in patients who have progressive, severe, or irreversible intestinal failure with associated liver disease. Other considerations might be a lack of venous access, recurrent life-threatening central venous catheter-associated sepsis, complete mesenteric thrombosis, slow growing tumors of the hepatic hilum or root of mesentery, or extremely short residual bowel with no chance of achieving enteral autonomy in patients who prefer transplantation over lifelong PN dependence [54]. Small bowel transplantation has a 5-year graft survival rate of 48% with lifelong immunosuppressant medications. Types of transplantation include isolated intestine, isolated liver, combined liver and intestine, and multi-visceral. Complications are rejection, infection, graft-versus-host disease, and posttransplant lymphoproliferative disease. Overall, one year patient and intestine graft survival is 89%, being 79% in intestine and 72% in liver-intestine graft recipients. Patient and intestine graft survival falls to 46% by 10 years. At 10 years the survival of intestine only recipients is 29%, whereas, that of liver-intestine recipients 39-42%. More recently, living donor intestinal transplantation has been done successfully in pediatric patients which eliminates waiting time.

9.6 Intestinal rehabilitation

This requires a multidisciplinary approach. The focus is on optimizing enteral feeding and weaning from PN with judicious use of pharmacotherapy and surgical interventions. The approach is associated with improved survival and achievement of independence from PN.

10. Complications

The acute complications of NEC are sepsis, meningitis, peritonitis, intraabdominal abscess formation, DIC, thrombocytopenia, hypotension, shock, respiratory failure, metabolic or combined acidosis, hyponatremia, hyperglycemia, or less often hypoglycemia. Late complications are stricture formation, short bowel syndrome, and intestinal failure [55]. Rarely enterocele, enterocolic fistula, and intraabdominal abscess formation may be encountered. About 24% (95% CI 17–31%) of infants treated medically or surgically develop strictures in bowel which is unrelated to the severity of NEC or gestational age. The commonest location is in the colon, followed by the ileum and jejunum. Multiple sites strictures are seen. It can appear within 2 to 3 months of the acute episode and as late as 20 months. Stricture may lead to local bacterial overgrowth resulting in repeated infections, bloody stools, failure to thrive, and symptoms of bowel obstruction. Strictures are more common following enterostomy; therefore contrast enemas should be performed 4–6 weeks after the occurrence of NEC and prior to surgical closure of enterostomy with reanastomosis or if and when feeding intolerance develops. Recurrent NEC may occur in 8% and adhesion ileus in 6% cases of NEC. Overall intestinal failure happens in 13% of all cases of NEC, inclusive of medically and surgically treated infants.

11. Long-term outcomes

Approximately half of all cases of NEC display no long-term sequelae. This includes cases of stage I NEC from Bell's criteria. NEC is associated with significant impairment of growth and neurodevelopment [56–58]. Ten to thirteen percent of patients suffer from late gastrointestinal morbidity if resection is performed. Majority of infants who have had no extensive intestinal resection have normal gastrointestinal function at 1–10 years of age.

11.1 Growth and neurodevelopment

In a large multicenter study from the National Institute of Child Health and Human Development (NICHD) Neonatal Research Network, extremely low birth weight (ELBW) infants (BW <1000 g) who required surgical care were more likely to have significant growth delay and poorer developmental outcome at 18–22 months compared with infants without NEC [56]. ELBW treated medically or surgically suffer from significant growth failure until 22 months, and in a lesser percentage beyond that age [57], while those who were medically treated do not differ in growth or developmental testing compared with those without NEC [58]. Infants with NEC are at increased risk for cerebral palsy and cognitive and severe visual impairment. At 7 years of age, survivors with NEC compared to controls demonstrate a higher rate of neurologic functional impairment.

11.2 Mortality

Overall survival in cases with NEC is 70–80%, being >95% in medical and 70–75% in surgical NEC [59]. Lower BW and GA and surgical intervention, such as laparotomy and peritoneal drainage, are independent predictors for mortality.

Other risk factors associated with death from NEC are mechanical ventilation, treatment with vasopressor agents, surgical intervention, and black ethnicity as per a retrospective multicenter review of data [60]. Two thirds of NEC deaths occur within 7 days of diagnosis, with a median time of death being 1 day from the day of onset. Infants who die within 7 days of diagnosis have higher BW, and more often they are on vasopressors and high-frequency ventilation at the time of diagnosis. Risk factors for fulminant NEC, defined as death within 48 h of onset, are presence of portal venous air, increase in feeding volume by >20 mL/kg per day, HCT <22%, I/T ratio > 0.5, and total lymphocyte count <4000/μL as demonstrated in a multicenter study [61].

11.3 Financial burden of NEC

The average total treatment cost of one case of NEC is US $500,000 [62, 63]. Total annual estimated cost of care of NEC in the United States is between $500 million and $1 billion. Infants with NEC are hospitalized for 60 days longer than unaffected preterm infants if surgery is performed and >20 days longer if surgery is not required. Bowel resection—one of the most severe complications of NEC—is the major cause of short bowel syndrome in pediatric patients, making 95% of all such cases. The total mean cost of care over a 5-year period for a child with the short bowel syndrome has been estimated to be nearly $1.5 million.

12. Prevention

Prevention is the primary strategy in this devastating disease with undetermined etiology. Breast milk feeding, prolonging gestation to avoid prematurity, antenatal steroid, and the use of probiotics/prebiotics are established prevention strategies in NEC [16]. Nonaggressive feeding is evidenced to be efficacious. The rate of advancement of feeding under 20 ml/kg/day is considered to be safe. Newer strategies, such as use of toll-like receptor agonist, glutamine, n-3 fatty acids, anti-cytokines, and growth factors are proposed preventive interventions, but most of these either lack evidence or have questionable safety. Compound CpG-DNA inhibit TLR4 signaling, thereby dramatically reducing the severity of NEC in mice. Clinically, the following measures are suggested to be practiced in order to reduce the risk of NEC: human milk (both mother's and donor's); standardized feeding guidelines, including early initiation with trophic feeds; the use of probiotics; antibiotic stewardship; optimization of enteral nutrition and growth; elimination of H2 blockers and acid pump suppressors; elimination of cow's milk products; transfusion protocols; and transfusion outcome monitoring. Avoidance of hyperosmolar agents, treatment of polycythemia, and delayed cord clamping are other interventions that are suggested to be followed. Prophylactic probiotics, although not yet universally applied due to uncertainties about its dose and duration of therapy, have been documented to reduce the incidence of NEC, especially that of severe cases (RR 0.75 95% CI −0.57 to 0.92) in infants <1500 g in multiple studies [64]. There are concerns about bacteremia and some aspects of quality control which restrict its use.

13. Future directions

NEC remains a major unsolved medical challenge for which no specific therapy exists. Recent research is concentrated on the role of TLR4 signaling within the intestinal epithelium and intestinal stem cells and modulation of the genetics and intestinal microbiome. Fecal microbiota transplantation (FMT) has been shown to reverse the severity of experimental necrotizing enterocolitis (NEC) via oxidative stress modulation [65]. FMT decreases the extent of TLR4-mediated pro-inflammatory signaling through TLR9 in the intestinal mucosa tissue. FMT also suppresses intestinal apoptosis and bacterial translocation across the intestinal barrier, which is accompanied by decreased inflammatory cytokine levels, altered bacterial microbiota, and regulated lymphocyte proportions. Research is needed to determine if the use of biomarkers along with specific clinical-biochemical indicators could lead to earlier intervention with modalities, such as peritoneal drainage or laparotomy that might decrease the severity of the disease process, thereby improving the long-term neurodevelopmental and growth outcomes. Improved care of short bowel syndrome with new surgical and medical approaches are additional subject for investigation. Tissue engineering techniques and techniques involving intestinal stem cells may represent unique, novel strategies for intestinal failure after severe NEC in the future.

Author details

Rita Prasad Verma* and Archana Kota
Department of Pediatrics, Nassau University Medical Center, East Meadow, NY, USA

*Address all correspondence to: rverma2@numc.edu

References

[1] Yee WH, Soraisham AS, Shah VS, et al. Incidence and timing of presentation of necrotizing enterocolitis in preterm infants. Pediatrics. 2012;**129**(2):e298-e304. DOI: 10.1542/peds.2011-2022

[2] Stoll BJ, Hansen NI, Bell EF, et al. Trends in care practices, morbidity, and mortality of extremely preterm neonates, 1993-2012. JAMA. 2015;**314**:1039

[3] Niño DF, Sodhi CP, Hackam DJ. Necrotizing enterocolitis: New insights into pathogenesis and mechanisms. Nature Reviews. Gastroenterology & Hepatology. 2016;**13**:590

[4] Sharma R, Tepas JJ 3rd, Hudak ML, et al. Neonatal gut barrier and multiple organ failure: Role of endotoxin and proinflammatory cytokines in sepsis and necrotizing enterocolitis. Journal of Pediatric Surgery. 2007;**42**(3):454-461

[5] Holman RC, Stoll BJ, Curns AT, et al. Necrotising enterocolitis hospitalisations among neonates in the United States. Paediatric and Perinatal Epidemiology. 2006;**20**:498

[6] Battersby B, Santhalingam T, Costeloe K, Modi N. Incidence of neonatal necrotising enterocolitis in high-income countries: A systematic review. Archives of Disease in Childhood: Fetal & Neonatal. 2018;**103**:F182-F189. DOI: 10.1136/archdischild-2017-313880

[7] Rees CM, Eaton S, Pierro A. National prospective surveillance study of necrotizing enterocolitis in neonatal intensive care units. Journal of Pediatric Surgery. 2010;**45**:1391-1397

[8] Henry MC, Moss LR. Surgical therapy for necrotizing enterocolitis: Bringing evidence to the bedside. Seminars in Pediatric Surgery. 2005;**14**:181-190

[9] Guillet R, Stoll BJ, Cotten CM, et al. Association of H2-blocker therapy and higher incidence of necrotizing enterocolitis in very low birth weight infants. Pediatrics. 2006;**117**:e137-e142

[10] Stoll BJ, Hansen NI, Bell EF, et al. Neonatal outcomes of extremely preterm infants from the NICHD Neonatal Research Network. Pediatrics. 2010;**126**:443-456

[11] Lin HC, Wu SF, Underwood M. Necrotizing enterocolitis. The New England Journal of Medicine. 2011;**364**:1878-1879

[12] Fanaroff AA, Stoll BJ, Wright LL, Carlo WA, Ehrenkranz RA, Stark AR, et al. Trends in neonatal morbidity and mortality for very low birthweight infants. American Journal of Obstetrics and Gynecology. 2007;**196**(2):147

[13] Hull MA, Fisher JG, Gutierrez IM, Jones BA, Kang KH, Kenny M, et al. Mortality and management of surgical necrotizing enterocolitis in very low birth weight neonates: A prospective cohort study. Journal of the American College of Surgeons. 2014;**18**(6):1148-1155

[14] Reese CM, Pierro A, Eaton S. Neurodevelopmental outcomes of neonates with medically and surgically treated necrotizing enterocolitis. Archives of Disease in Childhood: Fetal and Neonatal Edition. 2007;**92**(3):F193-F198

[15] Robinson JR, Rellinger EJ, Hatch LD, Weitkamp J, Speck E, Danko M, et al. Surgical necrotizing enterocolitis. Seminars in Perinatology. 2017;**41**(1):70-79

[16] Patel AL, Panagos PG, Silvestri JM. Reducing incidence of necrotizing enterocolitis. Clinics in Perinatology. 2017;**44**:683-700

[17] Uauy RD, Fanaroff AA, Korones SB, et al. Necrotizing enterocolitis in very low birth weight infants: Biodemographic and clinical correlates. National Institute of Child Health and Human Development Neonatal Research Network. Journal of Pediatrics. 1991;**119**:630

[18] Berseth CL. Feeding strategies and necrotizing enterocolitis. Current Opinion in Pediatrics. 2005;**17**:170

[19] Gephart SM, Spitzer AR, Effken JA, Dodd E, Halpern M, McGrath JM. Discrimination of GutCheck (NEC): A clinical risk index for necrotizing enterocolitis. Journal of Perinatology. 2014;**34**(6):468-475

[20] Lambert DK, Christensen RD, Henry E, et al. Necrotizing enterocolitis in term neonates: Data from a multihospital health-care system. Journal of Perinatology. 2007;**27**:437-443

[21] Neu J. The 'myth' of asphyxia and hypoxia-ischemia as primary causes of necrotizing enterocolitis. Biology of the Neonate. 2005;**87**:97-98

[22] Liu Z, Li N, Neu J. Tight junctions, leaky intestines, and pediatric diseases. Acta Paediatrica. 2005;**94**(4):386-393

[23] Neu J, Walker WA. Necrotizing enterocolitis. The New England Journal of Medicine. 2011;**364**(3):255-264

[24] Ballance WA, Dahms BB, Shenker N, Kliegman RM. Pathology of neonatal necrotizing enterocolitis: A ten year experience. The Journal of Pediatrics. 1990;**117**:S6-S13

[25] Frost BL, Modi BP, Jaksic T, Caplan MS. New medical and surgical insights into neonatal necrotizing enterocolitis: A review. JAMA Pediatrics. 2017;**171**(1):83-88

[26] Treszl A, Tulassay T, Vasarhelyi B. Genetic basis for necrotizing enterocolitis—Risk factors and their relations to genetic polymorphisms. Frontiers in Bioscience. 2006;**11**(2006):570-580

[27] Sharma R, Young C, Neu J. Molecular modulation of intestinal epithelial barrier: Contribution of microbiota. Journal of Biomedicine & Biotechnology. 2010:305879. DOI: 10.1155/2010/305879. [Epub 2010 Jan 31]

[28] Lin PW, Nasr TR, Stoll BJ. Necrotizing enterocolitis: Recent scientific advances in pathophysiology and prevention. Seminars in Perinatology. 2008;**32**(2):70-82

[29] Hunter CJ, Upperman JS, Ford HR, Camerini V. Understanding the susceptibility of the premature infant to necrotizing enterocolitis (NEC). Pediatric Research. 2008;**63**:117-123

[30] Denning TL, Bhatia AM, Kane AF, et al. Pathogenesis of NEC: Role of the innate and adaptive immune response. Seminars in Perinatology. 2017;**41**:15-28

[31] Tanner SM, Berryhill TF, Eelenburg JL, et al. Pathogenesis of NEC: Modelling the innate immune response. American Journal of Pathology. 2015;**185**(1):4-16

[32] Maheshwari A, Schelonka RL, Dimmitt RA, et al. Cytokines associated with necrotizing enterocolitis in extremely-low-birth-weight infants. Pediatric Research. 2014;**76**(1):100-108

[33] Sodhi CP et al. Toll-like receptor-4 inhibits enterocyte proliferation via impaired β-catenin signaling in necrotizing enterocolitis. Gastroenterology. 2010;**138**:185-196

[34] Lu P, Sodhi CP, Hackam DJ. Toll-like receptor regulation of intestinal development and inflammation in the pathogenesis of necrotizing enterocolitis. Pathophysiology. 2014;**21**:81-93

[35] Yazji I et al. Endothelial TLR4 activation impairs intestinal microcirculatory perfusion in necrotizing enterocolitis via eNOS-NO-nitrite signaling. Proceedings of the National Academy of Sciences of the United States of America. 2013;**110**:9451-9456

[36] Ostlie DJ, Spilde TL, St Peter SD, et al. Necrotizing enterocolitis in full-term infants. Journal of Pediatric Surgery. 2003;**38**:1039-1042

[37] Walsh MC, Kliegman RM. Necrotizing enterocolitis: Treatment based on staging criteria. Pediatric Clinics of North America. 1986;**33**:179-201

[38] Fortune PM, Wagstaff M, Petros AJ. Cerebro-splanchnic oxygenation ratio (CSOR) using near infrared spectroscopy may be able to predict splanchnic ischaemia in neonates. Intensive Care Medicine. 2001;**27**:1401-1407

[39] Munaco AJ, Veenstra MA, Brownie E, Danielson LA, Nagappala KB, Klein MD. Timing of optimal surgical intervention for neonates with necrotizing enterocolitis. The American Surgeon. 2015;**81**:438-443

[40] Zani A, Eaton S, Puri P, et al. International survey on the management of necrotizing enterocolitis. European Journal of Pediatric Surgery. 2015;**25**:27-33

[41] Aydemir O, Aydemir C, Sarikabadayi YU, et al. Fecal calprotectin levels are increased in infants with necrotizing enterocolitis. The Journal of Maternal-Fetal & Neonatal Medicine. 2012;**25**:2237-2241

[42] Benkoe T, Reck C, Gleiss A, et al. Interleukin 8 correlates with intestinal involvement in surgically treated infants with necrotizing enterocolitis. Journal of Pediatric Surgery. 2012;**47**:1548-1554

[43] Benkoe T, Reck C, Pones M, et al. Interleukin-8 predicts 60-day mortality in premature infants with necrotizing enterocolitis. Journal of Pediatric Surgery. 2014;**49**:385-389

[44] Gaudin A, Farnoux C, Bonnard A, et al. Necrotizing enterocolitis (NEC) and the risk of intestinal stricture: The value of C-reactive protein. PLoS One. 2013;**8**:e76858

[45] Guthmann F, Borchers T, Wolfrum C, Wustrack T, Bartholomaus S, Spener F. Plasma concentration of intestinal- and liver-FABP in neonates suffering from necrotizing enterocolitis and in healthy preterm neonates. Molecular and Cellular Biochemistry. 2002;**239**:227-234

[46] Tepas JJ 3rd, Sharma R, Leaphart CL, Celso BG, Pieper P, Esquivia-Lee V. Timing of surgical intervention in necrotizing enterocolitis can be determined by trajectory of metabolic derangement. Journal of Pediatric Surgery. 2010;**45**:310-313

[47] Lacher M, Kuebler FK, Dingemann J, Ure BM. Minimal invasive surgery in the newborn: Current status and evidence. Seminars in Pediatric Surgery. 2014;**23**:249-256

[48] Smith J, Thyoka M. What role does laparoscopy play in the diagnosis and immediate treatment of infants with necrotizing enterocolitis? Journal of Laparoendoscopic & Advanced Surgical Techniques. 2013;**4**:397-401

[49] Rao SC, Basani L, Simmer K, Samnakay N, Deshpande G. Peritoneal drainage versus laparotomy as initial surgical treatment for perforated necrotizing enterocolitis or spontaneous intestinal perforation in preterm low birth weight infants. Cochrane Database of Systematic Reviews. 2011;**6**:CD006182. DOI: 10.1002/14651858.CD006182.pub2

[50] Rees CM, Eaton S, Kiely EM, et al. Peritoneal drainage or laparotomy for neonatal bowel perforation? A randomized controlled trial. Annals of Surgery. 2008;**248**:444-491

[51] Blakely ML, Tyson JE, Lally KP, et al. Laparotomy versus peritoneal drainage for necrotizing enterocolitis or isolated intestinal perforation in extremely low birth weight infants: Outcomes through 18 months adjusted age. Pediatrics. 2006;**117**:e680

[52] Cole CR, Hansen NI, Higgins RD, Ziegler TR, Stoll BJ. Very low birth weight preterm infants with surgical short bowel syndrome: Incidence, morbidity and mortality, and growth outcomes at 18 to 22 months. Pediatrics. 2008;**122**:e573-e582

[53] Duro D, Kalish LA, Johnston P, et al. Risk factors for intestinal failure in infants with necrotizing enterocolitis: A Glaser Pediatric Research Network study. Journal of Pediatrics. 2010;**157**(2):203-208.e1

[54] Amin SC, Pappas C, Iyengar H, Maheshwari A. Short bowel syndrome in the NICU. Clinics in Perinatology. 2013;**40**(1):53-68

[55] Schwartz MZ, Richardson CJ, Hayden CK, et al. Intestinal stenosis following successful medical management of necrotizing enterocolitis. Journal of Pediatric Surgery. 1980;**15**:890

[56] Hintz SR, Kendrick DE, Stoll BJ, et al. Neurodevelopmental and growth outcomes of extremely low birth weight infants after necrotizing enterocolitis. Pediatrics. 2005;**115**:696

[57] Hong CR, Fullerton BS, Mercier CE, et al. Growth morbidity in extremely low birth weight survivors of necrotizing enterocolitis at discharge and two-year follow-up. Journal of Pediatric Surgery. 2018;**53**:1197-1202

[58] Schulzke SM, Deshpande GC, Patole SK. Neurodevelopmental outcomes of very low-birth-weight infants with necrotizing enterocolitis: A systematic review of observational studies. Archives of Pediatrics & Adolescent Medicine. 2007;**161**:583

[59] Fitzgibbons SC, Ching Y, Yu D, et al. Mortality of necrotizing enterocolitis expressed by birth weight categories. Journal of Pediatric Surgery. 2009;**44**:1072-1075

[60] Clark RH, Gordon P, Walker WM, Laughon M, Smith PB, Spitzer AR. Characteristics of patients who die of necrotizing enterocolitis. Journal of Perinatology. 2011;**32**(3):199-204

[61] Lambert DK, Christensen RD, Baer VL, et al. Fulminant necrotizing enterocolitis in a multihospital healthcare system. Journal of Perinatology. 2012;**32**:194

[62] Stey A et al. Outcomes and costs of surgical treatments of necrotizing enterocolitis. Pediatrics. 2015;**135**:e1190-e1197

[63] Bisquera JA, Cooper TR, Berseth CL. Impact of necrotizing enterocolitis on length of stay and hospital charges in very low birth weight infants. Pediatrics. 2002;**109**:423-428

[64] Thomas JP, Raine T, Reddy S, Belteki G. Probiotics for the prevention of necrotising enterocolitis in very low-birth-weight infants: a meta-analysis and systematic review. Acta Paediatr 2017;**106**:1729-1741

[65] Li X, Li X, Shang Q, Gao Z, Hao F, Guo H, et al. Fecal microbiota transplantation (FMT) could reverse the severity of experimental necrotizing enterocolitis (NEC) via oxidative stress modulation. Free Radical Biology & Medicine. 2017;**108**:32-43

Chapter 3

Oesophageal Atresia: Drowning a Child in His/Her Own Saliva

Samuel Osei-Nketiah and William Appeadu-Mensah

Abstract

Oesophageal atresia (OA) is a congenital anomaly characterised by absence or loss of a segment of the oesophagus. This commonly affects the thoracic portion of the oesophagus, leaving upper and lower oesophageal segments. Loss of the oesophageal luminal continuity leads to impaired in utero swallowing of amniotic fluid as well as postnatal swallowing of saliva and food. Besides the loss of oesophageal continuity, most of the patients tend to have a connection between the trachea and the lower oesophageal segment and a few between the trachea and the upper oesophageal segment, a condition called tracheo-oesophageal fistula (TOF). In view of these, the main principles guiding the definitive surgical management of OA are (1) to disconnect any TOF and (2) to establish a conduit for swallowing, preferably using the native oesophageal segments. This chapter seeks to discuss OA by focusing on the embryology, anatomy and physiology of the oesophagus, stressing on the embryological basis of OA. Other areas to cover include aetiology, pathogenesis, epidemiology, pathologic classification, associated anomalies, pathophysiology, clinical presentation and diagnosis. Further discussion will focus on prognostic classification of patients, management and post-operative complications.

Keywords: oesophageal atresia, pathology, associated anomalies, pathophysiology, clinical presentation, diagnosis, pre-operative management, surgical management, outcome, prognosis

1. Introduction

Oesophageal atresia (OA), a congenital anomaly characterised by absence or loss of a segment of the oesophagus, commonly affects the thoracic portion of the oesophagus, leaving upper and lower oesophageal segments. Loss of the oesophageal luminal continuity leads to impaired in utero swallowing of amniotic fluid as well as postnatal swallowing of saliva and food. Besides the loss of oesophageal continuity, most of the patients tend to have a connection between the trachea and the lower oesophageal segment and a few between the trachea and the upper oesophageal segment, a condition called tracheo-oesophageal fistula (TOF). In view of these, the main principles guiding the definitive surgical management of oesophageal atresia are (1) to disconnect any tracheo-oesophageal fistula and (2) to establish a conduit for swallowing, preferably using the native oesophageal segments.

During the early years, the surgical management of oesophageal atresia was associated with lots of challenges and high mortality [1–4]. Over the past two to three decades, however, the surgical outcome has improved significantly in most centres in the developed countries. This improvement is attributed to advances

IntechOpen

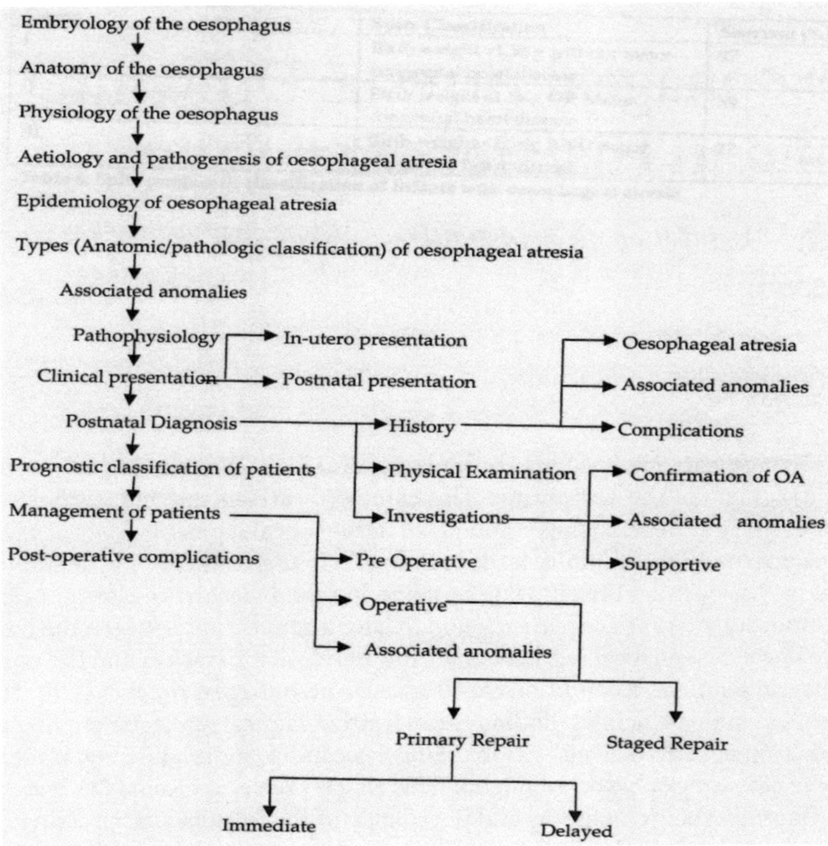

Figure 1.
Flow chart showing various topics to be discussed under oesophageal atresia.

in neonatal anaesthesia, well-established neonatal intensive care units (NICU), availability of total parental nutrition (TPN) and refined surgical skills [1, 5–8]. Conversely, the surgical outcome of oesophageal atresia in developing countries still remains very poor due to lack of the aforementioned facilities, in addition to late presentation [9–11].

This chapter seeks to discuss OA by focusing on the topics shown in **Figure 1**.

2. Embryology of the oesophagus

The oesophagus develops from the primitive foregut as a continuation of the pharynx. It is said to be present by the fifth week of gestation, and it attains its final foetal length (8–10 cm) during the 7th week of gestation [12]. Thus, the length of the oesophagus at birth is 8–10 cm, and this doubles during the first few years of life [12].

The normal embryology of the foregut, as found in most reports and textbooks of embryology, is divided into five developmental steps [13]:

1. During the first step, the endoderm (epithelium) of the primitive foregut differentiates into a ventral area called the *lung field* and a dorsal area called *oesophageal area*. The epithelium of the ventral area (lung field) of the primitive foregut consists of 3–4 cell layers, while that of the dorsal area (oesophageal area) has only one cell layer. This phase occurs when the embryo is about 22–23 days old.

2. Lung (tracheal) bud develops at the caudal end of the lung field.

3. During the third step, beginning caudally at the area of the lung bud, the lateral walls of the foregut start to approximate, developing longitudinal ridges inside the lumen of the foregut. This clearly separates the ventral lung field and the dorsal oesophageal area.

4. Epithelial tracheo-oesophageal septum develops during the fourth step; and it is assumed that this process also starts caudally and ends cranially close to the laryngeal primordium. This process is described by most investigators in four steps: (i) the epithelium of the longitudinal ridges starts to proliferate; (ii) the ridges, therefore, fuse in the midline of the primitive foregut and form an epithelial septum; (iii) cell death takes place in the central areas of the septum, noticeable by the appearance of nuclei pyknosis and (iv) as a result, mesenchymal tissue then expands into the area between the trachea and the oesophagus.

5. Separation of the respiratory tract from the oesophagus becomes definitive between the sixth and the seventh weeks of gestation through the formation of a mesenchymal septum called tracheo-oesophageal septum.

It should be noted that most steps in this schematic description of the foregut embryology lack clear evidence [13].

Other developmental features of the oesophagus include [12]:

Mesenchymal circular coat (muscle) develops early in the sixth week of gestation. The longitudinal muscle forms between the ninth and twelfth weeks of gestation, and the muscularis mucosa develops at approximately the fourth month of gestation [12].

Blood vessels enter the oesophageal wall during the seventh month of gestation and lymph capillaries between the third and fourth months of life [12]. The most important embryologic structure for blood supply to the oesophagus is the fourth branchial arch. The arch produces the subclavian artery and its branches, including the inferior thyroid artery which supplies the cervical oesophagus. The fourth branchial arch also produces the aorta, from which vessels spring to supply the thoracic oesophagus.

The formation of the oesophageal epithelium is peculiar; it "changes face" four times. The epithelium is stratified columnar at the start of embryonic life, becoming cuboidal later. In foetal life, it is ciliated columnar, and, finally, it becomes stratified squamous soon after birth. Innervation of the oesophageal wall is received from sympathetic nerve fibres from the thoracic trunk and celiac plexus and parasympathetic innervation from the vagus nerve.

The oesophageal wall is formed from endoderm and mesoderm (**Figure 2**). The endoderm produces the oesophageal epithelium and glands, whereas the mesoderm produces the connective tissue, muscular coat, and angioblasts. Splanchnic mesenchyme surrounds the oesophagus and trachea. The splanchnic mesenchyme forms the smooth muscle of the lower oesophagus.

The causal branchial arches (4 and 6) are responsible for the formation of the striated musculature of the upper oesophagus and pharynx. They are innervated by the vagus nerve (nerve to the fourth arch) and the recurrent laryngeal nerve branch of the vagus nerve (nerve to the sixth arch) [12].

The oesophageal lumen is almost filled with vacuolated cells from proliferation of oesophageal epithelium during the seven–eighth weeks of gestation. The filling is never complete, and hence the so-called solid stage does not exist. At 10 weeks' gestation, the lumen of the oesophagus is restored as the vacuolated cells disappear.

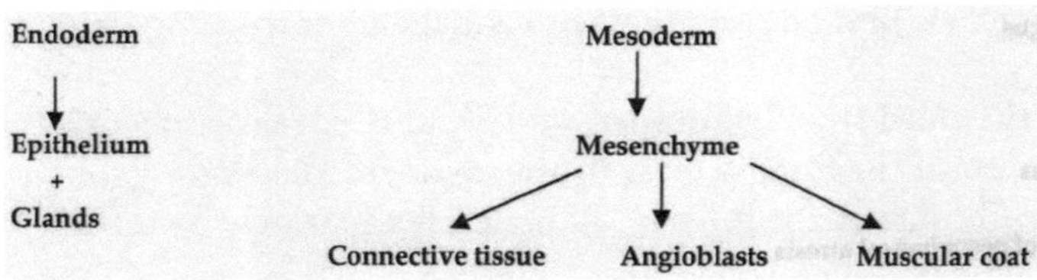

Figure 2.
Embryologic duo responsible for genesis of the oesophagus.

2.1 Anatomy of the oesophagus

The oesophagus is a muscular tube connecting the pharynx to the stomach. At birth, the length of the oesophagus is about 8–10 cm, and this doubles in the first few years of life. The length of the oesophagus in the adult is about 25 cm. It extends from the lower border of the cricoid cartilage (at the level of the C6 vertebra) to the cardiac orifice of the stomach at the level of T11 vertebra. The upper limit in the newborn is found at the level of the fourth or fifth cervical vertebra and ends higher at the level of the T9 vertebra [14, 15].

The oesophageal wall is composed of mucosa, submucosa, muscularis propria and adventitia, lacking a distinct serosa. The mucosa is the strongest layer of the oesophageal wall. Hence, meticulous approximation of the oesophageal mucosa is essential for a technically sound anastomosis.

The oesophagus is divided into three segments—*cervical, thoracic and abdominal segments*. The cervical portion is somewhat curved, with its convex side to the left, thereby projecting to the left of the trachea. Incisions for approaching the cervical oesophagus are commonly made on this side. Anteriorly, the cervical oesophagus is covered by the trachea.

The arterial blood supply to the oesophagus is generally considered with regard to the cervical, thoracic and abdominal segments of the oesophagus. The arterial blood supply to the pharyngo-oesophageal junction and the cervical oesophagus is derived from branches of the inferior thyroid artery. In addition, the pharyngo-oesophageal junctional area of the oesophagus is supplied by small arterial branches of the subclavian (artery of Luschka), common carotid, vertebral, superior thyroid and costocervical trunk vessels [12, 16]. The thoracic oesophagus is supplied from oesophageal branches of the aorta, the bronchial arteries and the right intercostal arteries. Accessory oesophageal branches are also present directly from the internal mammary, common carotid and superior intercostal arteries [12, 17]. The left gastric artery provides oesophageal blood supply to the abdominal segment of the oesophagus in most individuals. Rarely, oesophageal arteries will arise from an accessory left hepatic artery. In less than one-half of individuals, the oesophagus receives arterial blood via the left inferior phrenic artery and rarely from the right inferior phrenic artery [16]. A well-developed subepithelial network of capillaries is present in the oesophageal mucosa and submucosa [18, 19]. The excellent submucosa plexus of the proximal oesophagus allows for extensive mobilization without compromise to the blood supply, whereas caution should be taken distally because of the segmental lower oesophageal blood supply.

Venous drainage from the oesophagus includes intrinsic and extrinsic vessels. The intrinsic system includes subepithelial and submucosal veins that join gastric veins and perforating veins that join with the extrinsic system of veins. The extrinsic veins include larger longitudinal vessels that run on the outer surface of the oesophagus and are close to the vagus nerves. These vessels connect the left gastric vein to the azygous or hemiazygous veins either directly or indirectly via the posterior bronchial veins. Extrinsic veins drain into the inferior thyroid, vertebral and deep cervical veins in the cervical region. Oesophageal veins at the level of the cardia join the phrenic and abdominal oesophageal veins to drain primarily into the left gastric vein, as well as the gastroepiploic and splenic veins [20]. This may be a point of importance when dealing with a patient with portal hypertension.

The oesophageal lymphatics form plexuses in the mucosa (lamina propria), submucosa, muscularis, and adventitia with interconnectivity [12]. Collecting trunks originate in the submucosa and empty into the nearest lymph nodes.

In the oesophageal wall are two plexuses of nerves for intrinsic nerve supply: (i) Meissner's plexus in the submucosa and (ii) Auerbach's plexus in the connective tissue between the circular and longitudinal muscularis externa [12]. These plexuses form networks of multipolar ganglion cells, the processes of which are in contact with one another and receive axons from the vagus. The oesophagus receives extrinsic nerve supply from three sources: the (a) cerebrospinal, (b) sympathetic and (c) parasympathetic (vagal) nervous systems [12].

The cricopharyngeal (CP) muscle, which is located at the pharyngo-oesophageal junction, attaches to the cricoid cartilage and forms a C-shaped muscular band. It is innervated by the pharyngeal plexus of the vagus nerve and the recurrent laryngeal nerve [21]. The main function of the CP muscle is to control luminal flow between the pharynx and oesophagus. The CP sphincter muscle is tonically contracted at rest and relaxes during swallowing. The major component of the upper oesophageal sphincter (UES) is the CP muscle, although the inferior pharyngeal constrictor and striated muscles of the proximal oesophagus also contribute [22].

The function of the lower oesophageal sphincter is abolished by total truncal vagotomy.

2.2 Physiology of the oesophagus

The main function of the oesophagus is for swallowing, and this is achieved through peristalsis. Functionally, the oesophagus is divided into three areas: (i) the upper oesophageal sphincter (UOS), (ii) the oesophageal body and (iii) the lower oesophageal sphincter (LOS). The coordinated activity of these three parts is essential to ensure propulsion of bolus from the pharynx to the stomach. The UOS plays a key role in controlling regurgitation of oesophageal content into the pharynx and the airways, while the LOS prevents reflux of gastric content into the oesophagus.

2.3 Aetiology and pathogenesis of oesophageal atresia

Various theories were developed in the past to explain the embryology of foregut anomalies. These theories are grouped into four [13]: (i) oesophageal occlusion theory, (ii) theories of spontaneous deviation of the tracheo-oesophageal septum, (iii) mechanical theories and (iv) not otherwise specified (NOS) theories.

Tandler postulated the theory of foregut occlusion in 1902 as a physiological occlusion during duodenal development [13]. Such physiological occlusion is also postulated to occur during oesophageal development; and that failure of recanalisation leads to oesophageal atresia [13]. Tracheo-oesophageal septal deviation is found to be another theory that explains the development of OA [13]. Various mechanisms have been used to explain the mechanical theory [13]. These include ventral pressure on the developing oesophagus by a very big anlage of the heart and aberrant vessels. The NOS theories include the development of a very large tracheal field that uses too much tissue to form the trachea, resulting in a shortage of dorsal tissue. Abnormal septation, combined with a disturbance in the organ inducing field, is believed to account for OA with TOF. Isolated TOF is speculated to result from a loss of epithelial proliferation or through an excessive necrosis in the area of the epithelial tracheo-oesophageal septum [13].

Aetiologically, various genetic defects have been found to be associated with oesophageal atresia. Important genes related to the pathogenesis of OA, and mostly involved in developmental pathways, include vitamin A effectors, retinoic acid receptors a and b (Rara and Rarb), sonic hedgehog pathway effectors (Shh, Gli2, Gli3 and Foxf1) and other homeobox containing transcription factors (Hoxc4, Ttf-1 and Pcsk5) [23]. Various environmental teratogens have also been implicated in the pathogenesis of OA-TOF [23]. Infants born to mothers with prolonged exposure to contraceptive pills (exposure to progesterone and oestrogen) during pregnancy have high risk. Oesophageal atresia has also been reported in some infants of hyperthyroid and uncontrolled diabetic mothers. Intrauterine exposure to thalidomide and diethylstilbestrol are also found to be associated with OA.

2.4 Epidemiology of oesophageal atresia

The incidence of OA, with or without TOF, is reported to be 1:3500 live-born infants. This, however, varies geographically [23] from 1 in 2440 births in Finland to 1 in 4500 births in the United States and Australia. In a European study, 62% of infants with OA-TOF were male, whereas a California database found considerable variations in the male-to-female ratios between types of OA-TOF defects [23]. Mothers of white ethnicity have a higher (>60%) prevalence of OA-TOF than non-white populations do [23]. First pregnancy and increasing maternal age have been found to be associated with an increased risk OA-TOF [23]. The risk is reported to be twofold for women 35–40 years old and threefold for those older than this age [23]. Offspring of in vitro fertilization patients also have a significantly increased risk of developing OA (OR 3.65:CI 2/53–5/26) [23].

2.5 Anatomic (pathologic) classification of oesophageal atresia

Various systems of classifications have been used to classify OA. The two most frequently used ones are shown in **Table 1** [24].

2.6 Associated anomalies

About 50–70% of patients with oesophageal atresia have associated congenital anomalies [23]. Cases without tracheo-oesophageal fistula tend to be most commonly associated with other anomalies, while those with the H-type are less commonly associated with other anomalies. Associated anomalies may negatively affect patient management and overall outcome of patients.

Anatomic Description	Gross type	Vogt type	Approximate Incidence (%)41
Oesophageal Agenesis	-	I	
Oesophageal Atresia without tracheo-oesophageal fistula	A	II	6
Oesophageal atresia with proximal tracheo-oesophageal fistula	B	IIIa	2
Oesophageal atresia with distal tracheo-oesophageal fistula	C	IIIb	85
Oesophageal atresia with both proximal and distal tracheo-oesophageal fistulae	D	IIIc	1
Tracheo-oesophageal fistula without oesophageal atresia	E	IV	6

Table 1.
Types of oesophageal atresia—anatomic (pathologic) classification of oesophageal atresia.

About 50% of patients with associated anomalies have recognizable syndromes, sequences, and associations [23]. VACTERL (vertebral, anorectal malformation, cardiac, tracheo-oesophageal, renal, limb) association is found in 20% of cases [25]. These syndromes, sequences, and associations usually result from chromosomal anomalies or single gene mutations (**Tables 2** and **3**) [23, 26].

Patients with oesophageal atresia have trisomies 18 and 21 in about 7% of patients. In trisomy 21 (Down syndrome), the possibility of associated duodenal atresia, Hirschsprung's disease and congenital heart disease should be considered. In patients with clinically suspected trisomy 18, surgery should be postponed and chromosomal analysis done immediately since prognosis for trisomy 18 is very poor.

The common associated anomalies in non-syndromic oesophageal atresia include the cardiovascular system (CVS), genitourinary tract (GUT), gastrointestinal tract (GIT), musculoskeletal system (MSS), and central nervous system (CNS) (**Table 4**). Cardiovascular anomalies tend to occur most frequently (**Table 4**) [23, 25, 27]. This is followed by the GUT, GIT, MSS, and CNS (neurologic anomalies). A review of cases seen at our centre in Accra Korle-Bu, however, showed overall incidence of associated anomalies of 32.5%, with GIT system being the most commonly affected, followed by the CVS [9].

The most common CVS anomalies are ventricular septal defect (VSD) and atrial septal defect (ASD). Other CVS defects include tetralogy of Fallot, patent ductus arteriosus (PDA), and coarctation of the aorta. A few patients tend to have the descending thoracic aorta on the right side. Renal agenesis or hypoplasia, undescended testis, cystic renal disease, hydronephrosis, vesicoureteric reflux (VUR) and ureteric duplication are some of the GUT anomalies associated with oesophageal atresia. Other GUT anomalies include pelvi-ureteric junction (PUJ) obstruction, vesicoureteric junction (VUJ) obstruction, urachal anomalies, ambiguous genitalia, bladder exstrophy and cloacal exstrophy. The GIT anomalies found in oesophageal atresia include anorectal malformation (ARM), duodenal atresia, intestinal malrotation, ileal atresia, annular pancreas and pyloric stenosis. Vertebral and radial abnormalities are the usual MSS defects associated with oesophageal atresia. The CNS defects found in oesophageal atresia include neural tube defects, hydrocephalus, holoprosencephaly and anophthalmia or microphthalmia.

2.7 Pathophysiology of oesophageal atresia

The discontinuation of the oesophageal lumen prevents swallowed amniotic fluid by the foetus from reaching the stomach and hence the intestine. In view of this, the physiological control of amniotic fluid volume by the foetus, through swallowing and absorption, is impaired, leading to polyhydramnios. This would in turn lead to premature rupture of membrane, umbilical cord prolapse and premature delivery.

Chromosomal Defect	Resultant Syndrome
Trisomy 21	Down syndrome
Trisomy 18	Edward syndrome
Trisomy 13	Patau syndrome
Chromosome 22q deletion	1. DiGeorge syndrome 2. Autosomal dominant Opitz G/BBB syndrome
Chromosome 17q deletion	Chromosome 17q deletion syndrome, including renal cyst and diabetes (RCAD) syndrome and Mayer-Rokitansky-Kuster-Hauser syndrome
Chromosome 16q deletion	Chromosome 16q deletion syndrome, including Townes-Brocks syndrome
Chromosome 13q deletion	Chromosome 13q deletion syndrome

Table 2.
Chromosomal abnormalities associated with oesophageal atresia.

Single Gene Mutation (Chromosomal location)	Resultant Syndrome, Sequence and Associations
MYCN (2p24.1)	Feingold syndrome (ODED syndrome – Oculo-digito-esophageal-duodenal syndrome)
CHD7 (8q12)	CHARGE (Coloboma, Heart defects, Atresia of nasal choanae, Retarded growth/development, Genitourinary abnormalities, Ear anomalies) syndrome
SOX2 (3q26.33)	AEG (Anolphthalmos-Esophageal-Genital) syndrome
GLI3 (7p13)	Pallister-Hall syndrome
FANCA (16q24.3)	Fanconi anaemia
TBX5 (12q24.21)	Holt-Oram syndrome (Heart-hand syndrome)
Multifactorial	Goldenhar syndrome (Oculo-auriculo-vertebral syndrome)
RFX6 (6q22.1)	Martinez-Frias syndrome
FANCB (Xp22.2); FANCC (9q22.3); FANCD1 (13q12.3); FANCD2 (3p25.3); FANCG (9p13.3); PTEN (10q23.31)	VACTERL Association with hydrocephalus (VACTERL-H)
MID1 (Xp22.2)	X-linked Opitz G/BBB

Table 3.
Single gene mutations associated with oesophageal atresia.

Postnatally, the neonate is not able to swallow saliva and food. This leads to accumulation of saliva and food in the upper oesophageal segment (pouch). The accumulated saliva and food then spill over into the lungs through the larynx and trachea. Patients are therefore prone to the development of aspiration pneumonia. Patients with distal tracheo-oesophageal fistula also tend to aspirate gastric secretions into the lungs, especially if lying in a head-down position.

The distal tracheo-oesophageal fistula also allows air to escape from the trachea to the stomach and hence the intestines. Consequently, patients can develop gross distention of the stomach and intestine, especially if patient is resuscitated using an Ambu bag. The distended stomach can then splint the diaphragm, impairing diaphragmatic excursion and thereby causing respiratory distress. The distended stomach can also rupture leading to chemical peritonitis.

In patients with delayed diagnosis, the constant regurgitation of swallowed food leads to malnutrition. Such patients tend to have poor surgical outcome and overall survival.

Associated congenital anomalies, especially severe cardiac and renal anomalies, also affect management and survival of patients. Low birth weight that may result from premature delivery owing to polyhydramnios also tends to affect management and survival.

2.8 Clinical presentation

Oesophageal atresia may be detected prenatally or postnatally.

2.8.1 Prenatal presentation and diagnosis

Prenatal diagnosis helps in planning of delivery and possible prenatal referral to centres that have the facilities to manage such patients.

Oesophageal atresia should be suspected prenatally in patients with evidence of polyhydramnios. Polyhydramnios will present with symphysio-fundal height

Associated anomaly	Incidence (%)
CVS	24
GUT	21
GIT	21
MSS	14
CNS	7

Table 4.
Common associated anomalies in non-syndromic oesophageal atresia.

of more than the expected for gestational age. This is confirmed with antenatal ultrasonography with amniotic fluid index (AFI) of more than 24 cm.

Antenatal ultrasonographic features of polyhydramnios, a small stomach, a distended upper oesophageal pouch and abnormal swallowing should raise the suspicion of oesophageal atresia [28–31].

2.8.2 Postnatal presentation and diagnosis

2.8.2.1 History

Postnatally, patients with oesophageal atresia present with drooling of saliva (excessive salivation). A history of antenatal polyhydramnios gives more credence to the diagnosis of oesophageal atresia. Delayed diagnosis leads to aspiration of saliva from the upper oesophageal pouch, causing aspiration pneumonia with cough, cyanosis and fever. Feeding leads to worsening of the aspiration pneumonia. Hence, early detection and avoidance of oral feeds helps to promote good outcome of patients.

Patients with distal tracheo-oesophageal fistula are also at risk of aspiration of gastric secretions into the lungs. In addition, swallowed air passes through the distal tracheo-oesophageal fistula into the stomach. This can lead to gross gastric distention, especially following Ambu bagging, resulting in diaphragmatic splinting and sometimes gastric rupture. They may thus present with respiratory distress, gross abdominal distention and sometimes peritonitis.

Patients with tracheo-oesophageal fistula without oesophageal atresia are usually diagnosed late. They present with recurrent cough associated with feeding and recurrent episodes of pneumonia.

Other symptoms would depend on associated congenital anomalies. Patients with cardiac anomalies may present with cyanosis. Patients with renal agenesis will have a history of anuria.

During history taking, one should seek for a maternal history of uncontrolled diabetes mellitus and the use of drugs such as oral contraceptives, antithyroid drugs (carbimazole and methimazole) and thalidomide. These are risk factors for oesophageal atresia.

The history of the maturity and weight of the baby at birth are also important considerations.

2.8.2.2 Physical examination

The principles of physical examination of a patient with suspected oesophageal atresia are to confirm the diagnosis, assess for aspiration pneumonia and evaluate for associated congenital anomalies.

To confirm the diagnosis, a stiff radiopaque 10-gauge French catheter is passed through the mouth into the oesophagus. The tube is not passed through the nose because it may traumatize the nasal passages. The diagnosis of oesophageal atresia is heightened if the tube fails to reach the stomach by getting arrested in the proximal oesophageal pouch at about 10 cm from the alveolar margin. A soft and smaller tube may coil in the upper oesophageal pouch, giving an impression of reaching the stomach. The secretions sucked through the tube can be tested with litmus paper to differentiate between saliva (basic) in the upper oesophageal pouch and gastric secretions (acidic).

The presence of fever, respiratory distress, reduced air entry in the lungs (especially on the right side) and crepitations in the lungs are an indication of aspiration pneumonia. However, patients in heart failure will have similar chest findings, and these are usually bilateral. Gastric distention and gastric rupture will be associated with respiratory distress, abdominal distention and abdominal signs of peritonitis.

Meticulous examination for associated anomalies is done. The presence of cyanosis may be due to cyanotic heart disease. The chest is examined for heart murmurs and crepitations. The abdomen is examined for any palpable flank mass. The perineum is examined for ARM. The spine and the limbs are also examined for any anomaly. Indeed, the VACTERL association could be used as a guide to take history, examine and investigate for any associated congenital anomaly.

2.8.2.3 Investigations

Investigations are also done to confirm the diagnosis, to assess for complications (aspiration pneumonitis and gastric rupture) and to evaluate for associated anomalies.

Oesophageal atresia is confirmed by taking a plain X-ray of the neck, chest, and abdomen with a radiopaque tube passed through the mouth in situ. In the presence of oesophageal atresia, the X-ray will show the tube arrested in the upper oesophageal pouch or coiled in the upper pouch. The same X-ray is also evaluated for evidence of associated aspiration pneumonia, cardiac enlargement, dextrocardia and vertebral anomalies.

The abdominal portion will help to determine the presence of air in the stomach and intestine. The presence of air in the stomach and intestine indicates the presence of a distal tracheo-oesophageal fistula. Pneumoperitoneum indicates gastric rupture. A gasless abdomen implies the absence of a distal tracheo-oesophageal fistula. Such a patient may either have no tracheo-oesophageal fistula or a proximal fistula. The proximal fistula can be identified with the aid of bronchoscopy [32]. **Table 5** summarises the important diagnostic features of OA.

Abdominal ultrasound to assess the kidneys, ureters and the urinary bladder is also done. Patients with bilateral renal agenesis or severe multicystic dysplastic kidneys will need no further management since such patients will not survive. Renal scintigraphy will confirm non-functioning kidneys.

Ultrasonography (USG) of the spine is used to assess the spinal cord for anomalies, including tethered cord. The USG of the spinal cord should be done before 3 months of age since the bones become ossified after this age, rendering the use of USG impossible. Magnetic resonance imaging (MRI) may be used to evaluate the spinal cord. It is, however, very expensive and implies the need for general anaesthesia in a new born with a relatively high anaesthetic risk. It is not readily available at most centres, especially in the developing countries.

	Prenatal	Postnatal
Clinical Features	• Polyhydramnios	• Drooling of saliva (Excessive salivation) • Cough, Fever, chest crepitations (Due to associated aspiration pneumonitis) • Choking during feeding • Prenatal history of polyhydramnios • Cynosis due to aspiration pneumonitis and/or associated cyanotic heart disease • Stiff radio-opaque 10-French catheter fails to reach the stomach (Arrested at about 10cm from the alveolar margin)
Imaging Features	Ultrasound: • Dilated upper oesophageal pouch • Small stomach • Abnormal swallowing	Plain X-Ray of the neck, chest and abdomen with the stiff radio-opaque 10-French catheter insitu: • Catheter found arrested (sometimes curled up/coiled up) in the upper oesophageal pouch • Air in stomach and intestine indicates distal tracheo-oesophageal fistula • Gasless abdomen implies no distal trachea-oesophageal fistula

Table 5.
Important diagnostic features of oesophageal atresia.

Echocardiogram is used to evaluate the heart for a congenital heart disease and the direction of the arch of the aorta. The direction of the arch of the aorta (normally to the left) is utilised in deciding the side of the thoracotomy incision (usually on the right side since the arch is normally to the left). At our centre, echocardiogram is not routinely done for every patient since it is expensive and not readily available. Hence, we selectively use it for only patients with clinical evidence of congenital heart disease.

Patients with suspected chromosomal and genetic anomalies are evaluated to confirm the anomaly. However, this is not available at most centres in developing centres, including our centre. Patients with confirmed trisomy 18 (Edwards syndrome) should have any planned surgical intervention abandoned since prognosis for these patients is very poor.

Patients with Down syndrome should be evaluated for the possibility of associated duodenal atresia, congenital heart disease and Hirschsprung's disease.

Other investigations that are supportive are full blood count (FBC) and blood urea, electrolytes, and creatinine (BUE&Cr). Blood gases may be analysed in patients who are critically ill.

2.9 Clinical prognostic classification of patients

Prognostic classification is done based on risk factors that affect survival of infants with OA. It is used to guide operative treatment and to compare case outcomes over time and between centres. The first prognostic risk stratification of patients with OA was developed in 1962 (Waterston classification) [4]. This is based on birth weight, the presence of pneumonia and associated congenital anomalies (**Table 6**). It has provided important contribution to the care of infants with OA. Patients in group A (good-risk category) are offered immediate primary repair of the defect. Those in group B (moderate-risk category) are treated with delayed primary repair, while those in group C (high-risk category) are managed by staged repair.

Several new classification schemes have been developed because of improvement in neonatal intensive care and availability of more treatment options for multiple congenital anomalies. These new schemes include refinement of the Waterston classification by Randolf and colleagues in 1989 [33]. This is based on the overall physiologic status of the patient. Poenaru et al. [34] also developed a new prognostic classification based on severe pulmonary dysfunction with preoperative mechanical ventilation and severe associated anomalies. Spitz et al. [35] developed a new risk classification based on birth weight and major cardiac anomaly (**Table 7**). Currently, the Spitz classification is the most commonly used system [36, 37]. Another new prognostic classification system has been developed by adding preoperative respiratory distress syndrome and pneumonia to the Spitz classification [38].

Category	Waterston Classification	Survival (%)
A	Birth weight > 2.5Kg and otherwise healthy	100
B	(i) Birth weight 1.8-2.5Kg and well; OR (ii) Birth weight >2.5Kg with moderate pneumonia or moderate congenital anomaly	85
C	(i) Birth weight <1.8Kg; OR (ii) Birth weight >1.8Kg with severe pneumonia or Severe congenital anomaly	65

Table 6.
Waterston prognostic classification of oesophageal atresia infants.

Group	Spitz Classification	Survival (%)
I	Birth weight >1.5Kg without major congenital heart disease	97
II	Birth weight <1.5Kg **OR** Major congenital heart disease	59
III	Birth weight <1.5Kg **AND** major congenital heart disease	22

Table 7.
Spitz prognostic classification of infants with oesophageal atresia.

2.10 Management of patients

2.10.1 Pre-operative management

The aim of preoperative management is to make patient stable before surgical management of the oesophageal atresia. This involves prevention of complications, treatment of life-threatening complications, management of life-threatening associated congenital anomalies and general supportive measures.

Complications to be prevented are mainly aspiration and diaphragmatic splinting by gaseous distention of the stomach and intestines. Maintaining the child in a partly upright position and by repeated or continuous suctioning of the upper oesophageal pouch prevents aspiration. These measures keep the proximal oesophagus empty and reduce the likelihood of overflow of saliva into the lungs. The repeated suctioning of the upper oesophageal pouch should be done every 10 min or more often if the child appears to have excessive mucus or air bubbles. The best tube for suctioning, especially for continuous suctioning, is the Replogle tube. The partial upright position prevents aspiration of stomach secretions. Infants with OA should not be fed to prevent aspiration. The child should have minimal handling to prevent excessive crying and consequent filling of stomach with air. In addition, vigorous resuscitation by Ambu bagging should be avoided to prevent gastric distention.

The main life-threatening complication is respiratory distress. Respiratory distress may be due to prematurity, other congenital abnormalities, aspiration pneumonia, or diaphragmatic splinting. Diaphragmatic splinting in patients with OA results from excessive escape of air through the distal fistula into the stomach, causing distention of the stomach and intestines and, in some cases, causing gastric rupture. Thorough evaluation of the infant to determine the underlying cause and prompt management is paramount. Gross gastric distension and perforation, causing pneumoperitoneum and elevation of the diaphragm, can cause major morbidity by worsening ventilation. Prompt needle decompression of the abdomen should be offered. This is followed by urgent laparotomy to control the air leakage. This involves insertion of a Foley catheter through the gastric perforation into the lower oesophagus, thereby occluding the distal TOF and allowing thoracotomy to proceed, at which time the distal TOF is divided. Blood gases should be monitored, but if monitoring facilities are not available, the infant must be kept pink at all times, and pulse oximetry for monitoring is considered standard.

Patients with duct-dependent congenital heart disease should be stabilised, by keeping the duct (patent ductus arteriosus) patent with prostaglandin E1 infusion, before surgery is done.

General supportive measures include keeping the child warm, vitamin K administration, provision of IV fluids/parenteral nutrition and administration of broad-spectrum antibiotics.

2.10.2 Operative management of oesophageal atresia

The operative management may be immediate primary repair, delayed primary repair or staged repair; and this depends on the prognostic category of the patient and the gap between the upper and the lower oesophageal segments. Patients with pneumonia and duct-dependent congenital heart disease need to be stabilised and planned for delayed primary repair. Patients with long-gap oesophageal atresia could also be managed with delayed primary repair. Further growth of the upper oesophageal pouch tends to occur if primary repair is delayed for about 3 months. Hence, the role of total parenteral nutrition (TPN) becomes significantly important. No consensus has been reached for the definition of long-gap OA. However, long gap is defined by some authorities as a gap of ≥3 vertebral bodies or ≥5 cm [39].

Primary repair is achieved mostly through a right thoracotomy (readers should read operative textbooks for details of the surgical procedure). However, in patients with right-sided arch of aorta, left thoracotomy is done. The patient is placed at the right side uppermost and with a towel folded underneath the left chest to give lateral flexion. The right arm is extended above the head and the head slightly flexed. A transverse incision is centred on the inferior angle of the scapula, and the chest is entered through the fourth intercostal space. Approach to the oesophagus may be extrapleural or transpleural. The extrapleural approach is favoured because of the less likelihood of developing empyema following an anastomotic leak. The pleura is swept off the chest wall to identify the structures of the posterior mediastinum. The azygous vein is then ligated and divided.

Any distal TOF is identified and divided close to the trachea. The fistula is then closed with interrupted absorbable sutures such as 4/0 Vicryl, PDS, or Monocryl. Care should be taken to avoid damage to the vagal fibres and blood supply to the distal oesophageal segment.

The upper oesophagus is identified with the aid of a tube passed through the mouth or nose by the anaesthetist. It is then mobilised enough to allow an end-to-end, one-layer, interrupted oesophageal anastomosis, ensuring that the mucosa and the submucosa are included. The upper oesophageal segment can be extensively mobilized along its full length without risk of significant ischemia. If extensive mobilization of the proximal oesophagus fails to provide adequate length, the lower oesophagus may be mobilized to prevent undue tension on the anastomosis. Mobilising the lower oesophagus without complete disruption of its segmental vascular supply is possible. However, care should be taken to avoid excessive or rough handling of the oesophagus. If, despite extensive mobilisation of the two oesophageal segments, an anastomosis cannot be performed without excessive tension, an oesophageal myotomy (Levaditis procedure) can be performed. Myotomy (circular or spiral myotomy) is usually done using the upper pouch. It can cause significant damage to the nerve and blood supply distal to the myotomy and predisposes to diverticulum formation and strictures.

Patients with TOF without atresia have an oblique fistula running downward from the trachea to the oesophagus, usually at the level of T1–T3. This level is somewhat higher than what is seen in most patients with oesophageal atresia. In these patients, a cervical approach provides the best surgical access as most fistulas are in the root of the neck (at about the level of the second thoracic vertebra). Care should be taken to avoid damage to the recurrent laryngeal nerves, which lie in the grooves between the oesophagus and the trachea and closely related to the fistula, during operative dissection.

Staged repair of OA involves division of TOF, placement of feeding gastrostomy and cervical oesophagostomy. Disconnection of distal TOF is done at most centres through thoracotomy. At our centre, however, this is done by dividing the abdominal oesophagus during the placement of the feeding gastrostomy [27]. This helps to avoid the stress of thoracotomy that may negatively affect patient outcome. Patients who undergo staged repair are later offered oesophageal replacement surgery.

It should be noted that the surgical management of OA has been advanced into the realm of minimally invasive surgery (thoracoscopy) due to recent advances in surgical techniques. [40–49]. Thoracoscopic approach to the repair of OA is associated with early recovery and minimal chest wall musculoskeletal morbidity as compared with open surgery (thoracotomy).

2.11 Manoeuvres for managing long-gap OA to achieve primary repair

Various manoeuvres are used to narrow the gap between the upper and lower oesophageal segments [50]. These manoeuvres are classified as preoperative manoeuvres and intraoperative manoeuvres (**Table 8**).

Preoperative manoeuvres are those that are done before the surgery for primary repair is attempted; and they may be achieved thoracoscopically [45, 51]. These include external traction technique by Foker [50, 52, 53]; multistage, extrathoracic elongation technique by Kimura [52, 54]; bougienage of the upper oesophageal pouch, sometimes including the lower pouch; placement of magnets in the two ends of the oesophageal segments with patient placed in an electromagnetic field and delaying of surgery for some months to allow growth of the oesophagus.

In the Kimura technique, the upper part of the oesophagus is mobilised and brought out as an end-cervical oesophagostomy. The oesophagus and its cutaneous stoma are surgically mobilised and translocated down the anterior chest wall every 2–3 weeks. This is continued until enough length is achieved to perform an end-to-end oesophageal anastomosis. The Foker technique involves open or thoracoscopic placement of traction sutures on both the proximal and distal oesophageal pouches with the sutures exiting through the chest wall. These sutures are serially pulled in opposite directions until the pouches approximate. This external traction technique of Foker is reported to induce oesophageal growth and expedite approximation of the pouches.

Internal traction techniques have also been used to bridge long gaps [45, 55]. These include open or thoracoscopic suturing of the oesophageal segments to the prevertebral fascia or costal bone under tension.

Intra-operative manoeuvres include full mobilisation of the upper segment of the oesophagus; mobilisation of the distal segment; circular myotomy (Levaditis technique) or spiral myotomy, usually of the upper pouch and mobilisation of the stomach into the chest.

Other intraoperative techniques include full-thickness anterior flap of the upper pouch [56] and injection of Botox into the upper segment.

Figure 3 shows an algorithm for the management of patients with oesophageal atresia.

Pre-operative Maneuvers	Intra-operative Maneuvers
• Delaying surgery for about 3 months • Traction techniques - External traction technique by Foker - Internal traction technique (Suturing of oesophageal segments to prevertebral fascia or costal bone under tension) • Multistage extrathoracic oesophageal elongation technique by Kimura • Bougienage of oesophageal pouch • Magnetic elongation technique	• Extensive mobilisation of the upper oesophageal pouch; and sometimes the lower oesophageal pouch • Myotomy - Circular myotomy by Levaditis - Spiral myotomy • Full thickness anterior flap of the upper oesophageal pouch • Mobilisation of stomach into the chest • Injection of botox into the upper oesophageal segment

Table 8.
Pre-operative and intraoperative oesophageal elongation manoeuvres for long-gap oesophageal atresia.

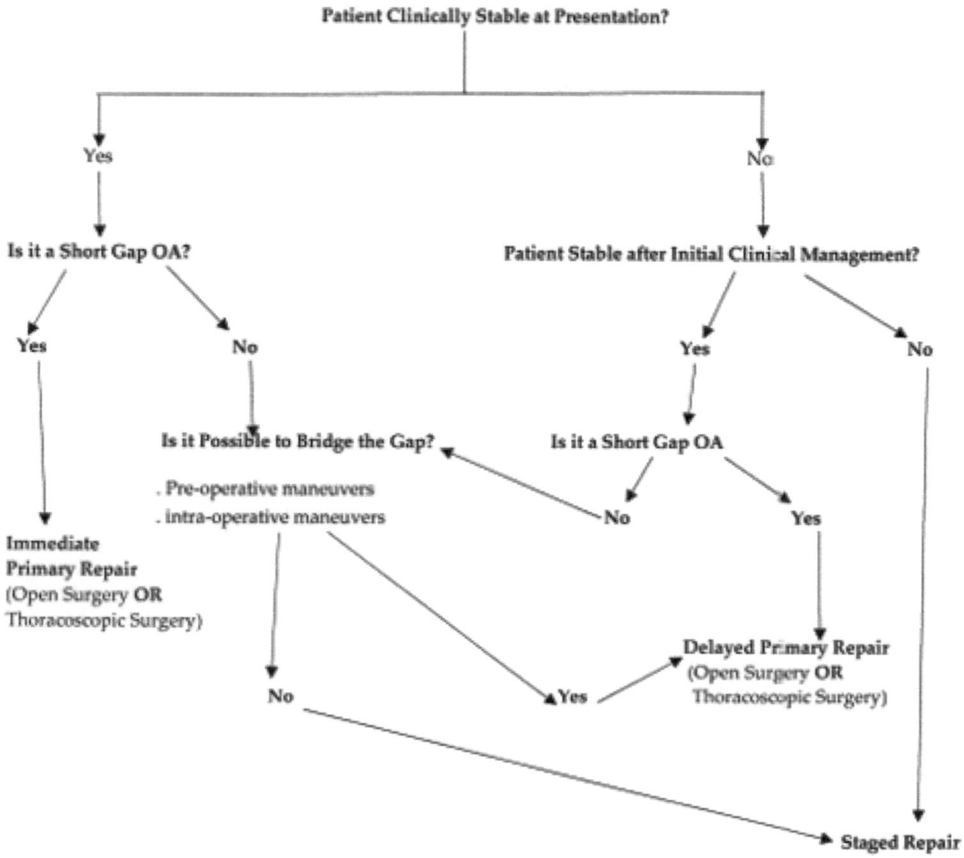

Figure 3.
Algorithm for the management of patients with oesophageal atresia.

2.12 Complications after repair of OA

Complications [57–59] resulting from repair of OA are generally grouped into two: early and late complications (**Table 9**). Early complications include anastomotic leak, anastomotic stricture, and recurrent tracheo-oesophageal fistula. Tracheomalacia, gastro-oesophageal reflux and oesophageal dysmotility are the late complications. Factors that promote postoperative complications include preoperative intubation, birth weight less than 2.5 kg, long-gap OA [60], post-operative intubation for more than 4 days, anastomotic leak and inability to feed orally for more than 1 month [61]. Management of the complications may involve a multidisciplinary approach.

2.12.1 Early complications

2.12.1.1 Anastomotic leak

Anastomotic leak at the oesophago-oesophagostomy is found in about 14–16% of patients after primary repair of OA. Most often, the leaks are clinically insignificant and can be managed with adequate drainage and nutritional support. Up to 95% of the leaks close spontaneously when a retropleural approach is undertaken and a patent mediastinal drain is in place [62]. Even in transpleural repair with leakage, spontaneous closure occurs with adequate drainage. Anastomotic breakdown

Early Complications	Late Complications
• Anastomotic leakage • Anastomotic stricture • Recurrent trachea-oesophageal fistula	• Gastro-oesophageal reflux • Tracheomalacia • Oesophageal dysmotility

Table 9.
Complications associated with oesophageal atresia repair.

usually leads to the formation of a stricture at the site and may be associated with a recurrent TOF. Only 3–5% of anastomotic leaks are known to result from major disruptions of the oesophageal anastomosis. They are found to be typically seen within 24–48 h after repair. Patients usually deteriorate as result of tension pneumothorax or mediastinitis. Hence, prompt reoperation with adequate drainage is imperative. Repair of the leak may be attempted, and this may be buttressed with the help of a pleural or pericardial patch, with or without intercostal muscle flap. Contributing factors to anastomotic leak include poor surgical technique, ischemia of the oesophageal ends, the use of myotomy and excessive tension at the anastomotic site [63, 64]. If reanastomosis is not possible, cervical oesophagostomy and delayed oesophageal replacement would be required.

2.12.1.2 Anastomotic stricture

Anastomotic stricture is found to be a common complication after repair of OA. It is characterised by dysphagia and recurrent respiratory problems due to aspiration or foreign body obstruction. The narrowing is noted on endoscopy or contrast oesophagography. Poor anastomotic technique (excessive tension, two-layered anastomosis and silk suture material), long gap, ischemia at the ends of the oesophagus, gastro-oesophageal reflux and anastomotic leak are factors implicated in the pathogenesis of oesophageal stricture.

Anastomotic stricture is treated by dilatation. However, a stricture resistant to repeated dilatations will require resection and reanastomosis or oesophageal replacement. Triamcinolone injection may be used at the stricture site. However, repeated injections may lead to adrenal suppression. Application of mitomycin C to the stricture under endoscopic control has also been reported to reduce stricture formation after dilation. It is important to determine whether the oesophageal stricture is associated with gastro-oesophageal reflux. This can be determined using contrast oesophagography, endoscopy, pH monitoring or a combination of these studies. The presence of gastro-oesophageal reflux is initially managed medically with proton pump inhibitors. Failure of medical management may warrant antireflux procedure.

2.12.1.3 Recurrent tracheo-oesophageal fistula

Recurrent TOF commonly results from anastomotic leak with local inflammation and erosion through the previous site of TOF repair. Recurrent TOF can be minimised by the use of a pleural flap, vascularized pericardial flap or azygous vein flap interposed between the oesophageal and tracheal suture lines. Symptoms of recurrent TOF can be typical of those seen with a congenital H-type TOF (coughing with feedings and recurrent respiratory distress). However, less obvious symptoms such as recurrent pulmonary infections are more common. Air-filled oesophagus on plain radiographs of the chest is suggestive of the diagnosis. As done in patients with congenital H-type fistula, contrast oesophagography performed in the prone position under videofluoroscopy is a reliable method of establishing the diagnosis. Another reliable diagnostic approach is bronchoscopy with cannulation of the fistula with a 2- to 3-French catheter. It is invaluable in locating the fistula during the operative procedure. About 50% of recurrent TOF is missed on routine contrast swallow studies. A recurrent TOF rarely closes spontaneously and usually requires surgical repair. Operation of choice is thoracotomy with fistula ligation, and division is the operation of choice. Pleura, intercostal muscle or pericardium should be interposed between the oesophagus and trachea to minimise recurrence. Endoscopic treatment of TOF by means of various chemicals or diathermy has also been reported. Various case reports and case series have reported the use of diathermy or laser deepithelialization followed by fibrin glue.

2.12.2 Late complications

2.12.2.1 Gastro-oesophageal reflux

Gastro-oesophageal reflux is a common complication after repair of OA [65]. It is probably related to shortening of the intra-abdominal portion of the oesophagus because of anastomotic tension and/or oesophageal motor dysfunction. The motor dysfunction may be intrinsic to the congenital anomaly or acquired from operative manipulation. Clinically, gastro-oesophageal reflux is suspected in patients with symptoms of vomiting, dysphagia and recurrent anastomotic stenosis. Episodes of foreign body or food bolus impaction may occur. Respiratory symptoms such as stridor, cyanotic spells, recurrent pneumonia and reactive airway disease are also suggestive of gastro-oesophageal reflux.

Upper gastrointestinal contrast study and 24-h pH probe data are diagnostic tools for gastro-oesophageal reflux. Multichannel oesophageal impedance combined with pH monitoring may emerge as a superior test. Abnormal oesophageal peristalsis and decreased lower oesophageal sphincter pressures after OA repair have been documented on oesophageal manometry. Medical management typically consists of thickening of feedings, positioning of the infant in a prone or upright posture, administration of acid reduction agents such as histamine-2 blockers, proton pump inhibitors and prokinetic agents. Antireflux operations are offered for patients with failed medical management, failure to thrive, chronic pulmonary infection, refractory anastomotic stricture or the development of a distal oesophageal stricture.

2.12.2.2 Tracheomalacia

Respiratory symptoms occurring after repair of OA can be due to tracheomalacia. Tracheomalacia is defined as generalized or localized weakness of the trachea that allows the anterior and posterior tracheal walls to come together during expiration or coughing.

Symptoms of tracheomalacia are often difficult to clinically distinguish from those of recurrent TOF, anastomotic leak, or gastro-oesophageal reflux. Embryologic events leading to TOF are believed to contribute to the development of tracheomalacia [61]. The tracheal cartilage is shorter than normal, thereby failing to provide the support necessary to maintain a patent airway [61]. The trachea may also be compressed between the aorta anteriorly and the often dilated upper oesophagus posteriorly after repair of OA; and such compression has been considered a significant contributor to the pathophysiology of tracheomalacia [61]. The tracheal collapse usually occurs in the region of or just above the original site of TOF in the distal third of the trachea which is generally at the level of the aortic arch; and severe tracheomalacia appears less common in infants with pure OA. Tracheomalacia has broad clinical manifestations, ranging from a "brassy" or "barking" cough in mild cases to recurrent pneumonia or acute, life-threatening apnoeic spells. Because of difficulty in breathing or cyanotic attacks during feeding, infants with tracheomalacia are often reluctant to feed. Life-threatening apnoeic and cyanotic spells occur during or within 5–10 min of a meal. They are characterized by cyanosis progressing to apnoea, bradycardia, and ultimately, cardiorespiratory arrest if not detected and managed promptly. Diagnosis is established by bronchoscopy with spontaneous ventilation. This reveals a slit-like lumen of the trachea at the involved area. However, because the symptoms overlap those of a stricture or gastro-oesophageal reflux, contrast oesophagogram is usually done as an initial investigation. Close attention to the tracheal air column on the lateral views during such a study will often reveal complete tracheal collapse during forced expiration (i.e., crying) or when contrast fills a distended upper oesophagus just above the anastomosis. Most mild to moderate symptoms of tracheomalacia tend to improve with time. Hence, operative intervention is not required. Operative treatment of choice for patients with severe symptoms, including acute life-threatening events, is aortopexy [46, 61, 66]. This is usually performed through a left anterior mediastinotomy (Chamberlain approach) or anterolateral thoracotomy [61]. The ascending aorta and arch are sutured to the posterior surface of the sternum after partial thymectomy [61]. The lifting of the aorta up in this fashion raises the anterior wall of the trachea and opens the tracheal lumen. In cases in which the aortic arch would not reach the posterior aspect of the sternum without undue tension, the use of a flap of pericardium based at the root of the aorta to be sutured to the sternum may be used [61]. Aortopexy and tracheopexy have also been done through anterior mediastinal approach via a low transverse cervical incision.

2.13 Oesophageal replacement

Oesophageal replacement surgery is usually done for patients with OA when primary repair fails or when primary repair is impossible. Various operative procedures have been described; and the most commonly used ones are colon or ileocolon interposition, reversed (antiperistalsis) gastric tube interposition, isoperistalsis gastric tube interposition, jejunum interposition and gastric transposition (gastric pull-up) [67] (**Table 10**).

Among the methods, colon replacement, or ileocolon, has been widely practiced for many years as a method of oesophageal replacement. This involves placement of the right or left colon substernally or behind the hilum of the lung on the right or left side. To avoid stricture or ulceration at the cologastric anastomosis, vagotomy and a gastric drainage procedure are typically performed. Complications after colonic interposition include cervical anastomotic leak, stricture and intrathoracic redundant colon with stasis, gastric reflux, respiratory problems and diarrhoea.

Reversed gastric tube as a substitute is preferred by some surgeons. A tubularised portion of the greater curvature is brought up to the cervical oesophagus in the substernal or retrohilar position. This procedure has similar complications as described for colonic interposition. A portion of the greater curvature of the stomach can be fashioned into a "free" tube graft based on the right gastroepiploic artery; and this is used as a modification of the reversed gastric tube for oesophageal replacement.

- Colon or ileocolon interposition
- Gastric tube interposition
    - Reversed (antiperistalsis)
    - Isoperistalsis
- Jejunum interposition
- Gastric transposition (gastric pull-up)

Table 10.
Commonly used oesophageal replacement techniques.

Oesophageal replacement can also be achieved using the jejunum, both in a Roux-en-Y fashion and as a free graft with microvascular anastomosis. Recently, a well-established method for oesophageal replacement is the use of gastric transposition.

2.14 Outcome and conclusion

During the early years, the surgical management of OA was associated with lots of challenges and high mortality [1–4]. Respiratory failure, inadequate resuscitation, and complications of prematurity resulted in most deaths in the past. Complications of the surgical repair of the oesophageal atresia itself, particularly sepsis after dehiscence of the oesophageal anastomosis, and prolonged poor nutrition are other major causes of mortality.

Over the past two to three decades, however, the surgical outcome has improved significantly in most centres in the developed countries. This improvement is attributed to advances in neonatal anaesthesia, well-established neonatal intensive care units (NICU), availability of total parental nutrition (TPN) and refined surgical skills [1, 5–8]. The current major cause of mortality in most developed countries is from associated major congenital abnormalities. Death from prematurity or oesophageal complications is now rare. In view of this, the previously used Waterston classification has little relevance in developed countries. The prognosis however remains poor in developing countries where late presentation is the norm. Waterston classification may remain relevant in these countries.

Gastro-oesophageal reflux and poor oesophageal clearance due to some degree of ongoing oesophageal dysmotility may limit long-term survival. Dysplastic changes in the lower oesophageal mucosa may predispose to oesophageal carcinoma. Ongoing gastro-oesophageal reflux is a significant risk fact for oesophageal carcinoma. Hence, regular surveillance in these patients is important.

Conflict of interest

Nil.

Author details

Samuel Osei-Nketiah* and William Appeadu-Mensah
Department of Surgery, University of Ghana School of Medicine and Dentistry, Accra, Ghana

*Address all correspondence to: oseivatican@yahoo.com

References

[1] Pinheiro PF, Simões e Silva AC, Pereira RM. Current knowledge on esophageal atresia. World Journal of Gastroenterology. 2012;**18**:3662-3672

[2] Spitz L. Oesophageal atresia. Orphanet Journal of Rare Diseases. 2007;**2**:24

[3] Lanman TH. Congenital atresia of the oesophagus: A study of thirty-two cases. Archives of Surgery. 1940;**7**:1060

[4] Waterston DJ, Carter RE, Aberdeen E. Oesophageal atresia: Tracheo-oesophageal fistula. A study of survival in 218 infants. Lancet. 1962;**1**:819-822

[5] Spitz L. Esophageal atresia. Lessons I have learned in a 40-year experience. Journal of Pediatric Surgery. 2006;**41**:1635-1640

[6] Grosfeld JL, Ladd AP. Congenital anomalies. In: Silva AC, Pereira RM, Pinheiro PF, editors. Pediatric Surgery—Clinical and Surgical Conduct. Rio de Janeiro: Guanabara Koogan; 2005. pp. 291-298

[7] Nakayana DK. Congenital abnormalities of the esophagus. In: O'Neill JA Jr, Grosfeld JL, Foukalsrud EW, Coran AG, Caldanone AA, editors. Principles of Pediatric Surgery. 2nd ed. St. Louis, MO: Mosby; 2003. pp. 385-394

[8] Goyal A, Jones MO, Couriel JM, Losty PD. Oesophageal atresia and tracheo-oesophageal fistula. Archives of Disease in Childhood. Fetal and Neonatal Edition. 2006;**91**:F381-F384

[9] Osei-Nketiah S, Hesse AA, Appeadu-Mensah W, Glover-Addy H, Etwire VK, Sarpong P. Management of oesophageal atresia in a developing country: Is primary repair forbidden? African Journal of Paediatric Surgery. 2016;**13**:114-119

[10] Karakus SC, Ozokutan BH, Bakal U, Ceylan H, Sarac M, Kul S, et al. Delayed diagnosis: An important prognostic factor for oesophageal atresia in developing countries. Journal of Paediatrics and Child Health. 2016;**52**(12):1090-1094

[11] Ameh EA, Dogo PM, Nmadu PT. Emergency neonatal surgery in a developing country. Pediatric Surgery International. 2001;**17**:448-451

[12] Skandalakis JE, Ellis H. Embryologic and anatomic basis of esophageal surgery. The Surgical Clinics of North America. 2000;**80**(1):85

[13] Kluth D, Fiegel H. The embryology of the forgut. Seminars in Pediatric Surgery. 2003;**12**(1):3-9

[14] Beasley P. Anatomy of the pharynx and esophagus. In: Kerr AG, Gleeson M, editors. Scott-Brown's Otolaryngology. 6th ed. Oxford, UK: Butterworth-Heinemann; 1997

[15] Postma GN, Seybt MW, Rees CJ. Esophagology. In: Snow JB, Wackym PA, editors. Ballinger's Otolaryngology Head & Neck Surgery. 17th ed. Shelton, Conn: BC Decker Inc; 2009. pp. 975-995

[16] Swigart LL. The esophageal arteries. Surgery, Gynecology & Obstetrics. 1950;**90**:234-243

[17] Geboes K, Geboes KP, Maleux G. Vascular anatomy of the gastrointestinal tract. Best Practice & Research. Clinical Gastroenterology. 2001;**15**(1):1-14

[18] Potter SE. Observations on the intrinsic blood supply of the esophagus. Archives of Surgery. 1950;**61**:944-948

[19] Shapiro AL. The esophageal arteries: Their configurational anatomy and variations in relation to surgery. Annals of Surgery. 1950;**131**:171-185

[20] Butler H. The veins of the oesophagus. Thorax. 1951;**6**:276-296

[21] Sasaki CT, Kim YH, Sims HS, et al. Motor innervation of the human cricopharyngeus muscle. Annals of Otology, Rhinology, and Laryngology. 1999;**108**(12):1132-1139

[22] Goyal RK, Martin SB, Shapiro J, et al. The role of cricopharyngeus muscle in pharyngoesophageal disorders. Dysphagia. 1993;**8**(3):252-258

[23] Harmon CM, Coran AG. Congenital anomalies of the esophagus. In: Coran AG, Adzick NS, Krummel TM, et al., editors. Pediatric Surgery. 7th ed. Vol. 1. Philadelphia, USA: Elsevier Saunders; p. 896 (chapter 69)

[24] Beasley SW. Esophageal atresia and tracheoesophageal fistula. In: Oldham KT, Colombani PM, Foglia RP, Skinner MA, editors. Principles and Practice of Pediatric Surgery. 4th ed. Vol. 2. Philadelphia, USA: Lippincott Williams & Wilkins; p. 1040 (chapter 65)

[25] Harmon CM, Coran AG. Congenital anomalies of the esophagus. In: Coran AG, Adzick NS, Krummel TM, et al., editors. Pediatric Surgery. 7th ed. Vol. 1. Philadelphia, USA: Elsevier Saunders; p. 897 (chapter 69)

[26] Brosens E, Marsch F, de Jong EM, et al. Copy number variations in 375 patients with oesophageal atresia and/or tracheoesophageal fistula. European Journal of Human Genetics. 2016;**24**(12):1715-1723

[27] Al-Salem AH, Tayeb M, Khogair S, et al. Esophageal atresia with or without tracheoesophageal fistula: Success and failure in 94 cases. Annals of Saudi Medicine. 2006;**26**(2):116-119

[28] Shulman A, Mazkereth R, Zalel Y, et al. Prenatal identification of oesophageal atresia: The role of ultrasonography for evaluation of functional anatomy. Prenatal Diagnosis. 2002;**22**(8):669-674

[29] Tröbs RB, Nissen M, Wald J. The upper pouch in oesophageal atresia shows proportional growth during late foetal life. Acta Paediatrica. 2018;**107**(9):1648-1649

[30] Garabedian C, Sfeir R, Langlois C, Bonnard A, Khen-Dunlop N, Gelas T, et al. Does prenatal diagnosis modify neonatal treatment and early outcome of children with esophageal atresia? American Journal of Obstetrics and Gynecology. 2015;**212**:e1-e7

[31] Bradshaw CJ, Thakkar H, Knutzen L, Marsh R, Pacilli M, Impey L, et al. Accuracy of prenatal detection of tracheoesophageal fistula and oesophageal atresia. Journal of Pediatric Surgery. 2016;**51**(8):1268-1272

[32] Summerour V, Stevens PS, Lander AD, Singh M, Soccorso G, Arul GS. Characterization of the upper pouch tracheo-oesophageal fistula in oesophageal atresia. Journal of Pediatric Surgery. 2017;**52**(2):231-234

[33] Randolf JG, Newman KD, Anderson KD. Current results in repair of esophageal atresia with tracheaoesophageal fistula using physiologic status as a guide to therapy. Annals of Surgery. 1989;**209**:526, discussion 530

[34] Poenaru D, Laberge JM, Neilson IR, et al. A new prognostic classification for esophageal atresia. Surgery. 1993;**113**:426

[35] Spitz L, Kiely EM, Morecroft JA, Drake DP. Esophageal atresia: At-risk groups for the 1990s. Journal of Pediatric Surgery. 1994;**29**:723

[36] Driver CP, Shanker KR, Jones MO, et al. Phenotypic presentation and outcome of esophageal atresia in the era of Spitz classification. Journal of Pediatric Surgery. 2001;**36**(9):1419-1421

[37] Konkin DE, O'Hali AW, Webber EM, Blair GK. Outcomes in esophageal

atresia and tracheoesophageal fistula. Journal of Pediatric Surgery. 2003;**38**(12):1726-1729

[38] Yagyu M, Gitter H, Richter B, et al. Esophageal atresia in Bremen, Germany—Evaluation of preoperative risk classification in esophageal atresia. Journal of Pediatric Surgery. 2000;**35**(4):584-587

[39] Barnhart DC, Area MJ, Coran AG. Esophageal atresia with or without tracheoesophageal fistula. In: Glick PL, Pearl RH, Irish MS, Caty MG, editors. Pediatric Surgery Secrets. Philadelphia, USA: Hanley & Belfus Inc.; 2001. p. 35

[40] Prakash KR, Bhardwaj N, Dwivedi D, et al. Thoracoscopic repair of esophageal atresia with tracheoesophageal fistula: Basics of technique and its nuances. Journal of Indian Association of Pediatric Surgeons. 2016;**21**(3):120-124

[41] Okuyama H, Koga H, Ishimaru T, et al. Current practice and outcomes of thoracoscopic esophageal atresia and tracheoesophageal fistula repair: A multi-institutional analysis in Japan. Journal of Laparoendoscopic & Advanced Surgical Techniques. Part A. 2015;**25**(5):441-444

[42] Lee S, Lee SK, Seo JM. Thoracoscopic repair of esophageal atresia with tracheoesophageal fistula: Overcoming the learning curve. Journal of Pediatric Surgery. 2014;**49**(11):1570-1572

[43] Rothenberg S. Thoracoscopic repair of esophageal atresia and tracheo-esophageal fistula in neonates: The current state of the art. Pediatric Surgery International. 2014;**30**(10):979-985

[44] Rothenberg SS, Flake AW. Experience with thoracoscopic repair of long gap esophageal atresia in neonates. Journal of Laparoendoscopic & Advanced Surgical Techniques. Part A. 2015;**25**(11):932-935

[45] Tainaka T, Uchida H, Tanano A, et al. Two-stage thoracoscopic repair of long-gap esophageal atresia using internal traction is safe and feasible. Journal of Laparoendoscopic & Advanced Surgical Techniques. Part A. 2017;**27**(1):71-75

[46] van der Zee DC, Tytgat SHA, van Herwaarden MYA. Esophageal atresia and tracheo-esophageal fistula. Seminars in Pediatric Surgery. 2017;**26**(2):67-71

[47] Holcomb GW 3rd. Thoracoscopic surgery for esophageal atresia. Pediatric Surgery International. 2017;**33**(4):475-481

[48] García LI, Olivos PM, Santos MM, Guelfand CHM. Thoracoscopic repair of esophageal atresia with and without tracheoesophageal fistula. Revista Chilena de Pediatría. 2014;**85**(4):443-447

[49] Woo S, Lau S, Yoo E, Shaul D, Sydorak R. Thoracoscopic versus open repair of tracheoesophageal fistulas and rates of vocal cord paresis. Journal of Pediatric Surgery. 2015;**50**(12):2016-2018

[50] Shieh HF, Jennings RW. Long-gap esophageal atresia. Seminars in Pediatric Surgery. 2017;**26**(2):72-77

[51] van der Zee DC, Gallo G, Tytgat SH. Thoracoscopic traction technique in long gap esophageal atresia: Entering a new era. Surgical Endoscopy. 2015;**29**(11):3324-3330

[52] Sroka M, Wachowiak R, Losin M, et al. The Foker Technique (FT) and Kimura Advancement (KA) for the treatment of children with long-gap esophageal atresia (LGEA): Lessons learned at two European centers. European Journal of Pediatric Surgery. 2013;**23**:3-7

[53] Bobanga ID, Barksdale EM. Foker technique for the management of pure esophageal atresia: Long-term outcomes at a single institution. European Journal of Pediatric Surgery. 2016;**26**(2):215-218

[54] Miyano G, Okuyama H, Koga H, et al. Type-A long-gap esophageal atresia treated by thoracoscopic esophagoesophagostomy after sequential extrathoracic esophageal elongation (Kimura's technique). Pediatric Surgery International. 2014;**29**(11):1171-1175

[55] Bogusz B, Patkowski D, Gerus S, et al. Staged thoracoscopic repair of long-gap esophageal atresia without temporary gastrostomy. Journal of Laparoendoscopic & Advanced Surgical Techniques. Part A. 2018;**28**(12):1510-1512

[56] Sharma AK, Mangal D. Simple technique of bridging wide gap in esophageal atresia with tracheoesophageal fistula—"Surgical innovation". Journal of Indian Association of Pediatric Surgeons. 2017;**22**(3):187-188

[57] Krishnan U, Faure C. Editorial: Oesophageal atresia-tracheoesophageal fistula. Frontiers in Pediatrics. 2017;**5**:190

[58] Sadreameli SC, McGrath-Morrow SA. Respiratory care of infants and children with congenital tracheo-oesophageal fistula and oesophageal atresia. Paediatric Respiratory Reviews. 2016;**17**:16-23

[59] Duvoisin G, Krishnan U. Gastric function in children with oesophageal atresia and tracheoesophageal fistula. Frontiers in Pediatrics. 2017;**5**:76

[60] Thakkar HS, Cooney J, Kumar N, Kiely E. Measured gap length and outcomes in oesophageal atresia. Journal of Pediatric Surgery. 2014;**49**(9):1343-1346

[61] Harmon CM, Coran AG. Congenital anomalies of the esophagus. In: Coran AG, Adzick NS, Krummel TM, et al., editors. Pediatric Surgery. 7th ed. Vol. 1. Philadelphia, USA: Elsevier Saunders; p. 911 (chapter 69)

[62] Manning PB, Morgan RA, Coran AG, et al. Fifty years experience with esophageal atresia and tracheoesophageal fistula. Beginning with Cameron Haight's first operation in 1935. Annals of Surgery. 1986;**204**:446

[63] Velligas-Alvarez F, Olvera-Duran J, Rodriguez-Aranda E, et al. Esophageal anastomotic failure: An experimental study. Archives of Medical Research. 2003;**34**:171

[64] Yanchar NL, Gordon R, Cooper M, et al. Significance of the clinical course of and early upper gastrointestinal studies in predicting complications associated with repair of esophageal atresia. Journal of Pediatric Surgery. 2001;**36**(5):815-822

[65] Svoboda E, Fruithof J, Widenmann-Grolig A, et al. A patient led, international study of long term outcomes of esophageal atresia: EAT 1. Journal of Pediatric Surgery. 2018;**53**(4):610-615

[66] Arnaud AP, Rex D, Elliott MJ, et al. Early experience of thoracoscopic aortopexy for severe tracheomalacia in infants after esophageal atresia and tracheo-esophageal fistula repair. Journal of Laparoendoscopic & Advanced Surgical Techniques. Part A. 2014;**24**(7):508-512

[67] Soccorso G, Parikh D. Esophageal replacement in children: Challenges and long-term outcomes. Journal of Indian Association of Pediatric Surgeons. 2016;**21**(3):98-105

Chapter 4

Meconium Ileus

Udefiagbon Omogiade

Abstract

Meconium ileus is a type of neonatal intestinal obstruction that occurs when abnormally thick meconium impacts in the ileum causing blockage of intestinal flow. Most infants with meconium ileus have cystic fibrosis, a congenital condition characterized by abnormally thick intestinal secretions and pancreatic insufficiency. The pathogenesis of meconium ileus is due to hyperviscous mucus secreted by abnormal intestinal glands, abnormal concentrating processes in the proximal small intestine, and pancreatic enzyme insufficiency. The clinical presentation of meconium ileus is that of abdominal distention, bilious vomiting, and failure to pass meconium. Cases of meconium ileus are usually evaluated with plain abdominal radiograph and contrast enema. Numerous air-filled loops of bowel on the supine view with characteristic absence of air-fluid levels are commonly seen on the radiograph, but the presence of calcification suggests intestinal perforation. Contrast enema examination is useful in cases with microcolon. Uncomplicated meconium ileus obstruction can be relieved by giving one or more dilute diatrizoate sodium enema (with Nacetylcysteine added) under fluoroscopy. Surgery is indicated when there is progressive distention or signs of clinical deterioration despite multiple enemas, as well as in complicated cases like meconium peritonitis, ileal atresia or stenosis, ileal perforation, and volvulus with or without pseudocyst formation.

Keywords: meconium ileus, cystic fibrosis, ileal obstruction, gastrografin enema, nonoperative treatment, enterotomy, enterostomy, resection and anastomosis

1. Introduction

Meconium ileus is a type of neonatal intestinal obstruction that occurs when abnormally thick and tenacious meconium becomes impacted, thus creating a blockage in a part of the distal small intestine, usually the ileum [1, 2]. It accounts for about 30–33% of cases of neonatal small intestinal obstruction [3]. Meconium ileus is a rare condition affecting only 1 in 25,000 babies [4]. It occurs in either a simple or a complicated form and is said to be the earliest clinical manifestation of cystic fibrosis occurring in approximately 16–20% of patients with cystic fibrosis [4]. Cystic fibrosis is a disease condition characterized by abnormally thick intestinal secretions and pancreatic insufficiency.

While majority of patients with meconium ileus have the disease cystic fibrosis (80–90%), a few of them do not have it; approximately 20% of one series of cases of meconium ileus did not have cystic fibrosis [5]. Preterm infants whose mothers had medications to slow down labor are sometimes associated with meconium ileus.

Meconium is the first series of stools that a newborn pass. It is formed during intrauterine life and consists of shed intestinal epithelial cells, bile, succus entericus, mucus, lanugo, and amniotic fluid ingested in utero. It is a dark olive green viscous and almost odorless substance that comprises the initial stools of the newborn. Meconium contains lactic acid-producing bacteria (e.g., *Lactobacillus*) and the so-called enteric bacteria family (e.g., *Escherichia coli*) [6]. It is usually evacuated within the first 24–48 hours after birth following which the usual yellowish feces are passed by the neonate. However, there might be in utero evacuation of meconium as a result of a vagal response due to perinatal stress to the fetus. Such newborn immediately after delivery may develop signs of respiratory distress from meconium aspiration syndrome.

Meconium ileus may be associated with complications such as meconium peritonitis, ileal atresia or stenosis, ileal perforation, and volvulus with or without pseudocyst formation [7–13]. The infants with cystic fibrosis are more likely to present with complicated meconium ileus [14].

2. Detailed overview of meconium ileus

An overview of meconium ileus in terms of etiology, pathophysiology, clinical features, investigations, and treatment will now be undertaken.

2.1 Etiology

Up to 20% of babies with cystic fibrosis are born with meconium ileus, and almost all babies with meconium ileus have cystic fibrosis [15, 16]. Cystic fibrosis is caused by gene mutations in the cystic fibrosis transmembrane conductance regulator (CFTR) encoding gene [17–19]. The loss of CFTR-mediated Cl– and/or HCO3– transport by the intestinal epithelium and/or from pancreatic dysfunction is postulated as the pathogenesis of meconium ileus [20–24]. Cystic fibrosis is characterized by the triad of chronic obstruction and infection of the respiratory tract, exocrine pancreatic insufficiency, and elevated sweat chloride levels.

The pathogenesis of meconium ileus is due to hyperviscous mucus secreted by abnormal intestinal glands, abnormal concentrating processes in the proximal small intestine, and pancreatic enzyme insufficiency.

The histology is characterized by the presence of distended goblet cells in the intestinal mucosa.

2.2 Pathophysiology

The simple form of meconium ileus is characterized by thickened sticky meconium obstructing the ileum with consequent proximal dilatation, bowel wall thickening, and congestion. Immediately beyond the level of the obstructing inspissated meconium in the terminal ileum, there may be a few separate gray-white globular meconium pellets. Further distally, the colon is narrow and empty—the microcolon.

The complicated form may result in volvulus, atresia, necrosis, perforation, meconium peritonitis, and pseudocyst formation. These complications may manifest as incidental findings on abdominal radiographs or with clinical features suggestive of bowel obstruction caused by reactive fibro-adhesive bands due to the meconium in the peritoneal cavity or as clinical features of peritonitis. If a neonate at birth manifests features of peritonitis, it is likely due to meconium peritonitis secondary to meconium ileus bowel perforation. This may also result in intestinal atresia, intraperitoneal calcifications, or ascites [25]. Meconium pseudocyst is formed when the extruded meconium becomes walled off; it is a cystic mass with rim calcification [26].

In utero, about 50% of meconium ileus cases may be complicated by intestinal perforation, meconium peritonitis, volvulus, and ischemic necrosis of the bowel that results in stenosis or atresia [4].

Meconium ileus patients are at risk for developing cholestasis, especially if they are on total parenteral nutrition. As such, alkaline phosphatase (ALP), alanine aminotransferase (ALT), aspartate aminotransferase (AST), and bilirubin levels should be monitored weekly in such infants.

2.3 Clinical features

At birth, the neonate may be apparently normal. However, with progression of time and feeding, the infant develops abdominal distention, bilious vomiting, and failure to pass meconium. Sometimes thickened distended bowel loops are observed through the abdominal wall filled with rubbery meconium which when palpated feel characteristically doughy [3]. Bowel sounds tend to be hypoactive, and digital rectal examination may be followed by passage of pale mucosal plugs. Meconium pellets might be palpated in the scrotum of some infants who had in utero bowel perforation. In cases complicated by peritonitis or when postnatal perforation has occurred, the infant presents with respiratory distress, marked abdominal distention with abdominal erythema, significant abdominal tenderness, and ascites.

2.4 Investigations

Cases of meconium ileus are usually evaluated with abdominal radiograph in which meconium might have a mottled appearance or be invisible [27].

Plain abdominal radiographs are routinely the first imaging done for cases of meconium ileus. They show numerous air-filled loops of bowel on the supine view with characteristic absence of air-fluid levels on the upright view due to the tenacious meconium and the abnormal mucous-gland secretion [5]. Although the absence of air-fluid levels strongly suggests meconium ileus, the presence of air-fluid levels does not exclude it as it may occasionally be demonstrated in some cases. In some cases of meconium ileus, the admixture of meconium and bowel gas gives a soap-bubble appearance usually in the right lower quadrant (Neuhauser sign). The presence of calcification, free air, or multiple air-fluid levels suggests intestinal perforation [4].

A contrast enema examination is useful in confirming the diagnosis of meconium ileus in which microcolon is seen; this differentiates it from meconium plug syndrome in which a normal or dilated colon is seen [25]. The microcolon, which represents the underused colon, could also be seen in other congenital conditions causing complete intrauterine obstruction of the distal small bowel such as ileal atresia; however for cases of meconium ileus, the presence of meconium pellets distending the distal ileum is usually identified when the contrast refluxes into the small bowel, and the diagnosis is confirmed (**Figure 1**).

Water-soluble agents are typically used in contrast evaluation of meconium ileus, and several of such contrast agents have been used. The hyperosmolar meglumine (GastrografinRx) diluted at ratio 1:3 to water used to be the mainstay, but some radiologists have stopped using it because of the occurrence of deaths

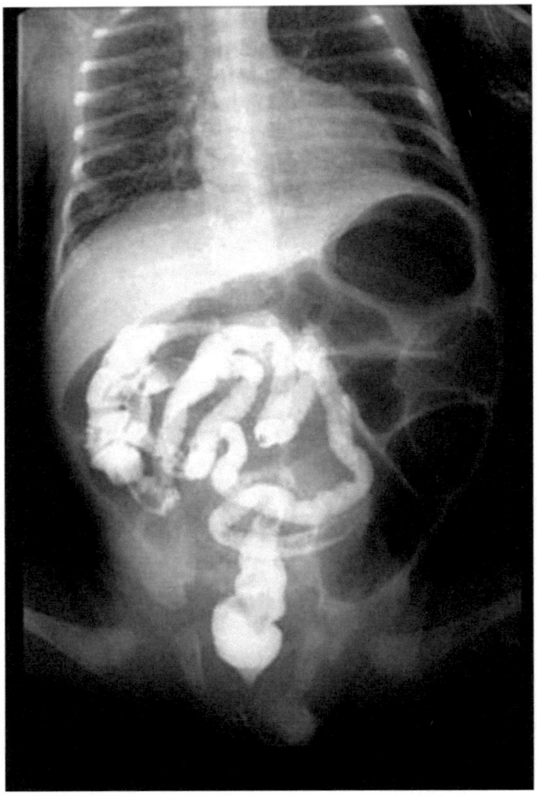

Figure 1.
Contrast enema showing microcolon and meconium pellets in the terminal ileum [courtesy Radiopaedia].

from fulminant colitis and dehydration sometimes reported with its use [28]. Also, the report of the Cystic Fibrosis Foundation Consensus Conference on gastrointestinal disorders concluded that there is no scientific evidence that hyperosmolar Gastrografin enema is any better than an iso-osmolar or hypo-osmolar enema. Nevertheless, many radiologists use it safely by ensuring appropriate dilution ratios. Adequate monitoring of fluid and electrolyte balance before, during, and after the contrast study is essential to avert potential fluid shifts with consequent hypovolemia which is worsened when bowel perforation and contrast leak occur. Nonionic contrast agents like Hypaque and Omnipaque are becoming popular with many radiologists since they have less risk of dehydration or colitis. Because of the tenacious and sticky nature of meconium, mucolytic agents like acetylcysteine are sometimes mixed with the contrast enema solution to aid passage of the meconium.

Meconium peritonitis may be an incidental abdominal radiograph finding in which the extruded meconium may be calcified or the radiograph may only suggest fluid in the abdomen when no calcification is present. When the calcification appears amorphous and curvilinear suggesting cystic loculation of the peritoneum, the term cystic or pseudocystic meconium peritonitis is used [5].

Prenatal ultrasound scan done at 17–18 weeks gestational age may show signs suggestive of meconium ileus; this include enlarged bowel loops or a mass with proximal bowel distention (likely cystic meconium peritonitis) [11, 12]. Also, calcified meconium may be seen if meconium peritonitis has already occurred. Also there might be polyhydramnios.

Postnatal ultrasound scan is seldom necessary for meconium peritonitis, as the findings on plain radiographs are usually diagnostic. However, ultrasonography may be useful when cystic masses are present. The cystic masses often appear circumscribed and heterogeneous with sonolucent areas seen within the cyst suggestive of fluid. They demonstrate increased echogenicity resulting from debris and calcifications, and loops of fluid-filled bowel bound to the matrix of the associated adhesions may be noted. The cyst wall may be thick or thin. Multiple speckled echoes are seen with free-floating meconium in the abdomen, and these result in the snowstorm configuration.

Zangheri et al. created the following classification system related to perinatal outcome [29]:

- Grade 0: isolated intra-abdominal calcifications (IAC)
- Grade I: IAC and one of the following: ascites, pseudocyst, or bowel dilatation
- Grade II: IAC and two of the following: ascites, pseudocyst, or bowel dilatation
- Grade III: all of the above (IAC, ascites, pseudocyst, and bowel dilatation)

Patients diagnosed with meconium ileus should be tested for cystic fibrosis; the sweat chloride test should be done [25].

2.5 Treatment

2.5.1 Initial medical management

Meconium ileus cases, both simple and complicated, are approached as intestinal obstruction and as such would require urgent initial resuscitative measures. These include intravenous fluid resuscitation, nasogastric decompression, urethral catheterization for hourly urinary monitoring, multiparameter vital sign monitoring, intravenous antibiotic therapy, laboratory evaluation of full blood count, coagulation work-up, and serum electrolytes, urea, and creatinine with necessary corrections instituted. Where necessary, mechanical respiratory support is provided. Once the infant has been optimized, the decision for nonoperative or operative management is taken based on the presentation.

2.5.2 Nonoperative treatment

Nonoperative management can be achieved by diatrizoate meglumine enemas as first described by Noblett in 1969 [30]. Variations on his approach have been established as effective first-line treatment for uncomplicated meconium ileus.

Uncomplicated meconium ileus obstruction can be relieved by giving one or more dilute diatrizoate sodium or diatrizoate (gastrografin) enema (with N-acetylcysteine added) under fluoroscopic guidance. The hyperosmolar nature of this compound increases the influx of fluid into the bowel lumen to liquefy the viscid meconium and thus facilitate its expulsion with consequent large gastrointestinal water losses. While carrying out this procedure, therefore, adequate intravenous fluid administration must be ensured to prevent hypovolemia.

2.5.3 Treatment algorithm

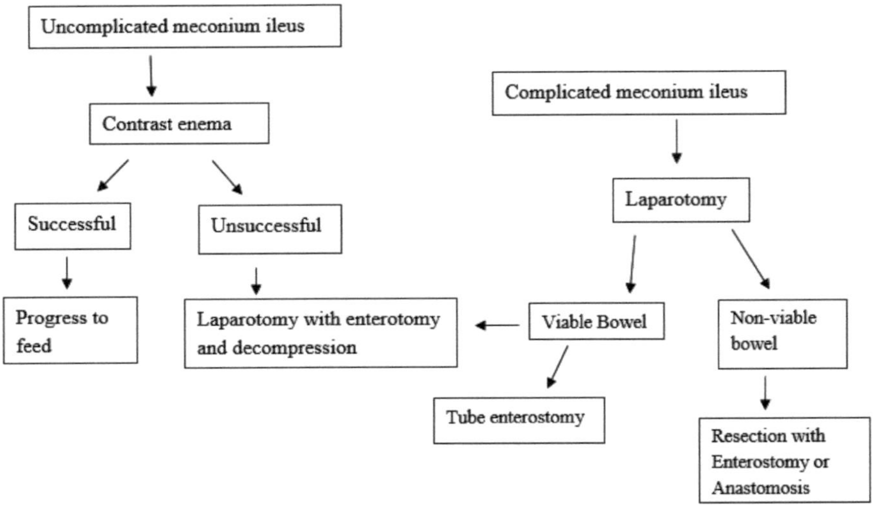

Diatrizoate meglumine (GastrografinRx) is a hyperosmolar, water-soluble, radiopaque solution containing 0.1% polysorbate 80 (Tween 80) and 37% organically bound iodine with osmolarity of 1900 mOsm/L. Success rate of 63–83% have been reported for gastrografin enemas for patients with uncomplicated meconium ileus [31].

Noblett's criteria for nonoperative gastrografin enema therapy [30]:

- Other causes of neonatal distal intestinal obstruction must first be excluded.
- There should be no clinical or radiologic signs of complications like volvulus, gangrene, perforation, peritonitis, and atresia of the small bowel.
- Ensure adequate fluid and electrolyte replacement and correction of hypothermia as preparatory measures before the enema.
- Provision for adequate resuscitation and hydration in anticipation of transient osmotic fluid losses associated with the hyperosmolar enema.
- The enema must be carried out under fluoroscopic guidance.
- Intravenous antibiotics should be administered to the infant.
- Assurance of close surgical supervision from the initial evaluation through the hospital course.

To carry out the enema, a two-way Foley's catheter is inserted into the rectum through which a 25–50% solution of gastrografin is slowly infused at low hydrostatic pressure under fluoroscopic control. The balloon of the catheter should not be inflated to minimize the risk of rectal perforation. Upon instillation, fluid is drawn into the intestinal lumen by osmosis, and this hydrates and softens the meconium mass. For very inspissated meconium, 1% N-acetylcysteine may be added to the enema solution for better deconcentration. The procedure is usually followed by rapid passage of loose meconium (liquefied to some extent), and this continues for the next 24–48 hours.

Although the perforation that occurs during enema administration can usually be seen on fluoroscopy, it is important to obtain an immediate abdominal radiograph after completion of the gastrografin enema to rule out bowel perforation and a late abdominal radiograph (8–12 hours later or as clinically indicated) to confirm evacuation of the obstruction and to exclude late perforation [31].

Sometimes a second gastrografin enema or serial gastrografin enemas can be performed at 6–24 hour intervals if evacuation is incomplete or if the first attempt at gastrografin evacuation does not reflux contrast into dilated bowel. Administration of a 10% N-acetylcysteine solution (5 mL q6h) through a nasogastric tube to liquefy upper gastrointestinal secretions as suggested by Noblett is also useful in such cases [30]. The potential complications associated with the gastrografin enema procedure include perforation, hypovolemic shock, and ischemia.

The risk of perforation during the procedure increases with repeated enemas. Late perforations, usually occurring 12–48 hours after the enema, may be due to direct injury to the bowel mucosa by the contrast medium, severe bowel distention by fluid osmotically drawn into the intestine, or extensive bowel necrosis.

Nonoperative treatment can be done for infants with peritoneal (or scrotal) calcifications on radiography who are presumed to have had meconium peritonitis in utero but who show no signs of obstruction and are passing meconium without difficulty [32].

In nonoperative management, if the enema was successful and the features of bowel obstruction have resolved, usually within 48 hours, the infant is commenced on feeds with pancreatic enzyme supplements added for infants with confirmed cystic fibrosis.

2.5.4 Surgical treatment

In uncomplicated meconium ileus, surgical exploration is indicated when there is progressive distention or signs of clinical deterioration or peritonitis despite multiple enemas. Whereas in complicated cases (e.g., meconium peritonitis, ileal atresia or stenosis, ileal perforation, and volvulus with or without pseudocyst formation), surgery is always indicated.

Indications for surgical management in meconium ileus [31]:

- Persistent or worsening abdominal distension
- Persistent bowel obstruction
- Enlarging abdominal mass
- Intestinal atresia
- Volvulus
- Perforation
- Meconium cyst formation with peritonitis
- Bowel necrosis
- Conditions associated with cystic fibrosis and meconium Ileus

In the operative management of simple uncomplicated meconium ileus, the aim is to evacuate meconium from the intestine without resecting any bowel segment; however, this might be inevitable in certain instances. On the other hand, complicated meconium ileus requires resection more often and may necessitate the use of temporary stomas.

The fibrous wall of the pseudocyst is debrided without sacrificing viable intestine. Extensive adhesiolysis is required for adhesive obstruction due to meconium peritonitis; these adhesions are typically dense and very vascular. It is not necessary to perform a radical debridement of all meconium calcified plaque encountered, as long as the obstruction is relieved [32].

The surgical approach for treatment of uncomplicated meconium ileus should be individualized for each infant, although many procedures have been proposed over the years with variable success rates achieved. In all cases, uncomplicated or complicated, the following procedures are commonly done:

- Enterotomy and decompression
- Enterostomy (with or without tube) with subsequent irrigation
- Resection and enterostomy
- Resection and anastomosis

2.5.5 Enterotomy and decompression

An enterotomy is made on the antimesenteric border of the dilated ileum for instillation of irrigation solution (dilute acetylcysteine or saline solution) which help to loosen the inspissated meconium and liquefy it for effective evacuation through the enterotomy. The irrigation solution is introduced using a size 10 French catheter, and both the proximal and distal loops of bowel are irrigated. After complete decompression of inspissated meconium, the enterotomy is closed transversely. An appendectomy is performed with the specimen sent for histologic examination to detect the presence of ganglion cells, as well as possible presence of mucous plugging of the crypts and exuberant intraluminal mucinous material, which are suggestive of cystic fibrosis. Postoperatively, a gentle anal dilatation and rectal irrigation may sometimes be required for further evacuation of large amount of meconium passed distally into the colon during intraoperative irrigation. Enterotomy and decompression are usually indicated for simple uncomplicated meconium ileus. A supraumbilical transverse incision or transverse right lower abdominal incision can be used for the procedure.

2.5.6 Enterostomy with subsequent irrigation

In cases where the irrigation done after an enterotomy cannot effectively evacuate the inspissated meconium despite a patient approach, an indwelling ostomy tube (e.g., T-tube) can be inserted for postoperative bowel irrigation decompression. The irrigations are started on the first postoperative day and continued for 7–14 days. After successfully evacuating the inspissated meconium, the tube is removed, and the enterocutaneous fistula thus formed is allowed to close spontaneously. T-tube enterostomy was first described by Harberg et al. in 1981 [33]. Enterostomy for postoperative irrigation can also be done without using tube; in which case the ileal opening is sutured to skin and the bowel tacked to the fascia in standard fashion.

2.5.7 Resection with enterostomy or anastomosis

Bowel resection is indicated when meconium ileus is associated with a nonviable bowel, bowel perforation, atresia, volvulus, and the like. Resection is usually combined with enterostomy procedure, but primary anastomosis may be done if the intraoperative findings and the patient's general condition are favorable. The disadvantages of the procedures involving resection and stoma(s) or anastomosis are potential postoperative fluid losses through high-volume stomas, bowel shortening by resection, and the need for a second procedure to reestablish intestinal continuity [25, 31]. Hence, they are rarely used today.

Various stoma operations have been described with the most widespread being the Bishop-Koop-type anastomosis. This is a Roux-en-Y construct in which the distal limb is brought out as an end stoma and the proximal bowel is anastomosed end-to-side approximately 4 cm from the opening of the distal segment (**Figure 2**). Normal gastrointestinal transit is permitted by this technique, and should distal obstruction occur, it provides a means for management through the ileostomy [25, 31].

The reverse of the Bishop-Koop enterostomy is the proximal enterostomy, described by Santulli and Blanc in 1961 [25, 31]. In this technique, the end of the distal limb is anastomosed to the side of the proximal limb after resection, while the end of the proximal limb is brought out as the enterostomy (**Figure 2**). This arrangement enhances proximal irrigation and decompression, thus making intraoperative evacuation of the dilated proximal bowel loop unnecessary. A catheter can be inserted into the distal limb through the stoma for irrigation of the distal bowel. The proximal stoma created in this technique predisposes to high-output losses with inherent risk of dehydration.

The Mikulicz enterostomy, first reported by Gross in 1953, consists of a double-barrel stoma in which the two ends are sutured together side to side for some length

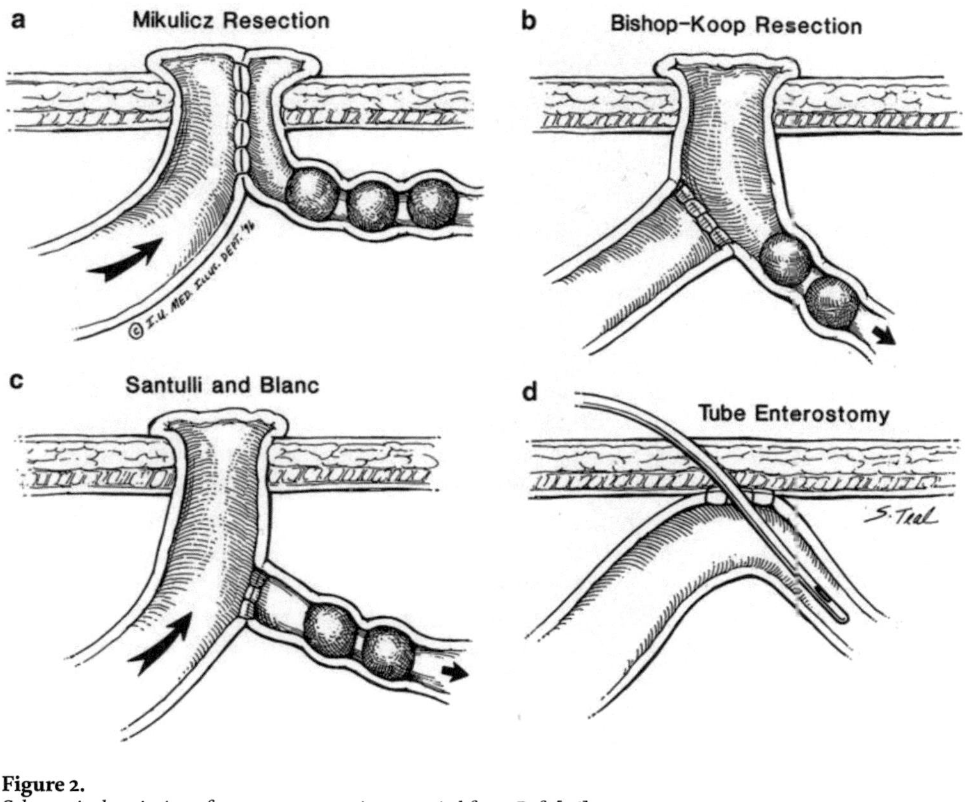

Figure 2.
Schematic description of some enterostomies as copied from Ref. [36].

proximal to the end of the stoma (**Figure 2**) [25, 31]. It was designed for bedside stoma closure in which the common wall was crushed and obliterated with a specially designed clamp and the bowel ends were closed over the top. It has the following distinct advantages:

- The procedures reduce operating and anesthetic times because complete evacuation of inspissated meconium is unnecessary.
- The procedures avoid intra-abdominal anastomosis, which eliminates the risk of anastomotic leakage.
- The bowel can be opened after complete closure of the abdominal wound; this reduces the risk of intraperitoneal contamination.

Swenson was the first to suggest resection with primary anastomosis in 1962 [25, 31]. Anastomotic leakage was initially a major issue with such operation; however some authors have reported improved results with adequate resection of the compromised bowel, complete evacuation of proximal and distal meconium, and preserving an adequate blood supply to the anastomosis [34, 35].

2.6 Postoperative care

Immediately postoperatively, management involves ongoing resuscitation with special attention given to replacement of the fluid losses caused by surgery and preoperative hyperosmolar enemas (if attempted), as well as correction of ongoing losses (i.e., losses from nasogastric suction and ileostomy) [31]. Also, the infant is initially on bowel rest with general supportive care provided after any major laparotomy. The oral gastric tube is maintained until bowel function returns, and further acetylcysteine irrigations can be done via the tube as described for nonoperative management. Combining this with rectal irrigations may further aid passage of retained meconium in the distal loop as well. Most infants will need central venous access for parenteral nutrition during this period. If cystic fibrosis has not been confirmed preoperatively, the sweat chloride test should be done to confirm or rule it out. Close attention has to be given to pulmonary care in infants with cystic fibrosis. Multiple pediatric subspecialists including gastroenterologists, geneticists, pulmonologists, and pediatric surgeons are required for a good outcome of management in infants with meconium ileus, more so when they have cystic fibrosis. Once they have established a normal stooling pattern (usually within 1–2 weeks postoperative), they are commenced on graded oral feedings with pancreatic enzyme supplementation. Infants with uncomplicated meconium ileus and cystic fibrosis may receive breast milk or routine infant formula, enzymes, and vitamins, while complicated cases would benefit from predigested infant formulas (e.g., Alimentum and Pregestimil), for enteral feeding [31]. For those with stomas, administering of ostomy-drip feeds of glutamine-enriched formula at low volumes enhances bowel growth and helps prevent bacterial translocation [31]. After 4–6 weeks, when symptoms would have resolved and the infant attained an adequate weight gain, the stomas can be taken down. It is advisable to perform a distal contrast study to rule out obstruction before embarking on this procedure of reanastomosis.

2.7 Postoperative complications

Short-term complications are uncommon in infants with simple meconium ileus.

Infants who have had significant (i.e., >33%) bowel resection may develop short bowel syndrome, especially if the ileocecal valve has been resected.

Short bowel syndrome predisposes to acidic intestinal environment that inactivates pancreatic enzymes and prevents dissolution of enteric-coated microcapsules. As such, histamine 2 receptor blockers are useful adjunct to pancreatic enzyme therapy in patients with significant bowel resections.

There are excessive fluid and sodium losses in those with stomas.

Mucus plugging and atelectasis can occur postoperatively, hence the need to initiate vigorous prophylactic pulmonary care with chest physiotherapy.

High-dose pancreatic enzyme supplementation has been associated with the development of colonic strictures and distal intestinal obstruction syndrome.

Long-term complications are mostly common to patients with cystic fibrosis.

Some infants, especially those who had meconium peritonitis may present years later with bowel obstruction due to adhesions or segmental volvulus.

Some older patients have been known to develop bowel obstruction from inspissated stools in the ileum and colon; this condition is known as "meconium ileus equivalent" [32].

3. Conclusion

Meconium ileus is a cause of neonatal small intestinal obstruction which mainly affects the ileum and common in infants with cystic fibrosis. Contrast (gastrografin) enema is usually diagnostic and may sometimes be therapeutic. Infants who have unsuccessful management with enemas and those with complications related to the obstruction, including volvulus, perforation, or atresia, require operative intervention.

At laparotomy, a small enterotomy is done for those with simple meconium ileus to irrigate the bowel lumen with acetylcysteine solution and thus promote effective evacuation of the highly viscous meconium. Patients with complicated meconium ileus may require bowel resection with anastomosis or tube enterostomy or creation of a stoma. Various types of stomas have been described over the years for management of the disease, but the Bishop-Koop enterostomy seems to be widespread.

Most patients respond well to therapy in the short-term but need to be followed closely for long-term complications like bowel obstruction, which has many potential causes in these patients. Advances in perinatal diagnosis and management of meconium ileus and cystic fibrosis have vastly improved the outlook for affected infants.

Conflict of interest

There is no "conflict of interest."

Notes/thanks/other declarations

None.

Author details

Udefiagbon Omogiade
Department of Pediatric Surgery, Irrua Specialist Teaching Hospital, Irrua, Nigeria

*Address all correspondence to: dokernie11@gmail.com

References

[1] Carlyle BE, Borowitz DS, Glick PL. A review of pathophysiology and management of foetuses and neonates with meconium ileus for the pediatric surgeon. Journal of Pediatric Surgery. 2012;**47**:772-781

[2] Copeland DR, St Peter SD, Sharp S, et al. Diminishing role of contrast enema in simple meconium ileus. Journal of Pediatric Surgery. 2009;**44**:2130-2132

[3] Cochran WJ. Meconium ileus. Merck Manuals. Kenilworth, NJ, USA: Merck & Co., Inc.; 2018

[4] Leung AKC, Wong AL, Kao P. Meconium ileus: Causes and complications. Modern Medicine Network Special Report; 2005

[5] Hekmatnia A, Mc Hugh K, Hiorns MP. Meconium Ileus Imaging. In: Lin EC, Chief Editor; 2019. Medscape ©. Web MD LLC

[6] Jimenez E et al. Is meconium from healthy newborns actually sterile? Research in Microbiology;**159**(3):187-193

[7] Burge D, Drewett. Meconium plug obstruction. Pediatric Surgery International. 2004;**20**(2):108-110

[8] Fakhoury K, Durie PR, Levison H. Meconium ileus in the absence of cystic fibrosis. Archives of Disease in Childhood. 1992;**67**(10 Spec):1204-1206

[9] Lang I, Daneman A, Cutz E, et al. Abdominal calcification in cystic fibrosis with meconium ileus: Radiologic-pathologic correlation. Pediatric Radiology. 1997;**27**(6):523-527

[10] Lim CT, Yip CH, Chang KW. Meconium ileus–A rare cause of neonatal intestinal obstruction in Malaysia. Singapore Medical Journal. 1994;**35**(1):74-76

[11] Boczar M, Sawicka E, Zybert K. Meconium ileus in newborns with cystic fibrosis–Results of treatment in the group of patients operated on in the years 2000-2014. Developmental Period Medicine. 2015;**19**(1):32-40

[12] Takacs ZF, Meier CM, Solomayer G. Prenatal diagnosis and management of an intestinal volvulus with meconium ileus and peritonitis. Archives of Gynecology and Obstetrics. 2014;**290**(2):385-387

[13] Jerdee T, Newman B, Rubesova E. Meconium in perinatal imaging: Associations and clinical significance. Seminars in Ultrasound, CT, and MR. 2015;**36**(2):161-177

[14] Burke MS, Ragi JM, Karamanoukian HL, et al. New strategies in the nonoperative management of meconium ileus. Journal of Pediatric Surgery. 2002;**37**:760-764

[15] van der Doef HP, Kokke FT, van der Ent CK, Houwen RH. Intestinal obstruction syndromes in cystic fibrosis: Meconium ileus, distal intestinal obstruction syndrome, and constipation. Current Gastroenterology Reports. 2011;**13**(3):265-270. DOI: 10.1007/s11894-011-0185-9

[16] Gelfond D, Borowitz D. Gastrointestinal complications of cystic fibrosis. Clinical Gastroenterology and Hepatology. 2013;**11**(4):333-342. DOI: 10.1016/j.cgh.2012.11.006

[17] Welsh MJ, Ramsey BW, Accurso F, Cutting GR. The metabolic and molecular basis of inherited disease. In: Scriver CR, Beaudet AL, Sly WS, Valle D, Childs B, Vogelstein B, editors. Cystic Fibrosis. 8th ed. New York, New York, USA: McGraw-Hill; 2001. pp. 5121-5189

[18] Rowe SM, Miller S, Sorscher EJ. Cystic fibrosis. The New England Journal

of Medicine. 2005;**352**(19): 1992-2001. DOI: 10.1056/NEJMra043184

[19] Quinton P. Physiological basis of cystic fibrosis: A historical perspective. Physiological Reviews. 1999;**79**(suppl 1): S3-S22

[20] Clarke LL, Harline MC. Dual role of CFTR in cAMP-stimulated HCO3- secretion across murine duodenum. American Journal of Physiology. Cell Physiology. 1998;**274**(4 pt 1):G718-G726

[21] Clarke LL, Stien X, Walker NM. Intestinal bicarbonate secretion in cystic fibrosis mice. Journal of the Pancreas: JOP. 2001;**2**(4 suppl):263-267

[22] Harmon GS et al. Pharmacological correction of a defect in PPAR-gamma signaling ameliorates disease severity in Cftr-deficient mice. Nature Medicine. 2010;**16**(3):313-318. DOI: 10.1038/nm.2101

[23] Garcia MA, Yang N, Quinton PM. Normal mouse intestinal mucus release requires cystic fibrosis transmembrane regulator-dependent bicarbonate secretion. The Journal of Clinical Investigation. 2009;**119**(9):2613-2622. DOI: 10.1172/JCI38662

[24] Kristidis P et al. Genetic determination of exocrine pancreatic function in cystic fibrosis. American Journal of Human Genetics. 1992;**50**(6):1178-1184

[25] Ziegler MM. Meconium ileus. In: Coran AG, Adzick NS, Krummel TM, Laberge J-M, Shamberger RC, Caldamone AA, editors. Pediatric Surgery. 7th ed. Philadelphia, PA: Saunders, an imprint of Elsevier Inc; 2012. pp. 1073-1083

[26] Lee GS, Chandran S, Rajadurai VS. Calcified meconium pseudocyst: X-ray diagnosis of meconium peritonitis at birth. BML Case Reports. July 7, 2015:1

[27] Swischuk LE. Imaging of the Newborn Infant and Young Child. 4th ed. Philadelphia: Lippincott, Williams and Wilkins; 1997

[28] O'Halloran SM, Gilbert J, McKendrick OM, Carty HM, Heaf DP. Gastrografin in acute meconium ileus equivalent. Archives of Disease in Childhood. 1986;**61**(11):1128-1130

[29] Zangheri G, Andreani M, Ciriello E, Urban G, Incerti M, Vergani P. Fetal intra-abdominal calcifications from meconium peritonitis: Sonographic predictors of postnatal surgery. Prenatal Diagnosis. 2007;**27**(10):960-963

[30] Noblett HR. Treatment of uncomplicated meconium ileus by Gastrografin enema: A preliminary report. Journal of Pediatric Surgery. 1969;**4**(2):190-197

[31] Irish M, Bovet PM. Surgical Aspects of Cystic Fibrosis and Meconium Ileus. In: Minkes RK, Chief Editor, 2019. Medscape©, Web MD LLC

[32] Mattei P. Meconium ileus. In: Mattei P, editor. Fundamentals of Pediatric Surgery. New York, NY, USA: Springer Science+Business Media, LLC; 2011. pp. 395-400

[33] Harberg FJ, Senekjian EK, Pokorny WJ. Treatment of uncomplicated meconium ileus via T-tube ileostomy. Journal of Pediatric Surgery. 1981;**16**(1):61-63

[34] Chappell JS. Management of meconium ileus by resection and end-to-end anastomosis. South African Medical Journal. 1977;**52**(27):1093-1094

[35] Mabogunje OA, Wang CI, Mahour H. Improved survival of neonates with meconium ileus. Archives of Surgery. 1982;**117**(1):37-40

[36] Rescorla FJ, Grosfeld JL. Contemporary management of meconium ileus. World Journal of Surgery. 1993;**17**:381

Section 3

Hepatobiliary

Chapter 5

Pediatric Choledochal Cysts: Unknowns are Decreasing

Hasan Özkan Gezer

Abstract

Choledochal cysts (CCs) are congenital cystic dilatation of extrahepatic and/or intrahepatic bile ducts. CCs are more common in Asian population, the cause is still unknown. Although the etiology is controversial, the main elements in the natural historical emergence of the type I and type IV, which make up the majority of all types, have become clearer. The majority of CCs are diagnosed in childhood. Clinical presentation varies from jaundice in young patients to nonspecific abdominal pain in older, but morbidity increases with complications such as cholangitis, pancreatitis, perforation, hepatitis, liver failure, and malignancy in delayed diagnosed patients. MRCP is considered the current gold standard diagnostic modality that is able to accurately assess biliary anatomy. Although the treatment approach has been formed over the years, it still has not reached the last state. Eventually, the removal of the entire cyst and the reconstruction of the remaining biliary tract to drainage is the current treatment approach. But the dilemma is the way of reconstruction procedure (hepaticoduodenostomy or hepaticojejunostomy). All patients should be followed up for a long period of time, regardless of the surgery method.

Keywords: choledochal cyst, children, hepaticoduodenostomy, Roux-en-Y hepaticojejunostomy, common bile duct

1. Introduction

Choledochal cysts (CCs) are congenital dilatations of extrahepatic and/or intrahepatic bile ducts defined by Vater and Ezler in 1723. It is a rare biliary entity with an estimated incidence of 1:100–150,000 live births in Western countries. In the Asian population, the incidence can be as high as 1:1000 live births. CC is primarily a childhood disease—up to 80% of patients are diagnosed before 10 years of age. The original classification, first described by Alanso-Lej and colleagues in 1959, was changed in 1977 by Todani and colleagues that classified the CCs as five types. In addition, isolated cystic dilatation of the cystic canal was identified subsequently and proposed as type VI, apart from the revised Todani classification. Although the etiology is controversial, the main elements in the natural historical emergence of the type I and type IV, which make up the majority of all types, have become clearer. A common symptom is nonspecific abdominal pain in older children. When the cyst is complicated, the diagnosis is delayed, the treatment becomes complex, and the results are affected. External drainage (ED), internal drainage (ID), total cyst excision (CE) + hepaticoduodenostomy (HD), and total CE + hepaticojejunostomy (HJ) were defined according to historical development of treatment. Resection is considered that is necessary to prevent further complications and long-term sequel.

IntechOpen

2. History

The anatomist Abraham Vater first described the normal anatomy of the bile ducts and the fusiform dilatation of the common bile duct (CBD) in 1723 [1]. Then, Doctor Halliday Douglas first described clinically CBD dilatation in 1852. Douglas had detected a large tenderness cystic mass on the right upper quadrant by physical examination of a 17-year-old girl who had an intermittent right-sided pain, obstructive jaundice, and fever complaints in her history. Despite performing external drainage promptly, she died within 1 month. Subsequently, Douglas detected a CC with her autopsy [2]. In 1894, British surgeon William Swain performed the first successful operation in a 17-year-old girl presented with CC, by anastomosing the jejunum to a giant CC. This patient had been reported 2 months later with no jaundice. In 1922, Golder McWhorter underwent hepaticoduodenostomy after excising the CC in a 49-year-old patient who had complaints since infancy. In 1959, Alanso-Lej and colleagues first published the series of CCs. In this publication, they reviewed 94 cases, published previously, together with their own 2 cases and classified the congenital cystic dilatations of the bile ducts anatomically for the first time [3]. In 1977, Todani and colleagues modified the classification of CCs according to cholangiographic images [4–8].

3. Incidence

CCs are more common in Asian populations with an incidence of 1 in 13,000, even 1:1000 in Japan [9], versus 1 in 100,000–150,000 in Western populations [10]. The reason for this Asian preponderance is still unknown [11]. Although predominately diagnosed in children, CCs are found with increasing frequency in adults such that adults comprise the majority of patients in recent series [12, 13], which in part may be due to the increased use of diagnostic imaging [14]. In both adult and children [15], females are higher risk for the disease with a nearly 4:1 female preponderance [10, 16]. Nearly, 80% of CCs are diagnosed in early infancy [10, 17].

4. Pathology

Grossly, CCs appear as a diffuse dilatation of the bile ducts [18]. In the congenital dilatations of the bile ducts, the cyst wall thickness is between 2 and 7 mm in diameter and usually involves an inflammatory reaction (80%) [18] that becomes severe after 10 years of age. Cysts, especially infected, are usually being adherent to the surrounding tissues. Bile ducts and columnar epithelium can be seen in the microscopic examination of the cyst wall. Choledochocele that is covered with duodenal mucosa appears different from other types of CCs according to epithelial histology. Liver biopsy findings usually vary with the age in patients with CC. Although, newborn liver is mostly normal, mild periportal fibrosis may be seen in older children. Varying degrees of histological hepatic changes severity may be seen in most patients with CC when it is diagnosed [19]. Higher degree of liver damage associates with the presence of an anomalous pancreaticobiliary ductal union (APBDU), more severe symptoms, type IVa CC, and younger age [19–21]. It has been observed by investigating liver biopsies that most of these changes resolve after surgical excision; however, preoperative portal fibrosis and central venous distension may remain stable or increase in severity [19]. It is considered that carcinoma of the cyst wall may develop due to recurrent chronic inflammation attacks.

However, it can also be seen in non-APBDU-associated CC patients. Additionally, the cancer can develop from anywhere such as the cyst wall, the gall bladder, or the common channel junction nearly pancreas, as a consequence of chronic inflammation due to cholangitis [22, 23].

5. Etiology

Despite the existence of numerous theories and laboratory works to explain the etiology of the disease, the exact etiology remains incompletely understood. Initial theories, put forward in this regard, were congenital weakness of the choledochal wall, distal obstruction, oligoganglionosis, and disturbances in the process of recanalization. However, more accepted theories have been produced parallel to the progress in radiological imaging methods [24, 25]. Today, there are two main theories that are widely accepted; (1) reflux of trypsin and other pancreatic enzymes to the bile ducts due to an APBDU; (2) obstruction of distal CBD [26–28]. The idea that the choledochal and pancreatic ducts' abnormality about joint and angle was first reviewed by Babbitt in 1969, and subsequently many number of studies, supporting this view, were made [22, 23, 29–32]. A normal pancreaticobiliary junction usually has an acute angle between the CBD and the pancreatic duct [33] and is located within the duodenal wall [34]. The common channel (distance from between the junction of the CBD and the pancreatic duct to ampulla Vater) length is 4 mm or less, normally. In patients with CCs, this distance (common channel length) increases 5–20 mm [22, 23, 35, 36] that makes the common channel longer [37]. Okada defined it as "common channel syndrome" [36, 38]. It is considered that an abnormal long common channel (especially >15 mm proximal to ampullary sphincter) [39, 40] causes the pancreatic duct communicating with the choledochal duct without the support of ampulla Vater's circular muscular layer (sphincter of Oddi) [41], which protects the biliary tree from reflux of pancreatic enzymes and bile [34]. Another observation is that the junction angle of the two ducts that should be acute normally, however, is close to 90° in these patients. It also causes the pancreatic fluids to flow into the CBD due to the higher pressure of pancreatic duct (**Figure 1**) [41]. Eventually, it is considered that APBDU has a tendency to cause reflux of the pancreatic enzyme into biliary tree with consequent biliary duct inflammation and increased duct pressure, leading to duct wall damage and cystic changes [42, 43]. In animal models of murine APBDU, this mechanism has also been demonstrated [44, 45]. APBDU is seen in up to 90% of patients with CC [25, 46], compared with 2% in the general population [10] and this seems to have important clinical implications. In a comparison of APBDU-associated CC versus non-APBDU-associated CC, APBDU-associated CC patients were significantly more likely to have evidence of pathologically confirmed inflammation including hepatitis, cholangitis, and pancreatitis [47, 48]. However, APBDU is not enough to explain the etiology of all CCs, such as diverticular cyst (type II), where the bile ducts were normal except cyst and the cyst is considered to be a sequel of an intrauterine CC rupture, such as meconium pseudocyst [28]. Additionally, type V CCs are possibly due to dysfunctional remodeling of the ductal plate during embryogenesis [40, 49].

In addition, it is considered that primary strictures of the CBD may also play a role in the development of CCs. The types of the CCs are determined according to the location, severity, and length of the stricture. Detection of these strictures preoperatively is important because treating the CC without addressing the stricture may lead to recurrent episodes of cholangitis. This mechanism has been under estimated and is now believed to be more significant in the pathophysiology of CCs [50].

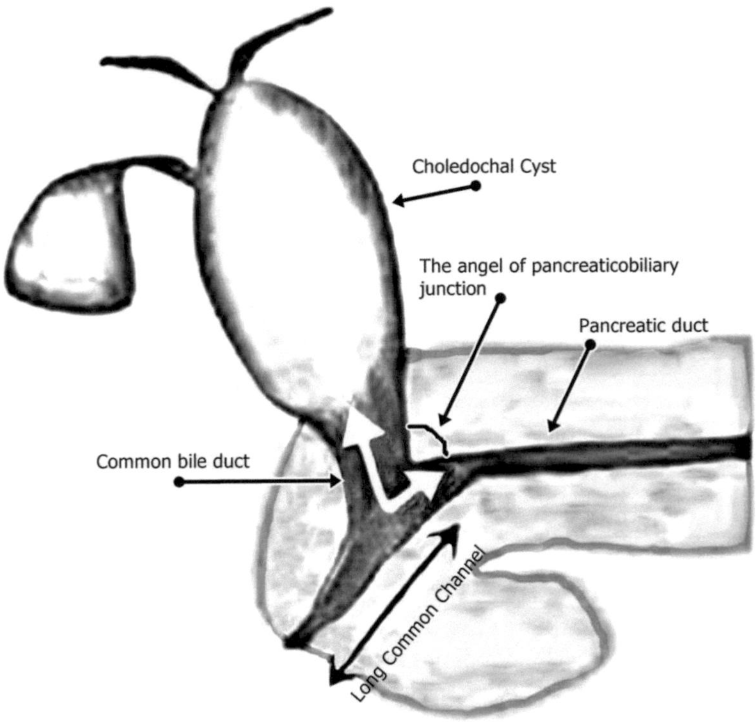

Figure 1.
Anomalous pancreaticobiliary union.

The association of CC with congenital anomalies remains ambiguous. Previous reports have demonstrated an association of pediatric CC and congenital anomalies. Murphy et al. reported in 2012 that screening for cardiac anomalies may be prudent in CC patients [51]. Other reports have postulated an association of CC with duodenal atresia, colonic atresia, gastroschisis, annular pancreas, and pancreatic cysts [10, 52–57].

6. Classification

CCs are first classified in 1959 by Alanso-Lej and colleagues [58]. The original classification identified four types of biliary cysts (types I–IV). In 1977, Todani and colleagues [8] modified this classification and added a fifth category of CC, type V biliary cysts or Carol disease (**Figure 2**) [10]. Apart from types I–V included in the revised Todani classification, isolated cystic dilatation of the cystic duct has been described and suggested as type VI [59].

Type I CC, most commonly seen, 80–90% of all CC, is a dilatation of the extrahepatic biliary tree. Importantly, the intrahepatic biliary tree is sometimes dilated secondarily due to biliary stasis. Type I cyst can be further subdivided into type Ia, Ib, and Ic cysts [10, 60]. Type Ia CCs are composed of the gallbladder arising directly from the CC, dilated extrahepatic biliary tree, and a nondilated intrahepatic tree. Type Ib CCs are focal segmental dilatation of the CBD and contain no evidence of APBDU [50, 60]. Finally, type Ic CCs are represented by a fusiform dilatation of the common hepatic duct and CBD in the presence of APBDU [10, 50, 60], and often also a low-grade stricture at the distal CBD [50]. In type I CC, usually, gallbladder is involved in cyst structure, and cyst extends from hepatic bifurcation to duodenum [61]. Most commonly, the ducts above (right, left, and

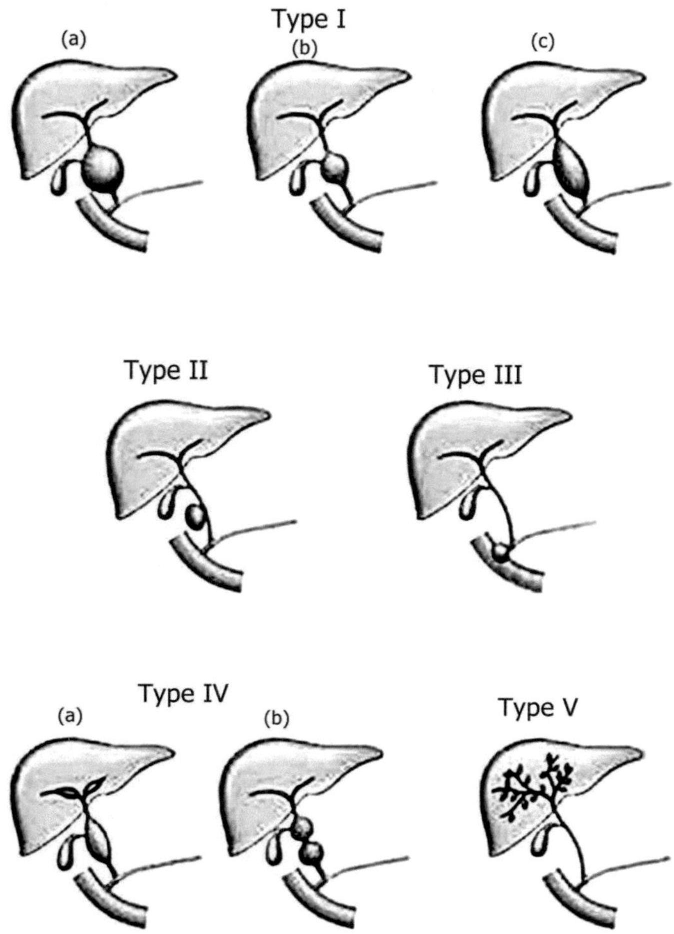

Figure 2.
Types of choledochal cysts, classified by Todani et al.

intrahepatic ducts) and below of the CC are not dilated [14], except type Ic. In type Ic, cyst extends continuously to the common hepatic duct or intrahepatic ducts [62]. Type I CCs, along with type IV cysts, have the highest risk of malignancy [10]. This is not surprising because both of them have extrahepatic involvement associated with APBDU [63].

Type II CCs (2% of all CCs) consist of a diverticular dilatation of the extrahepatic bile duct system and is considered true diverticulum. During the diagnostic cholangiography study, the diverticulum is filled with radiopaque substance and can be confused with the gall bladder duplication seen rarely [10].

Type III CCs (choledochoceles), 4% of all CCs, are characterized by distal (located at the pancreaticobiliary junction) CBD dilatation, confined to the wall of the duodenum and often bulging into the duodenal lumen [25]. Type III choledochal cysts are dissimilar to other types of CCs, with features such as appearing in both sexes equally and low malignancy incidence [10, 64]. Cysts are mostly not associated with APBDU. Because of all these characteristics, it has been suggested that type III CCs should not be classified as a type of CCs revised by Todani [25, 64, 65]. In addition, Ziegler et al. reported that choledochoceles occur more frequently in older male patients presenting with acute pancreatitis [64].

Type IV CCs, the second most common (15–20% of all), are multiple cysts which can involve both the intrahepatic and extrahepatic biliary trees. Type IV CC can be further subdivided into type IVa and IVb cysts depending on intrahepatic involvement. Type IVa CC refers to multiple segmental communicating biliary dilatations located in the intra- and extrahepatic biliary tracts, and relative stricture at the junction that is used to distinguish the true type IVa CC from type I [11]. Type IVa CCs are usually associated with APBDU [50]. Type IVb CC refers to multiple extrahepatic biliary cysts without intrahepatic involvement [25]. Some recent studies have shown that intrahepatic ductal dilatations seen on preoperative imaging are thought to have been caused by distal obstruction and not true intrahepatic biliary duct disease [11]. Additionally, the question of "Is the distinguishing type I from type IVa really necessary preoperatively?" has not answered yet. Because distinguishing between types I and IVa CCs is controversial for some authors due to complete excision of the extrahepatic bile ducts, and intensive long-term follow-up still remains standard of care for both types [11].

Type V CC or Carol disease, added by Todani, is characterized by multifocal segmental intrahepatic biliary ductal dilatation [14] without the evidence of extrahepatic dilatation [66]. Caroli disease is uncommon, accounting for less than 10% of cases. Patients often present in adolescence or early adulthood with recurrent cholangitis, abdominal pain, or jaundice. However, they may present later with the sequel of portal hypertension and cirrhosis [67]. Renal abnormalities, such as medullary sponge kidney, autosomal dominant polycystic kidney disease, and medullary cystic disease can be seen in Caroli disease [49]. Some authors call Caroli disease as Caroli syndrome when congenital hepatic fibrosis is also seen, as in half of the patients [68, 69].

Type VI CC, isolated cystic dilatation of the cystic duct, is rare with only several case reports describing it. Although it is not officially part of the revised Todani classification, it has been proposed to be called type VI CC [70]. If the cyst emerges from the cystic duct near a level close to the CBD, it can be confused with type II CCs. In such cases, the relation of the cyst with the cystic duct should be thoroughly evaluated to differentiate them [59].

7. Clinical presentation

Type IC cysts are the earliest cysts that can be detected by 15-gestational week fetal ultrasonography [71, 72]. There are two clinical forms of disease: adult and infant. In infant form, symptoms such as obstructive jaundice, clay colored stools, and hepatomegaly make it difficult to distinguish from biliary atresia. Adult form of CCs is also congenital, although they usually remain silent until the age of 2 years. There are three main symptoms in the classical clinical triad: recurrent jaundice 69–75%, right upper quadrant pain 47–60%, and right upper quadrant mass 47–80%. But the classic triad only presents in 10% of cases (6–25%) [46, 73, 74].

Abdominal pain is the most common symptom (93.8%) [75], especially in older patients and presents with colic pattern which has a variable interval time (between attacks) up to several years. When investigating the cause of CBD dilatation and differential diagnosis of unclear upper abdominal pain, jaundice, and pancreatitis in children, CCs must be considered [76]. Unfortunately, 29–62% of pediatric patients with CC have been reported that they have choledocholithiasis [77, 78], that is, distinguishing this two situation (CC-associated choledocholithiasis and -nonassociated choledocholithiasis) may be difficult. Choledocholithiasis can also lead to CBD dilatation which can be misdiagnosed as a CC [79].

In 1–2% of cases, especially in infants, CCs may present with rupture and biliary peritonitis prompting emergency biliary drainage [80, 81]. It is not a surprise in diagnosing pancreatitis in patients with CC, because of association of the presence of APBDU [10, 46, 82].

The risk for development of biliary carcinoma in the general population starts after the fourth decade and the incidence increase with age to 0.15% after the eighth decade. However, the risk for the development of carcinoma in patients with a CC starts in childhood and shows a significant increase with age. Interestingly, the age of biliary carcinoma development in patients who have undergone internal drainage without cyst excision has been reported to be 15 years earlier on average than patients who have never had surgery. This is thought to be associated with intestinal bacterial contamination and pancreatic enzymes added to biliary stasis [83]. The malignancy incidence in resected bile duct material has been reported as 7.5% for all age groups, and 0.4 and 11.4% for those under and over the age of 18, respectively. The incidence has been reported to gradually increase every decade to 38.2% over the age of 60, possibly related to chronic inflammation [5]. The incidence of a biliary malignancy development following CC excision is reported as 0.7–5.4%. The malignancy can arise from anywhere such as the porta hepatis, pancreas, or the intrahepatic bile ducts. The time to onset after primary surgical intervention is reported to be 1–34 years. The total excision of the cyst significantly decreases the probability of a malignancy although it does not eliminate it completely [84, 85].

8. Diagnostic evaluation

Ultimately, multimodality imaging techniques are often utilized including computed tomography (CT), magnetic resonance imaging (MRI), and/or endoscopic retrograde cholangiopancreatography (ERCP) to confirm the extent of ductal involvement or the presence of extrahepatic disease [25]. Frequently, further imaging techniques are used to differentiate type I CC from type IVa, in the presence of intrahepatic biliary dilatation [11]. A cyst, presenting in the porta hepatitis, separated from the gallbladder and continuing with enlarged biliary ducts can be shown by ultrasound (US). Additionally, fusiform dilatation of choledoch, intrahepatic biliary dilatation (60–80%), biliary stones, and state of liver parenchyma can be shown by US [86].

Other intraabdominal cysts, such as pancreatic pseudocysts, echinococcal cysts, or biliary cystadenomas should also be differentiated from CCs, whether the cyst has continuity with the biliary tree or not [40]. CT is not only useful for demonstrating continuity of the cyst with the biliary tree, but also demonstrates relation of the cyst with the surrounding structures and the presence of associated malignancy [87]. In order to correctly plan surgery, CT cholangiography can be used to identify the full anatomy of the biliary tree but unfortunately it has been reported to be less sensitive for imaging the pancreatic duct which is responsible for the reflux of contrast into the biliary ducts [87]. As it is well known today, the nephro-hepatotoxicity of the contrast and the ionized radiation exposed are the restrictions of CT utilization in pediatric population (**Figure 3**) [62].

MRCP is noninvasive and highly sensitive (70–100%) and specific (90–100%) in the diagnosis of CCs [88, 89], so, is considered the current gold standard imaging even for initial evaluation [62]. Additionally, there is no irradiation, and modern scanners have alleviated the need for protracted breath-hold making it more amenable to the pediatric population [10, 90]. Although both ultrasound and CT are highly sensitive and specific in the diagnosis of CCs, MRCP can better identify the CCs subtypes and coexisting abnormalities [89]. For example, MRI can easily identify the pancreaticobiliary ductal anatomy, while ultrasound cannot accurately demonstrate the APBDU [89, 91]. Additionally, MRCP is preferred modality in the pediatric population due to invasive nature and inherent risks of endoscopic ultrasound and ERCP, despite their ability of detecting the abnormality of the common

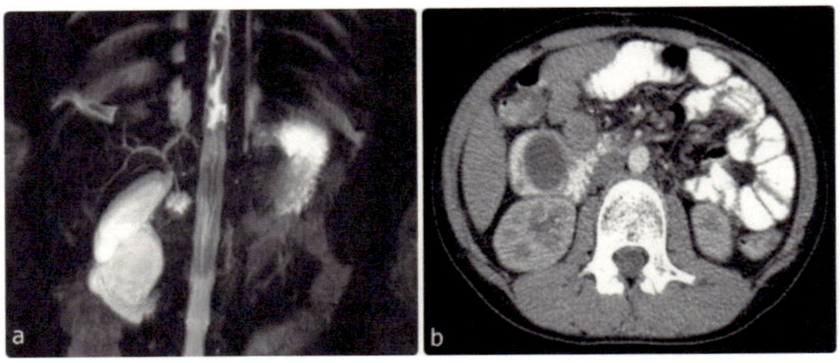

Figure 3.
Type III CC. (a) MRCP; (b) CT image.

channel [89]. MRCP has also been shown to be as effective as intraoperative cholangiography in planning surgery [18]. In addition, lower cost and morbidity compared to other imaging/diagnostic modalities, and reliability for detecting abnormalities associated with CCs such as cholangiocarcinoma and choledocholithiasis, are some of the favorable features of MRCP [89, 92]. Unfortunately, as seen often in patients with CCs, intraductal air, debris, stones, or protein plugs can interfere with the signal and alter visualization (**Figure 4**) [93].

Although it is highly sensitive, invasiveness and associated risks including cholangitis, bleeding, pancreatitis, and perforation makes percutaneous transhepatic cholangiography (PTC) or ERCP utilization less frequently [94]. Moreover, PTC and ERCP can be technically challenging and require general anesthesia in the pediatric population. A lot of surgeons are finding the use of diagnostic ERCP and PTC in CCs unnecessary due to advantages of both MRCP and perioperative cholangiography (performed in nearly almost patients and give highly detailed information about

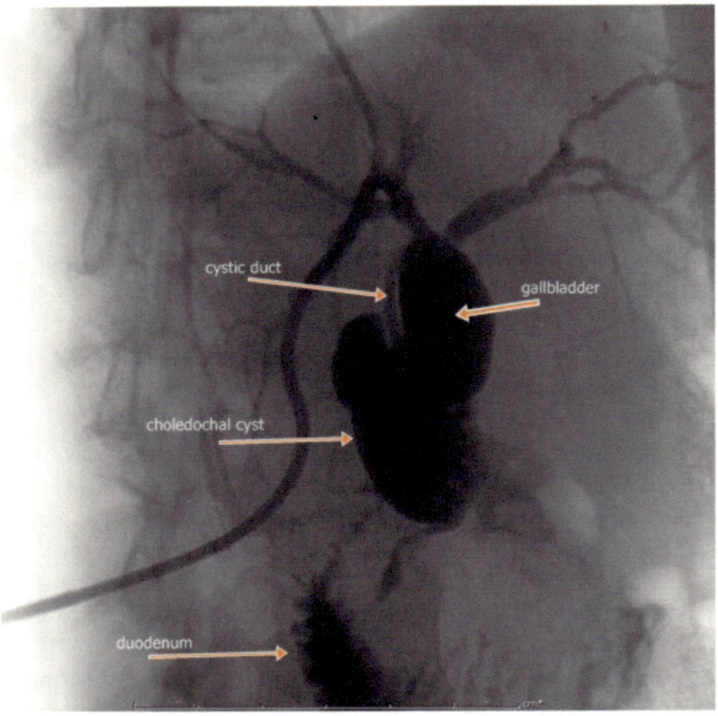

Figure 4.
PTC reveals the detailed anatomy of the biliary tracts and associated CC.

biliary anatomy) [10, 95, 96]. Contemporary, ERCP should only be performed in cases where the appropriate diagnosis cannot be made by other less-invasive examinations, or when therapeutic performance (complications such as cholangitis or biliary stone obstruction [97, 98] and stabilization of the patients with preparing them to the next definitive surgery) is required (**Figure 4**) [39, 99, 100].

Another method that is not preferred now for diagnostic purposes is hepatobiliary scintigraphy. Although it is possible to do it with all IDA variants, DISIDA is the best. The radio isotopic substance is collected in the liver and is normally thrown into the biliary tract, but accumulates in the cyst space in patients with CC [101, 102].

8.1 The differential diagnosis

There are many diseases including biliary atresia, infectious hepatitis, embryonal hepatic rhabdomyosarcoma, biliary lithiasis, pancreatitis, biliary hamartoma in the differential diagnosis of CCs, especially biliary atresia that is one of the two causes of neonatal obstructive jaundice in neonatal period [10]. Differentiating cystic biliary atresia (CBA), a subtype of biliary atresia and has an entirely different treatment approach, from CCs is particularly difficult. Therefore, prompt accurate diagnosis is critical [103]. While earlier presentation (<months of age), smaller cysts with less dilatation of the intrahepatic biliary system, and an atretic gallbladder with irregular and hypoplastic biliary radicles that is seen on ultrasound and cholangiography are characteristics of CBA patients [10, 20, 104, 105]; a dilated gallbladder communicated with the cyst in addition with a dilated intrahepatic biliary tree is mostly a determiner to infantile CC [104].

It is still important to differentiate biliary rhabdomyosarcoma, a rare soft tissue tumor that affects only 1% of children, from CC [106, 107]. In the presence of a mass or intraductal growth that causes obstructive jaundice, the possible diagnosis should return in favor of rhabdomyosarcoma in children and prompt evaluation is necessary [107].

"Children with CBD dilatation did not differ significantly in clinical characteristics compared with children who had obstructive CBD dilatation" said Oh and colleagues [78] by evaluating the cholangiographic characteristics of 85 children with CBD dilatation to differentiate obstructive and congenital CBD dilatation. Indeed, it can be difficult to distinguish them. Therefore, in the pediatric population with dilated biliary trees, ruling out a distal biliary obstruction that causes secondary biliary dilatation is prudent and essential [18].

As noted above, type I CC may present with intrahepatic biliary dilatation secondary to biliary stasis, thus resembling a type IVa CC. Some authors consider that this distinction is critical given the therapeutic implications and the need to include hepatic resection (in the case of type IVa CC) in addition to extrahepatic biliary tree excision [18], whereas the others consider that the need preoperatively distinguishing between type I and IVa CCs is controversial because for both, complete excision of the extrahepatic bile duct and intensive long-term follow-up remains standard of care [11].

9. Management

The treatment time of antenatal diagnosed of CCs has been still a matter of debate. Some reports say that they can be operated within 2–6 weeks, even if they are asymptomatic, due to a potential complication risk of cysts, whereas, the others suggest that they can be followed-up for a time of period with US and regular monitoring of liver functions [108, 109].

Surgical treatment of CCs should be performed electively except complicated ones such as cyst perforation. Children, who have acute problems related to liver and pancreas, should be initially received appropriate medical treatment to remove inflammation and associated obstruction at the pancreaticobiliary system before surgery [110].

In the first half of this century, treatment methods such as cyst aspiration, marsupialization, and external drainage (cholecystostomy, tube drainage) had been used more extensively in the surgical treatment of CCs. And as expected, high mortality and morbidity rates had been detected in patient's follow-up period. Surgical methods such as partial cyst excision and cystoduodenostomy were defined between 1920 and 1930 [111, 112]. Especially, cystoduodenostomy has been the preferred method by many surgeons until the early 1970s [113, 114] when the long-term morbidity was detected as higher (30–50%) [7]. Therefore, in those years, Roux-en-Y cystojejunostomy had identified with the idea of preventing the reflux of the duodenal contents into the bile ducts [7, 30, 115]. Indeed, the cholangitis had been significantly reduced with this method, but not completely eliminated [28]. After soon, it had been demonstrated that anastomosis with a large stoma, as possible as (at least 4 cm) is more important for protecting reflux-related cholangitis attacks than which intestinal segment it is performed (duodenum or jejunum) [116]. The recognition of the cancer development from the left cystic wall and Babbitt's APBDU theory made the idea of cyst excision popular soon after. It had been reported that carcinoma develops after the internal drainage procedures at a frequency of 2.5–17.5% several years later as a consequence of chronic inflammation of the cyst wall. Therefore, cyst excision had gain popularity in a very short time [116].

Contemporarily, the definitive treatment for CCs are total excision that has become preferred management strategy over the internal drainage procedures (choledochocystoduodenostomy or choledochocystojejunostomy), which have an only historical value today despite they had been used as a treatment method in the past although caused high morbidity (probably because of not relieving biliary stasis sufficiently) [117, 118]. Furthermore, only complete resection can fully decrease the risk of malignant degeneration: a critical point in the pediatric population with a large number of expectant life years. The general aim is to remove the cyst completely and restore biliary enteric drainage either into the duodenum by hepaticoduodenostomy (HD) or jejunum by Roux-en-Y hepaticojejunostomy (RYHJ), although specific approaches for types vary minimally. Surgical intervention should be elective and patients should be medically optimized prior to operative intervention. İf patient has a cholangitis or pancreatitis attack preoperatively, the infection should be adequately treated with broad-spectrum intravenous antibiotics or biliary decompression if needed [118].

Surgery for CC disease can be performed open or laparoscopically based on patient characteristics and surgeon preference.

HD and RYHJ are the two most commonly utilized techniques of reconstruction [119], although other replacement conduits such as jejunal interposition HD, valved jejunal interposition HD, nonrefluxing biliary appendicoduodenostomy, hepaticoenterostomy, and wide hilar hepaticojejunostomy have been reported [120–125]. HD has been favored by some groups [126, 127] but most series suggests significantly more bile reflux compared with RYHJ [121], which is currently the most commonly utilized reconstruction.

9.1 Open surgery

In all cases, cholangiography should be performed initially to obtain detailed anatomical information about the intra- and extrahepatic bile ducts, irrespective of preoperative examinations. Dissection of extrahepatic bile ducts starts from the gallbladder. The terminal end of the cyst opening to the duodenum should be isolated, clamped, cut, and transfixed, firstly. Some surgeons suggest that dissection should be continued until the appearance of pancreatic ducts, while the others not suggest. Additionally, some surgeons taking into account that dissection toward the lower end of the cyst may cause inevitable unplanned pancreatic duct injury that pancreaticoduodenectomy requirement should be in your mind, although very rarely [75]. After the distal portion of the cyst is ligated and cut, the posterior wall is dissected from the surface of the portal vein. In cases of marked inflammation, the cyst may be excised by leaving the posterior wall on the portal vein. The dissection should go on till the hepatic hilus. The best strategy to obtain a wide anastomosis stoma is to make a hepatic dissection more proximally until the left hepatic duct is seen. Although all parts of CCs need to be removed, sometimes residual proximal cyst walls can be left to facilitate biliary anastomosis [75]. Dilated bile ducts should be irrigated with heparinized saline to clear the gallstones before anastomosis. After the cyst is excised, one of the hepaticoenterostomy methods, such as hepaticojejunostomy, HD, jejunal interposition HD, valved jejunal interposition HD, nonrefluxing biliary appendicoduodenostomy, hepaticoenterostomy, and wide hilar hepaticojejunostomy [120–125] is performed for biliary reconstruction. In RYHJ, 40-cm jejunal loop replaces to the hepatic hilus. In RYHJ surgery, to avoid the elongation of a blind pouch as the child grows, an end-to-end anastomosis of the jejunum to the CBD is recommended if technically possible [128]. If an end-to-side anastomosis is required (in some cases, the bile duct is too small), it should be as close as possible to the closed end of the jejunal limb. Additionally, although it is not possible to predetermine the length of the Roux limb, it should be appropriate to the child's overall bowel length considering future growth. In HD, anastomosis is performed between the duodenum second part and the bile duct. The duodenum was mobilized to a limit. The duodenum is anchored to the liver at porta to avoid tension on the anastomosis (**Figure 5**).

The intraabdominal drain, kept in Morison's pouch, may be removed on the seventh postoperative day [124].

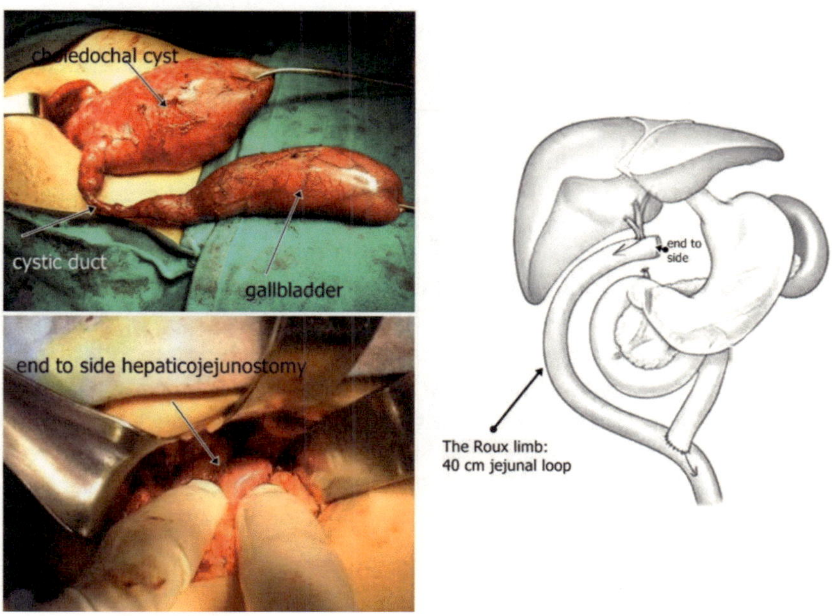

Figure 5.
Intraoperative pictures and drawn cartoon showing of the procedure.

9.2 Laparoscopic surgery

Laparoscopic treatment of choledochal cysts was first described in 1995 [129] and demonstrated that it could be performed in children as young as 3 months [130] and as small as 6 kg [131]. As with most surgical diseases, longer operating time and shorter hospital stay [132] were comparable with open surgical approaches, and in the absence of cholangitis or pancreatitis, it becomes more suitable treatment [132]. While four or five ports are typically used in the traditional laparoscopic approach [130, 133], the use of single-port laparoscopy [134] and robotic surgical system [135] has also been reported. In a prospective randomized study of 121 children undergoing laparoscopic cyst excision with RYHJ, routine postoperative drainage has been shown to be unnecessary [136].

9.3 The optimal technique for biliary reconstruction

The most commonly performed operations for biliary reconstruction after complete surgical resection of CCs are RYHJ or HD [124]. There is a debate regarding the optimal technique for biliary reconstruction [124]. RYHJ is considered as an ideal technique for the repair of CC, but HD has gained wide acceptance and favored by many surgeons open as well as laparoscopically because of its advantages over hepaticojejunostomy. HD is more physiologic, but theoretically, the closeness of hepaticoenterostomy to stomach makes HD to have greater chance of cholangitis and bile gastritis, but in a meta-analyzed study [137], it has been shown that while the incidence of bile gastritis after HD is even higher when examined endoscopically, interestingly, there is no difference of cholangitis between HD and RYHJ. Additionally, HD is simpler to perform and associated with fewer complications such as adhesive bowel obstruction, anastomotic leakage, and peptic ulcer as compared to RYHJ [138]. HD requires less operative time, allows faster recovery of bowel function, and produces fewer complications requiring reoperation [139]. If there is an anastomotic stricture following HD, it can be easily managed by endoscopy as against hepaticojejunostomy [124]. But, when the diameter of the common hepatic duct more than 10 mm that lets duodenal contents more likely to reflux easily into the intrahepatic bile ducts through the HD anastomosis or when the intrahepatic biliary dilatation is present that lets refluxed duodenal contents remain longer in the intrahepatic bile ducts, HD is not recommended because of higher risk of cholangitis or anastomotic stricture formation [124]. Some studies have demonstrated high incidence of secondary bile reflux proven by endoscopy after HD [121]. Recently, a patient with hilary bile duct carcinoma, who was performed HD for the biliary reconstruction at the age of 13 months, has been reported in the 19 years follow-up after the primary cyst excision. Reflux of duodenal contents (including activated pancreatic enzymes) into the intrahepatic bile ducts through the HD anastomosis is thought to be hazardous to the bile duct mucosa in this patient [124]. Adhesive bowel obstruction is seen with a higher incidence in RYHJ that comprises a Roux-en-Y jejuna limb and two anastomoses, compared with HD. Cholangitis, peptic ulcer, fat malabsorption, diarrhea, and malnutrition are the other complications [126]. A significant incidence of long-term complications requiring reoperation such as anastomosis stenosis has been observed with the follow-up studies of patients who underwent hepaticojejunostomy after cyst excision [138, 140], and a wide hilar hepaticojejunostomy extending into the left hepatic duct is advocated for the way to prevent it [125].

9.4 Treatment specifically for types

Treatment of type I CC includes excision of the extrahepatic biliary tract, cholecystectomy, and reconstruction of the biliary system. If the duct is dilated at the distal margin, the mucosa may be left behind to prevent damage to the pancreatico-biliary system and can be striped. Infrequently, because of recurrent episodes of the cholangitis, the cyst wall may densely adherent to the portal vein, precluding safe resection [141]. In such cases, resection of the anterior wall with careful fulguration of the mucosa of the posterior wall can be performed [141]. Hepatic bifurcation is carefully evaluated for stricture and inflammation before performing anastomosis during proximal transection. If one of them is seen, more proximal transection should be considered [18].

For type II CCs, mostly, diverticulectomy or simple cyst excision is enough for the treatment. Primary or over a T-tube closure can be performed, and reconstruction is occasionally required if there is significant luminal narrowing [18].

One of the methods such as endoscopic sphincterotomy, sphincteroplasty, sphincteroplasty with cyst excision, or pancreaticoduodenectomy may be used to manage pediatric patients with type III CCs (choledochoceles) [10, 25]. Various reports denote adequate symptom control with this approach [142, 143]; however, long-term follow-up is lacking. Cysts not amenable to endoscopic intervention may benefit from lateral duodenotomy with sphincteroplasty and unroofing or marsupialization of the cavity [18].

Type IV CC is approached differently based on the presence or absence and location of intrahepatic disease [15]. Type IVb cysts are treated in the same fashion as type I. Management for IVa disease differs due to the presence of intra- as well as extrahepatic involvement, as well as the presence of functional liver disease. Of foremost importance is the characterization of actual type IVa as opposed to type I with upstream ductal dilatation due to stasis and functional obstruction [50]. If the dilatation is anatomic and isolated (limited; i.e., left hemiliver), partial hepatectomy with reconstruction to the remaining hepatic ducts may be warranted due to the ongoing risk of malignant transformation in the intrahepatic biliary system [85]. However, not all patients are appropriate candidates for partial hepatectomy [144]. Those patients with obvious dilatations and stenosis of intrahepatic ducts, intrahepatic duct stones, or parenchymal atrophy may benefit from hepatectomy [144]. If hepatectomy is planned concomitantly with extrahepatic duct excision, the distribution should allow removal of all disease (of the vast majority of the severe disease) with adequate future liver remnant [15]. If the pattern is more diffuse or imaging is inconclusive, treatment in a type I paradigm with close postoperative surveillance to follow intrahepatic ducts has been utilized [145]. This approach is justified by studies demonstrating that patients who progress to malignancy most commonly develop extrahepatic cholangiocarcinoma or gallbladder cancer (approximately 85% of malignancy), whereas intrahepatic cholangiocarcinoma rarely occurs [144]. It is reported that the intrahepatic component has actually resolved in 3–6 months with adequate drainage [146]. To differentiate type IVa from type I, while in adults, preoperative percutaneous biliary drainage to decompress the intrahepatic biliary ductal system has been advocated [147], in children, this practice has not been reported probability due to the difficulty in maintaining the external tube. Although long-term results are not known, intrahepatic cystojejunostomy, in addition to hepaticojejunostomy, has been described as a way of preventing liver resection in type IVa cysts [148]. Complete extrahepatic excision with hepaticoenterostomy and drainage of the remaining cyst externally or internally should adequately ameliorate biliary stasis in the presence of bilobar unresectable intrahepatic cyst [18].

Management of patients with Caroli's disease can be particularly difficult given the location of the cysts and frequent necessity for surgery (considerable potential for cholangitis, liver complications, and biliary cirrhosis; moderate potential for neoplasia (7%)) [15]. In Caroli disease, intrahepatic cysts can be seen as limited disease restricted to a single segment/lobe or diffuse disease involving the entire intrahepatic biliary tree. If the patient has not developed cirrhosis and portal hypertension, the unilobar cystic disease should be treated with anatomic hepatectomy and biliary enteric bypass. However, bilobar disease should be treated with symptom-directed nonoperative treatment methods as including litholytic agents such as ursodiol, antibiotics, and percutaneous drainage if possible. Close follow-up is required for malignant transformation. Although there is no identification for prophylactically orthotopic liver transplantation in the treatment of the disease, it should be kept in mind for the choice of the treatment in patients who have diffuse symptomatic disease with cirrhosis or portal hypertension [149].

9.5 Follow-up

Patients should be monitored every 6 months during the postoperative 3 years and then annually. On initial follow-up, while all patients should be evaluated with complete blood count, liver function tests and abdominal US, on subsequent follow-up, investigations are done only in symptomatic ones. Long-term follow-up can be made by visits, telephonic conversations, and postal inquiry [124].

10. Outcomes and results

Resection of pediatric CC is generally well tolerated [18]. Despite recent advances in surgical techniques and perioperative management, short- and long-term complications are not rare in children, while they are more common in adults [6]. Complications such as recurrent cholangitis attacks, malignant transformation, intracystic or intrahepatic gallstone formation, cirrhosis development, and pancreatitis are common in patients who are not operated on. Complications such as anastomotic leakage, gastrointestinal or intraabdominal bleeding, acute pancreatitis, pancreatic leakage, wound infection, wound dehiscence, intraabdominal infection/abscess, intussusception can be seen in early postoperative period defined as short-term complications [150]. Most early complications can be treated conservatively [151].

However, most series are without early mortality and report rates of acute complications including wound infections from 0 to 17%, without significant difference between infants and children [46, 132].

Surgical inexperience and severe inflammation are often implicated in the development of anastomotic bile leakage [151]. The diagnosis of bile leakage is difficult and delayed in some cases due to nonspecific symptoms [151]. It may not always be possible to differentiate with the imaging findings of US and CT because not all of the intraabdominal fluid collection after surgery is associated with bile leakage, and so, this late diagnosis may result in mortality due to septicemia and septic shock [151]. However, it is reported that MRCP can be used to diagnose and accurately localize the site of bile leakage noninvasively [7, 151]. Bile leaks in the hepaticooenterostomy line can self-limited within a few weeks if they can be drained externally. If the bowel movement is sufficient during this period, the child can be fed by enterally. If the extracted bile is given back to the stomach with NG catheter, electrolyte losses can also be prevented. The bilirubin level of the child may remain high due to edema in the anastomosis line within the first 2 weeks, even if the operation has been successfully performed. If this takes longer, biliary tree, even anastomosis, can be evaluated with PTC [110]. Reoperation is considered only after the failure of conservative treatment [151]. The leakage can be repaired by a circumferential buried suture around the anastomotic site, peritoneal lavage, and effective drainage [151].

Gastrointestinal bleeding may be due to hepaticojejunostomy or stress ulcer.

Acute pancreatitis occurs in patients with CC, both preoperatively and due to injury of the pancreatic tissue during distal dissection of the cyst or to edema in the distal part of the pancreatic duct related postoperatively (4.2%) [151]. Therefore, it has been recovered with a conservative treatment for a short time period. Some reports say that CC excision without ligation of the distal stenotic stump decreases the incidence of pancreatic duct injury [75]. A probe inserted into the pancreatic duct through a duodenotomy may help to prevent pancreatic duct injury in difficult cases [75]. Additionally, Urushihara et al. [152] consider that using bipolar electro cautery to scrape pancreatic tissue away from the bile duct wall during the dissection of the intrapancreatic part of the bile duct causes minimal bleeding and enables clear identification of the narrow part of the CBD [151]. Eventually, complete resection of the distal portion of the cyst, removal of debris and protein plugs in the long common channel and pancreatic duct, and correction of anomalous arrangement of the pancreaticobiliary duct junction are essential to minimize pancreatic complications after the operations [151]. The pancreatic fistula occurs because of not closing the distal choledoch well after the cyst excision or injured pancreatic duct during the dissection. An external drainage of 3–4 weeks allows the fistulas closing.

Late/long-term complications (5–15%) [151] include anastomotic stricture, cholangitis, hepatolithiasis, ileus, cirrhosis, and malignancy. Benign anastomotic stricture with recurrent cholangitis is less common than in adults but is still seen in many as 10–25% of patients and can be associated with both intrahepatic and bile duct stone formation [117].

After intraabdominal surgery, small bowel obstructions, mostly due to adhesions, are common [154]. Patients should be closely monitored for any possible clinical deterioration [154]. If there is no improvement after 48 h of follow-up, there is a high risk of bowel resection due to bowel necrosis despite it has not been clearly defined [156]. Furthermore, it has been defined that during biliary reconstruction, the length and placement of the Roux loop is very important in adhesive bowel obstruction developing postoperatively [156].

In terms of anastomotic stricture, improvement of surgical skills, preservation of blood supply, no or mild inflammation cyst wall, and construction of wide (larger than 1 cm) and tension-free stoma are key factors to reduce anastomosis-related complication [138]. There should be no delay in surgical or endoscopic intervention once biliary obstruction develops postoperatively, but a great deal of planning and a thoughtful workup are required [151]. Kim et al. [155] reported that PTC with stone removal and balloon dilatation was useful in patients with anastomotic stricture. However, some investigators consider that recurrent anastomotic strictures may occur due to fibrosis even after balloon dilatation with PTCS, and repeated cholangitis may cause multiple intrahepatic biliary strictures, recurrent hepatic stones, and development of biliary carcinoma [152, 153]. Hence, especially in young patients, it is recommended that revision of the hepaticojejunostomy followed by ductoplasty, to create a wide stoma for sufficient bile drainage [152, 153].

Rigorous long-term follow-up after pediatric CC resection is limited, but the risk of biliary carcinoma (cholangiocarcinoma, squamous cell carcinoma, sarcoma, gallbladder cancer [12, 157], most often cholangiocarcinoma) clearly remains elevated even after CC excision compared to the general population [18]. The malignancy risk is considered to increase with age at surgery, and the cumulative biliary malignancy risk 25 years after primary surgery has been reported to be as high as 11% [75]. Malignant disease has been noted in up to 14% 0f patients after CC resection as a child [46]. In fact, cancer is the most frequent cause of late mortality in pediatric CC series [18]. Even after complete excision, patients are at higher risk for malignancy than general population [158]. Continued surveillance is, therefore, strongly recommended, though it is not known whether there are risk factors such as retained portion of cyst or not [18]. In those with known malignancy, oncologic principles should apply; patients who can undergo safe resection with negative margins are appropriate for operation [15]. Resection may include hepatectomy with regional lymphadenectomy, extirpation of extrahepatic bile ducts with regional lymphadenectomy (and cholecystectomy), or pancreaticoduodenectomy [15]. However, the 5-year survival rate for patients with CCs complicated by malignancy is high, up to 55% in patients with cholangiocarcinoma [159].

Author details

Hasan Özkan Gezer
Department of Pediatric Surgery, Başkent University Faculty of Medicine, Ankara, Turkey

*Address all correspondence to: hozkangezer@yahoo.com.tr

References

[1] Ando H, Ito T, Watanabe Y, Seo T, Kaneko K, Nagaya M. Spontaneous perforation of choledochal cyst. Journal of the American College of Surgeons. 1995;**181**(2):125-128

[2] Douglas AH. Case of dilatation of common bile duct. Monthly Journal of Medical Science (London). 1852;**14**:97

[3] Altın MA, Büyükpamukçu N, Hiçsönmez A. Çocukluk çağı koledok kistlerinin cerrahi tedavisi. Hacettepe Tıp Dergisi. 1985;**18**:186

[4] Caroli J. Diseases of intrahepatic bile ducts. Israel Journal of Medical Sciences. 1968;**4**(1):21-35

[5] Flanigan DP. Biliary cysts. Annals of Surgery. 1975;**182**:635-643

[6] Klotz D, Cohn BD, Kottmeier PK. Choledochal cysts: Diagnostic and therapeutic problems. Journal of Pediatric Surgery. 1973;**8**(2):271-283

[7] O'Neill JA Jr, Clatworthy HW Jr. Management of choledochal cysts: A fourteen-year follow-up. American Journal of Surgery. Apr 1971;**37**(4):230-237

[8] Todani T, Watanabe Y, Narusue M, Tabuchi K, Okajima K. Congenital bile duct cysts: Classification, operative procedures, and review of thirty-seven cases including cancer arising from choledochal cyst. American Journal of Surgery. 1977;**134**(2):263-269

[9] O'Neill JA Jr. Choledochalcyst. Current Problems in Surgery. 1992;**29**(6):361-410

[10] Soares KC, Arnaoutakis DJ, Kamel I, Rastegar N, Anders R, Maithel S, et al. Choledochal cysts: Presentation, clinical differentiation, and management. Journal of the American College of Surgeons. 2014;**219**(6):1167-1180. DOI: 10.1016/j.jamcollsurg.2014.04.023 [Epub Jun 27, 2014]

[11] Gezer HÖ, Oğuzkurt P, Temiz A, İnce E, Ezer SS, Hiçsönmez A. Choledochal cysts in children: Intrahepatic ductal dilatation does not indicate true intrahepatic biliary duct disease. Turkish Journal of Gastroenterology. Jan 2016;**27**(1):23-29. DOI: 10.5152/tjg.2015.150211 [Epub Nov 27, 2015]

[12] Edil BH, Cameron JL, Reddy S, Lum Y, Lipsett PA, Nathan H, et al. Choledochal cyst disease in children and adults: A 30-year single-institution experience. Journal of the American College of Surgeons. 2008;**206**(5):1000-1005; discussion 1005-8. DOI: 10.1016/j.jamcollsurg.2007.12.045 [Epub Mar 17, 2008]

[13] Xia HT, Yang T, Liang B, Zeng JP, Dong JH. Treatment and outcomes of adults with remnant intrapancreatic choledochal cysts. Surgery. 2016;**159**(2):418-425. DOI: 10.1016/j.surg.2015.04.042 [Epub Jun 27, 2015]

[14] Lewis VA, Adam SZ, Nikolaidis P, Wood C, Wu JG, Yaghmai V, et al. Imaging of choledochal cysts. Abdominal Imaging. 2015;**40**(6):1567-1580. DOI: 10.1007/s00261-015-0381-4

[15] Ronnekleiv-Kelly SM, Soares KC, Ejaz A, Pawlik TM. Management of choledochalcysts. Current Opinion in Gastroenterology. 2016;**32**(3):225-231. DOI: 10.1097/MOG.0000000000000256

[16] Lipsett PA, Pitt HA. Surgical treatment of choledochal cysts. Journal of Hepato-Biliary-Pancreatic Sciences. 2003;**10**(5):352-359

[17] Wiseman K, Buczkowski AK, Chung SW, Francoeur J, Schaeffer D, Scudamore CH. Epidemiology,

presentation, diagnosis, andoutcomes of choledochalcysts in adults in an urban environment. American Journal of Surgery. 2005;**189**(5):527-531; discussion 531

[18] Soares KC, Goldstein SD, Ghaseb MA, Kamel I, Hackam DJ, Pawlik TM. Pediatric choledochal cysts: Diagnosis and current management. Pediatric Surgery International. 2017;**33**(6):637-650. DOI: 10.1007/s00383-017-4083-6 [Epub Mar 31, 2017]

[19] Sugandhi N, Agarwala S, Bhatnagar V, Singh MK, Sharma R. Liverhistology in choledochal cyst-pathological changes and response to surgery: The over looked aspect? Pediatric Surgery International. 2014;**30**(2):205-211. DOI: 10.1007/s00383-013-3453-y

[20] Zhou LY, Guan BY, Li L, Xu ZF, Dai CP, Wang W, et al. Objective differential characteristics of cysticbiliary atresia and choledochal cysts in neonates and young infants: Sonographic findings. Journal of Ultrasound in Medicine. 2012;**31**(6):833-841

[21] Fumino S, Higuchi K, Aoi S, Furukawa T, Kimura O, Tajiri T.Clinic alanalysis of liver fibrosis in choledochal cyst.Pediatric Surgery International 2013;**29**(11):1097-1102. DOI: 10.1007/s00383-013-3368-7

[22] Guelrud M, Morera C, Rodriguez M, Prados JG, Jaén D. Normal and anomalous pancreaticobiliary union in children and adolescents. Gastrointestinal Endoscopy. 1999;**50**(2):189-193

[23] Iwai N, Yanagihara J, Tokiwa K, Shimotake T, Nakamura K. Congenital choledochal dilatation with emphasis on pathophysiology of the biliary tract. Annals of Surgery. 1992;**215**(1):27-30

[24] Kusunoki M, Saitoh N, Yamamura T, Fujita S, Takahashi T, Utsunomiya J. Choledochal cysts. Oligoganglionosis in the narrow portion of the choledochus. Archives of Surgery. 1988;**123**(8):984-986

[25] Martin RF. Biliary cysts: A review and simplified classification scheme. Surgical Clinics of North America. 2014;**94**(2):219-232. DOI: 10.1016/j.suc.2014.01.011

[26] Miyano T, Suruga K, Suda K. Abnormal choledocho-pancreatico ductal junction related to the etiology of infantile obstructive jaundice diseases. Journal of Pediatric Surgery. 1979;**14**(1):16-26

[27] Miyano T, Tsunoda S, suruga K, et al. A proposal of choledochopancreatic long common channnel disease. Japanese Journal of Pediatric Surgery. 1979;**11**:1111

[28] O'Neill JA Jr. Choledochal cyst. In: O'Neill JA Jr, Rowe MI, Grosfeld JL, Fonkalsrud EW, Coran AG, editors. Pediatric Surgery. 5th ed. Vol. 2. St Louis, Missouri; Mosby-Year Book, Inc; 1998; pp. 1483-1494

[29] Arima E, Akita H. Congenital biliary tract dilatation and anomalous junction of the pancreatico-biliary ductal system. Journal of Pediatric Surgery. 1979;**14**(1):9-15

[30] Babbitt DP. Congenital choledochal cysts: New etiological concept based on anomalous relationships of the common bile duct and pancreatic bulb.Annales de Radiologie (Paris) 1969;**12**(3):231-240

[31] Ikeda N. Experimental and clinical studies on anomalous relationship in the pancreaticobiliary duct. The Tokushima Journal of Experimental Medicine. 1978;**25**(1-2):47-57

[32] Ito T, Ando H, Nagaya M, Sugito T. Congenital dilatation of the common bile duct in children. The etiologic significance of the narrow segment

distal to the dilated common bile duct. Zeitschrift für Kinderchirurgie. 1984;**39**(1):40-45

[33] Lee HK, Park SJ, Yi BH, Lee AL, Moon JH, Chang YW. Imaging features of adult choledochal cysts: A pictorial review. Korean Journal of Radiology. 2009;**10**(1):71-80. DOI: 10.3348/kjr.2009.10.1.71

[34] Beltrán MA. Current knowledge on pancreaticobiliary reflux in normal pancreaticobiliary junction. International Journal of Surgery. 2012;**10**(4):190-193. DOI: 10.1016/j.ijsu.2012.02.009 [Epub Feb 20, 2012]

[35] Jona JZ, Babbitt DP, Starshak RJ, LaPorta AJ, Glicklich M, Cohen RD. Anatomic observations and etiologic and surgical considerations in choledochal cyst. Journal of Pediatric Surgery. 1979;**14**(3):315-320

[36] Okada A, Oguchi Y, Kamata S, Ikeda Y, Kawashima Y, Saito R. Common channel syndrome—Diagnosis with endoscopic retrograde cholangiopancreatography and surgical management. Surgery. 1983;**93**(5):634-642

[37] Li L, Yamataka A, Yian-Xia W, Da-Yong W, Segawa O, Lane GJ, et al. Ectopic distal location of the papilla of Vater in congenital biliary dilatation: Implications for pathogenesis. Journal of Pediatric Surgery. 2001;**36**(11):1617-1622

[38] Okada A, Nakamura T, Higaki J, Okumura K, Kamata S, Oguchi Y. Congenital dilatation of the bile duct in 100 instances and its relationship with anomalous junction. Surgery, Gynecology & Obstetrics. 1990;**171**(4):291-298

[39] Liu QY, Nguyen V. Endoscopic approach to the patient with congenital anomalies of the biliary tract. Gastrointestinal Endoscopy Clinics of North America. 2013;**23**(2):505-518. DOI: 10.1016/j.giec.2012.12.004 [Epub Jan 17, 2013]

[40] Levy AD, Rohrmann CA Jr. Biliary cystic disease. Current Problems in Diagnostic Radiology. 2003;**32**(6):233-263

[41] Iwai N, Tokiwa K, Tsuto T, et al. sphincter function of the bile duct in patients with congenital choledochal dilatation. Journal of the Japanese Society of Pediatric Surgeons. 1986;**22**:688

[42] Søreide K, Søreide JA. Bile duct cyst as precursor to biliary tract cancer. Annals of Surgical Oncology. 2007;**14**(3):1200-1211 [Epub Dec 23, 2006]

[43] Chang J, Jang JY, Kang MJ, Jung W, Shin YC, Kim SW. Clinicopathologic differences in patients with gallbladder cancer according to the presence of anomalous biliopancreatic junction. World Journal of Surgery. 2016;**40**(5):1211-1217. DOI: 10.1007/s00268-015-3359-z

[44] Yamashiro Y, Miyano T, Suruga K, Shimomura H, Suda K, Matsumoto M, et al. Experimental study of the pathogenesis of choledochal cyst and pancreatitis, with special reference to the role of bile acids and pancreatic enzymes in the anomalous choledocho-pancreatico ductal junction. Journal of Pediatric Gastroenterology and Nutrition. 1984;**3**(5):721-727

[45] Miyano T, Suruga K, Suda K. "The choledocho-pancreatic long common channel disorders" in relation to the etiology of congenital biliary dilatation and other biliary tract disease. Annals of the Academy of Medicine, Singapore. 1981;**10**(4):419-426

[46] de Vries JS, de Vries S, Aronson DC, Bosman DK, Rauws EA, Bosma A, et al. Choledochal cysts: Age of

presentation, symptoms, and late complications related to Todani's classification. Journal of Pediatric Surgery. 2002;**37**(11):1568-1573

[47] Park SW, Koh H, Oh JT, Han SJ, Kim S. Relationship between anomalous pancreaticobiliary ductal union and pathologic inflammation of bile duct in choledochal cyst. Pediatric Gastroenterology, Hepatology & Nutrition. 2014;**17**(3):170-177. DOI: 10.5223/pghn.2014.17.3.170 [Epub Sep 30, 2014]

[48] Song HK, Kim MH, Myung SJ, Lee SK, Kim HJ, Yoo KS, et al. Choledochal cyst associated the with anomalous union of pancreaticobiliary duct (AUPBD) has a more grave clinical course than choledochal cyst alone. The Korean Journal of Internal Medicine. 1999;**14**(2):1-8

[49] Fulcher AS, Turner MA, Sanyal AJ. Case 38: Caroli disease and renal tubular ectasia. Radiology. 2001;**220**(3):720-723

[50] Todani T, Watanabe Y, Toki A, Morotomi Y. Classification of congenital biliary cystic disease: Special reference to type Ic and IVA cysts with primary ductal stricture. Journal of Hepato-Biliary-Pancreatic Surgery. 2003;**10**(5):340-344

[51] Murphy AJ, Axt JR, Lovvorn HN 3rd. Associations between pediatric choledochal cysts, biliary atresia, and congenital cardiac anomalies. Journal of Surgical Research. 2012;**177**(2):e59-e63. DOI: 10.1016/j.jss.2012.04.018 [Epub May 1, 2012]

[52] Iwai A, Hamada Y, Takada K, Inagaki N, Nakatake R, Yanai H, et al. Choledochal cyst associated with duodenal atresia: Case report and review of the literature. Pediatric Surgery International. 2009;**25**(11):995-998. DOI: 10.1007/s00383-009-2462-3

[53] Shih HS, Ko SF, Chaung JH. Is there an association between duodenal atresia and choledochal cyst? Journal of Pediatric Gastroenterology and Nutrition. 2005;**40**(3):378-381

[54] Nijagal A, Ozgediz D, Feldstein VA, Lee H, Harrison MR. Colonic atresia and choledochal cyst: A rare combination. Pediatric Surgery International. 2009;**25**(1):113-115. DOI: 10.1007/s00383-008-2280-z [Epub Nov 5, 2008]

[55] Komuro H, Takahashi MI, Matoba K, Hori T, Hirai M, Gotoh C, et al. Rare association of severe hypoplasia of the abdominal aorta with imperforate anus, colonic atresia, and choledochal cyst. Pediatric Surgery International. 2006;**22**(3):289-292 [Epub Nov 26, 2005]

[56] Serber J, Stranzinger E, Geiger JD, Teitelbaum DH. Association of gastroschisis and choledochal cyst. Journal of Pediatric Surgery. 2009;**44**(3):e23-e26. DOI: 10.1016/j.jpedsurg.2008.12.005

[57] Komuro H, Makino S, Tahara K. Choledochal cyst associated with duodenal obstruction. Journal of Pediatric Surgery. 2000;**35**(8):1259-1262

[58] Alonso-lej F, Rever WB Jr, Pessagno DJ. Congenital choledochal cyst, with a report of 2, and an analysis of 94, cases. International Abstract of Surgery. 1959;**108**(1):1-30

[59] Serena Serradel AF, Santamaría Linares E, Herrera Goepfert R. Cystic dilatation of the cystic duct: A new type of biliary cyst. Surgery. 1991;**109** (3 Pt 1):320-322

[60] Rozel C, Garel L, Rypens F, Viremouneix L, Lapierre C, Décarie JC, et al. Imaging of biliary disorders in children. Pediatric Radiology. 2011;**41**(2):208-220. DOI: 10.1007/s00247-010-1829-x [Epub Sep 24, 2010]

[61] Spier LN, Crystal K, Kase DJ, Fagelman D, Spier N. Choledochocele: Newer concepts of origin and diagnosis. Surgery. 1995;**117**(4):476-478

[62] Drabek J, Keil R, Stovicek J, Lochmannova J, Hlava S, Snajdauf J, et al. The role of endoscopic retrograde cholangiopancreatography in choledochal cysts and/or abnormal pancreatobiliary junction in children. Przegląd Gastroenterologiczny. 2017;**12**(4):303-309. DOI: 10.5114/pg.2017.72107 [Epub Dec 14, 2017]

[63] Li L, Yamataka A, Wang YX, Wang DY, Wang K, Li ZX, et al. Anomalous pancreatic duct anatomy, ectopic distal location of the papilla of Vater and congenital biliary dilatation: A new developmental triad? Pediatric Surgery International. 2003;**19**(3):180-185 [Epub Apr 15, 2003]

[64] Ziegler KM, Pitt HA, Zyromski NJ, Chauhan A, Sherman S, Moffatt D, et al. Choledochoceles: Are they choledochal cysts? Annals of Surgery. 2010;**252**(4):683-690. DOI: 10.1097/SLA.0b013e3181f6931f

[65] Ziegler KM, Zyromski NJ. Choledochoceles: Are they choledochal cysts? Advances in Surgery. 2011;**45**:211-224

[66] Moslim MA, Gunasekaran G, Vogt D, Cruise M, Morris-Stiff G. Surgical management of Caroli's disease: Single center experience and review of the literature. Journal of Gastrointestinal Surgery. 2015;**19**(11):2019-2027. DOI: 10.1007/s11605-015-2918-9 [Epub Aug 25, 2015]

[67] Brancatelli G, Federle MP, Vilgrain V, Vullierme MP, Marin D, Lagalla R. Fibropolycystic liver disease: CT and MR imaging findings. Radiographics. 2005;**25**(3):659-670

[68] Mabrut JY, Bozio G, Hubert C, Gigot JF. Management of congenital bile duct cysts. Digestive Surgery. 2010;**27**(1):12-18. DOI: 10.1159/000268109 [Epub Apr 1, 2010]

[69] Santiago I, Loureiro R, Curvo-Semedo L, Marques C, Tardáguila F, Matos C, et al. Congenital cystic lesions of the biliary tree. American Journal of Roentgenology. 2012;**198**(4):825-835. DOI: 10.2214/AJR.11.7294

[70] Bode WE, Aust JB. Isolated cystic dilatation of the cystic duct. American Journal of Surgery. 1983;**145**(6):828-829

[71] Dewbury KC, Aluwihare AP, Birch SJ, Freeman NV. Prenatal ultrasound demonstration of a choledochal cyst. The British Journal of Radiology. 1980;**53**(633):906-907. DOI: 10.1259/0007-1285-53-633-906

[72] Howell CG, Templeton JM, Weiner S, Glassman M, Betts JM, Witzleben CL. Antenatal diagnosis and early surgery for choledochal cyst. Journal of Pediatric Surgery. 1983;**18**(4):387-393

[73] Goon HK, Tai A, Samad SA. congenital bile duct dilatation: Review of 35 cases. Pediatric Surgery International. 1992;7:332

[74] Miyano T, Yamataka A, Kato Y, Segawa O, Lane G, Takamizawa S, et al. Hepaticoenterostomy after excision of choledochal cyst in children: A 30-year experience with 180 cases. Journal of Pediatric Surgery. 1996;**31**(10):1417-1421

[75] Gadelhak N, Shehta A, Hamed H. Diagnosis and management of choledochal cyst: 20 years of single center experience. World Journal of Gastroenterology. 2014;**20**(22):7061-7066. DOI: 10.3748/wjg.v20.i22.7061

[76] Kim YA, Kim GM, Chun P, Hwang EH, Mun SW, Lee YJ, et al Management of pediatric patients presenting with acute abdomen accompanying dilatation of the common bile duct. Pediatric Gastroenterology, Hepatology &

Nutrition. 2018;**21**(3):203-208. DOI: 10.5223/pghn.2018.21.3.203 [Epub Jun 28, 2018]

[77] Huang CS, Huang CC, Chen DF. Choledochal cysts: Differences between pediatric and adult patients. Journal of Gastrointestinal Surgery. 2010;**14**(7):1105-1110. DOI: 10.1007/s11605-010-1209-8 [Epub Apr 27, 2010]

[78] Oh SH, Chang SH, Kim HJ, Cho JM, Hwang JH, Namgoong JM, et al. Cholangiographic characteristics of common bile duct dilatation in children. World Journal of Gastroenterology. 2015;**21**(20):6229-6235. DOI: 10.3748/wjg.v21.i20.6229

[79] Youn HS, Seo JH, Park CH, Cho JM, Park JJ. An infantile case of cholelithiasis initially misdiagnosed as choledochal cyst. Pediatrics International. 2012;**54**(1):168-169. DOI: 10.1111/j.1442-200X.2011.03546.x

[80] Yamaguchi M. Congenital choledochal cyst. Analysis of 1,433 patients in the Japanese literature. American Journal of Surgery. 1980;**140**(5):653-657

[81] Yamoto M, Urushihara N, Fukumoto K, Miyano G, Nouso H, Morita K, et al. Usefulness of laparoscopic cholecystostomy in children with complicated choledochal cyst. Asian Journal of Endoscopic Surgery. 2015;**8**(2):153-157. DOI: 10.1111/ases.12170 [Epub Feb 11, 2015]

[82] Diao M, Li L, Cheng W. Coagulopathy in a subtype of choledochal cyst and management strategy. World Journal of Gastroenterology. 2014;**20**(30): 10606-10612. DOI: 10.3748/wjg.v20.i30.10606

[83] Makin E, Davenport M. Understanding choledochal malformation. Archives of Disease in Childhood. 2012;**97**(1):69-72. DOI: 10.1136/adc.2010.195974 [Epub Mar 27, 2011]

[84] Ohashi T, Wakai T, Kubota M, Matsuda Y, Arai Y, Ohyama T, et al. Risk of subsequent biliary malignancy in patients undergoing cyst excision for congenital choledochal cysts. Journal of Gastroenterology and Hepatology. 2013;**28**:243-247

[85] He XD, Wang L, Liu W, Liu Q, Qu Q, Li BL, et al. The risk of carcinogenesis in congenital choledochal cyst patients: An analysis of 214 cases. Annals of Hepatology. 2014;**13**:819-826

[86] Hernanz-Schulman M, Ambrosino MM, Freeman PC, Quinn CB. Common bile duct in children: Sonographicdimensions. Radiology. 1995;**195**(1):193-195

[87] Lam WW, Lam TP, Saing H, Chan FL, Chan KL. MR cholangiography and CT cholangiography of pediatric patients with choledochal cysts. American Journal of Roentgenology. 1999;**173**(2):401-405

[88] Huang CT, Lee HC, Chen WT, Jiang CB, Shih SL, Yeung CY. Usefulness of magnetic resonance cholangiopancreatography in pancreatobiliary abnormalities in pediatric patients. Pediatrics & Neonatology. 2011;**52**(6):332-336. DOI: 10.1016/j.pedneo.2011.08.006 [Epub Nov 6, 2011]

[89] Sacher VY, Davis JS, Sleeman D, Casillas J. Role of magnetic resonance cholangiopancreatography in diagnosing choledochal cysts: Case series and review. World Journal of Radiology. 2013;**5**(8):304-312. DOI: 10.4329/wjr.v5.i8.304

[90] Suzuki M, Shimizu T, Kudo T, Suzuki R, Ohtsuka Y, Yamashiro Y, et al. Usefulness of nonbreath-hold 1-shot magnetic resonance

cholangiopancreatography for the evaluation of choledochal cyst in children. Journal of Pediatric Gastroenterology and Nutrition. 2006;**42**(5):539-544

[91] Guo WL, Huang SG, Wang J, Sheng M, Fang L. Imaging findings in 75 pediatric patients with pancreaticobiliary maljunction: A retrospective case study. Pediatric Surgery International. 2012;**28**(10): 983-938 [Epub Aug 15, 2012]

[92] Murphy AJ, Axt JR, Crapp SJ, Martin CA, Crane GL, Lovvorn HN 3rd. Concordance of imaging modalities and cost minimization in the diagnosis of pediatric choledochal cysts. Pediatric Surgery International. 2012;**28**(6): 615-621. DOI: 10.1007/s00383-012-3089-3 [Epub Apr 21, 2012]

[93] Arshanskiy Y, Vyas PK. Type IV choledochal cyst presenting with obstructive jaundice: Role of MR cholangiopancreatography in preoperative evaluation. American Journal of Roentgenology. 1998;**171**(2):457-459

[94] Saito T, Terui K, Mitsunaga T, Nakata M, Kuriyama Y, Higashimoto Y, et al. Role of pediatric endoscopic retrograde cholangiopancreatography in an era stressing less-invasive imaging modalities. Journal of Pediatric Gastroenterology and Nutrition. 2014;**59**(2):204-209. DOI: 10.1097/MPG.0000000000000399

[95] Park DH, Kim MH, Lee SK, Lee SS, Choi JS, Lee YS, et al. Can MRCP replace the diagnostic role of ERCP for patients with choledochal cysts? Gastrointestinal Endoscopy. 2005;**62**(3):360-366

[96] Sharma AK, Wakhlu A, Sharma SS. The role of endoscopic retrograde cholangiopancreatography in the management of choledochal cysts in children. Journal of Pediatric Surgery. 1995;**30**(1):65-67

[97] Schaefer JF, Kirschner HJ, Lichy M, Schlemmer HP, Schick F, Claussen CD, et al. Highly resolved free-breathing magnetic resonance cholangiopancreatography in the diagnostic workup of pancreaticobiliary diseases in infants and young children—Initial experiences. Journal of Pediatric Surgery. 2006;**41**(10):1645-1651

[98] Moyer V, Freese DK, Whitington PF, Olson AD, Brewer F, Colletti RB, et al. North American Society for Pediatric Gastroenterology, Hepatology and Nutrition. Guideline for the evaluation of cholestatic jaundice in infants: Recommendations of the North American Society for Pediatric Gastroenterology, Hepatology and Nutrition. Journal of Pediatric Gastroenterology and Nutrition. Aug 2004;**39**(2):115-128

[99] De Angelis P, Foschia F, Romeo E, Caldaro T, Rea F, di Abriola GF, et al. Role of endoscopic retrograde cholangiopancreatography in diagnosis and management of congenital choledochal cysts: 28 pediatric cases. Journal of Pediatric Surgery. 2012;**47**(5):885-888. DOI: 10.1016/j.jpedsurg.2012.01.040

[100] Otto AK, Neal MD, Slivka AN, Kane TD. An appraisal of endoscopic retrograde cholangiopancreatography (ERCP) for pancreaticobiliary disease in children: Our institutional experience in 231 cases. Surgical Endoscopy. 2011;**25**(8):2536-2540. DOI: 10.1007/s00464-011-1582-8 [Epub Feb 27, 2011]

[101] Dooms GC, Fisher MR, Higgins CB, Hricak H, Goldberg HI, Margulis AR. MR imaging of the dilated biliary tract. Radiology. 1986;**158**(2):337-341

[102] Riddlesberger MM Jr. Evaluation of the gastrointestinal tract in the child: CT, MRI, and isotopic studies. Pediatric Clinics of North America. 1988;**35**(2):281-310

[103] Hill SJ, Clifton MS, Derderian SC, Wulkan ML, Ricketts RR. Cystic biliary atresia: A wolf in sheep's clothing. The American Surgeon. 2013;**79**(9): 870-872

[104] Vijayaraghavan P, Lal R, Sikora SS, Poddar U, Yachha SK. Experience with choledochal cysts in infants. Pediatric Surgery International. 2006;**22**(10): 803-807 [Epub Sep 1, 2006]

[105] Kim WS, Kim IO, Yeon KM, Park KW, Seo JK, Kim CJ. Choledochal cyst with or without biliary atresia in neonates and young infants: US differentiation. Radiology. 1998;**209**(2):465-469

[106] Nakib G, Calcaterra V, Goruppi I, Romano P, Raffaele A, Schleef J, et al. Robotic-assisted surgery approach in a biliary rhabdomyosarcoma misdiagnosed as choledochal cyst. Rare Tumors. 2014;**6**(1):5173. DOI: 10.4081/rt.2014.5173 [eCollection Jan 23, 2014]

[107] Elwahab MA, Hamed H, Shehta A, Ali M, Zalata K. Hepatobiliaryrhabdomyosarcoma mimicking choledochal cyst: Lessons learned. International Journal of Surgery Case Reports. 2014;**5**(4): 196-199. DOI: 10.1016/j.ijscr.2014.01.020 [Epub Feb 7, 2014]

[108] Büyükyavuz I, Ekinci S, Ciftçi AO, Karnak I, Senocak ME, Tanyel FC, et al. A retrospective study of choledochal cyst: Clinical presentation, diagnosis and treatment. The Turkish Journal of Pediatrics. 2003;**45**(4):321-325

[109] Stringer MD, Dhawan A, Davenport M, Mieli-Vergani G, Mowat AP, Howard ER. Choledochal cysts: Lessons from a 20 year experience. Archives of Disease in Childhood. 1995;**73**(6):528-531

[110] Todani T, Watanabe Y, Toki A, Urushihara N. Carcinoma related to choledochal cysts with internal drainage operations. Surgery, Gynecology & Obstetrics. 1987;**164**(1):61-64

[111] Gross RE. Idiopathic dilatation of the common bile duct in children. The Journal of Pediatrics. 1933;**3**:730

[112] Mcworther GL. Congenital cystic dilatation of the common bile duct. Archives of Surgery. 1924;**8**:604

[113] Fonkalsrud EW, Boles ET. Choledochal cyst in infancy and childhood. Surgery, Gynecology & Obstetrics. 1965;**121**:733

[114] Madden JD, Gruwez JA, Tan PY. Obstructive (surgical) jaundice: an analysis of 140 consequtive cases and a consideration of choledocoduodenostomy in its treatment. American Journal of Surgery. 1965;**174**:711

[115] Spitz L. Choledochal cyst. Surgery, Gynecology & Obstetrics. 1978;**147**(3):444-452

[116] Başaklar AC. Bebek ve Çocukların Cerrahi ve Ürolojik Hastalıkları. Turkey: Palme yayıncılık; 2006. ISBN: 975-8982-83-4

[117] Schier F, Clausen M, Kouki M, Gdanietz K, Waldschmidt J. Late results in the management of choledochal cysts. European Journal of Pediatric Surgery. 1994;**4**(3):141-144

[118] Todani T, Watanabe Y, Toki A, Urushihara N, Sato Y. Reoperation for congenital choledochal cyst. Annals of Surgery. 1988;**207**(2):142-147

[119] Wei MF, Qi BQ, Xia GL, Yuan JY, Wang G, Weng YZ, et al. Use of the appendix to replace the choledochus. Pediatric Surgery International. 1998;**13**(7):494-496

[120] Todani T, Watanabe Y, Mizuguchi T, Fujii T, Toki

A. Hepaticoduodenostomy at the hepatic hilum after excision of choledochal cyst. American Journal of Surgery. 1981;**142**(5):584-587

[121] Shimotakahara A, Yamataka A, Yanai T, Kobayashi H, Okazaki T, Lane GJ, et al. Roux-en-Y hepaticojejunostomy or hepaticoduodenostomy for biliary reconstruction during the surgical treatment of choledochal cyst: Which is better? Pediatric Surgery International. 2005;**21**(1):5-7

[122] Narasimha Rao KL, Mitra SK, Kochher R, Thapa BR, Nagi B, Katariya S, et al. Jejunal interposition hepaticoduodenostomy for choledochal cyst. The American Journal of Gastroenterology. 1987;**82**(10):1042-1045

[123] Shamberger RC, Lund DP, Lillehei CW, Hendren WH 3rd. Interposed jejunal segment with nipple valve to prevent reflux in biliary reconstruction. Journal of the American College of Surgeons. 1995;**180**(1):10-15

[124] Patil V, Kanetkar V, Talpallikar MC. Hepaticoduodenostomy for biliary reconstruction after surgical resection of choledochal cyst: A 25-year experience. Indian Journal of Surgery. 2015;**77**(Suppl 2):240-244. DOI: 10.1007/s12262-012-0783-2 [Epub Dec 18, 2012]

[125] Stringer MD. Wide hilar hepaticojejunostomy: The optimum method of reconstruction after choledochal cyst excision. Pediatric Surgery International. 2007;**23**(6): 529-532 [Epub Apr 17, 2007]

[126] Schimpl G, Aigner R, Sorantin E, Mayr J, Sauer H. Comparison of hepaticoantrostomy and hepaticojejunostomy for biliary reconstruction after resection of a choledochal cyst. Pediatric Surgery International. 1997;**12**(4):271-275

[127] Yeung F, Chung PH, Wong KK, Tam PK. Biliary-enteric reconstruction with hepaticoduodenostomy following laparoscopic excision of choledochal cyst is associated with better postoperative outcomes: A single-centre experience. Pediatric Surgery International. 2015;**31**(2):149-153. DOI: 10.1007/s00383-014-3648-x [Epub Nov 30, 2014]

[128] Miyano T. Choledochal cysts. In: Stringer MD, Oldham KT, Mouriquand PDE, editors. Pediatric Surgery and Urology: Long-term Outcomes. Cambridge: Cambridge University Press. pp. 465-479

[129] Farello GA, Cerofolini A, Rebonato M, Bergamaschi G, Ferrari C, Chiappetta A. Congenital choledochal cyst: Video-guided laparoscopic treatment. Surgical Laparoscopy Endoscopy. 1995;**5**(5):354-358

[130] Le DM, Woo RK, Sylvester K, Krummel TM, Albanese CT. Laparoscopic resection of type 1 choledochal cysts in pediatric patients. Surgical Endoscopy. 2006;**20**(2):249-251 [Epub Dec 28, 2005]

[131] Lee JH, Kim SH, Kim HY, Choi YH, Jung SE, Park KW. Early experience of laparoscopic choledochal cyst excision in children. Journal of Korean Surgical Society. 2013;**85**(5):225-229. DOI: 10.4174/jkss.2013.85.5.225 [Epub Oct 25, 2013]

[132] Liuming H, Hongwu Z, Gang L, Jun J, Wenying H, KKY W, et al. The effect of laparoscopic excision vs open excision in children with choledochal cyst: A midterm follow-up study. Journal of Pediatric Surgery. 2011;**46**(4):662-665. DOI: 10.1016/j.jpedsurg.2010.10.012

[133] Margonis GA, Spolverato G, Kim Y, Marques H, Poultsides G, Maithel S, et al. Minimally invasive resection of choledochal cyst: A

feasible and safe surgical option. Journal of Gastrointestinal Surgery. 2015;**19**(5):858-865. DOI: 10.1007/s11605-014-2722-y [Epub Dec 18, 2014]

[134] Diao M, Li L, Cheng W. To drain or not to drain in Roux-en-Y hepatojejunostomy for children with choledochal cysts in the laparoscopic era: A prospective randomized study. Journal of Pediatric Surgery. 2012;**47**(8):1485-1489. DOI: 10.1016/j.jpedsurg.2011.10.066

[135] Chang EY, Hong YJ, Chang HK, Oh JT, Han SJ. Lessons and tips from the experience of pediatric robotic choledochal cyst resection. Journal of Laparoendoscopic & Advanced Surgical Techniques: Part A. 2012;**22**(6):609-614. DOI: 10.1089/lap.2011.0503 [Epub Jun 13, 2012]

[136] Diao M, Li L, Li Q, Ye M, Cheng W. Single-incision versus conventional laparoscopic cyst excision and Roux-Y hepaticojejunostomy for children with choledochal cysts: A case-control study. World Journal of Surgery. 2013;**37**(7):1707-1713. DOI: 10.1007/s00268-013-2012-y

[137] Narayanan SK, Chen Y, Narasimhan KL, Cohen RC. Hepaticoduodenostomy versus hepaticojejunostomy after resection of choledochal cyst: A systematic review and meta-analysis. Journal of Pediatric Surgery. 2013;**48**(11):2336-2342. DOI: 10.1016/j.jpedsurg.2013.07.020

[138] Todani T, Watanabe Y, Urushihara N, Noda T, Morotomi Y. Biliary complications after excisional procedure for choledochal cyst. Journal of Pediatric Surgery. 1995;**30**(3):478-481

[139] Santore MT, Behar BJ, Blinman TA, Doolin EJ, Hedrick HL, Mattei P, et al. Hepaticoduodenostomy vs hepaticojejunostomy for reconstruction after resection of choledochal cyst. Journal of Pediatric Surgery. 2011;**46**(1):209-213. DOI: 10.1016/j.jpedsurg.2010.09.092

[140] Yamataka A, Ohshiro K, Okada Y, Hosoda Y, Fujiwara T, Kohno S, et al. Complications after cyst excision with hepaticoenterostomy for choledochal cysts and their surgical management in children versus adults. Journal of Pediatric Surgery. 1997;**32**(7):1097-1102

[141] Senthilnathan P, Patel ND, Nair AS, Nalankilli VP, Vijay A, Palanivelu C. Laparoscopic management of choledochal cyst-technical modifications and outcome analysis. World Journal of Surgery. 2015;**39**(10):2550-2556. DOI: 10.1007/s00268-015-3111-8

[142] Saeki I, Takahashi Y, Matsuura T, Takahata S, Tanaka M, Taguchi T. Successful endoscopic unroofing for a pediatric choledochocele. Journal of Pediatric Surgery. 2009;**44**(8):1643-1645. DOI: 10.1016/j.jpedsurg.2009.03.042

[143] Dohmoto M, Kamiya T, Hünerbein M, Valdez H, Ibanegaray J, Prado J. Endoscopic treatment of a choledochocele in a 2-year-old child. Surgical Endoscopy. 1996;**10**(10):1016-1018

[144] Lee SE, Jang JY, Lee YJ, Choi DW, Lee WJ, Cho BH, Korean Pancreas Surgery Club et al. Choledochal cyst and associated malignant tumors in adults: A multicenter survey in South Korea. Archives of Surgery. 2011;**146**(10):1178-1184. DOI: 10.1001/archsurg.2011.243

[145] Acker SN, Bruny JL, Narkewicz MR, Roach JP, Rogers A, Karrer FM. Preoperative imaging does not predict intrahepatic involvement in choledochal cysts. Journal of Pediatric Surgery. 2013;**48**(12):2378-2382. DOI: 10.1016/j.jpedsurg.2013.08.008

[146] Joseph VT. Surgical techniques and long-term results in the treatment of choledochal cyst. Journal of Pediatric Surgery. 1990;**25**(7):782-787

[147] Savader SJ, Venbrux AC, Benenati JF, Mitchell SE, Widlus DM, Cameron JL, Osterman FA Jr. Choledochal cysts: Role of noninvasive imaging, percutaneous transhepatic cholangiography, and percutaneous biliary drainage in diagnosis and treatment. Journal of Vascular and Interventional Radiology 1991;**2**(3):379-385

[148] Urushihara N, Fukumoto K, Fukuzawa H, Tani M, Matsuoka T, Suzuki K, et al. Hepaticojejunostomy and intrahepatic cystojejunostomy for type IV-A choledochal cyst. Journal of Pediatric Surgery. 2007;**42**(10):1753-1756

[149] Shi LB, Peng SY, Meng XK, Peng CH, Liu YB, Chen XP, et al. Diagnosis and treatment of congenital choledochal cyst: 20 years' experience in China. World Journal of Gastroenterology. 2001;**7**(5):732-734

[150] Fujishiro J, Urita Y, Shinkai T, Gotoh C, Hoshino N, Ono K, et al. Clinical characteristics of liver fibrosis in patients with choledochal cysts. Journal of Pediatric Surgery. 2011;**46**(12):2296-2300. DOI: 10.1016/j.jpedsurg.2011.09.017

[151] Sheng Q, Lv Z, Xu W, Xiao X, Liu J, Wu Y. Reoperation after cyst excision with hepaticojejunostomy for choledochal cysts: Our experience in 18 cases. Medical Science Monitor. 2017;**23**:1371-1377

[152] Urushihara N, Fukumoto K, Fukuzawa H, Mitsunaga M, Watanabe K, Aoba T, et al. Long-term outcomes after excision of choledochal cysts in a single institution: Operative procedures and late complications. Journal of Pediatric Surgery. Dec 2012;**47**(12):2169-2174. DOI: 10.1016/j.jpedsurg.2012.09.001

[153] Edil BH, Olino K, Cameron JL. The current management of choledochal cysts. Advances in Surgery. 2009;**43**:221-232

[154] Lautz TB, Barsness KA. Adhesive small bowel obstruction—Acute management and treatment in children. Seminars in Pediatric Surgery. 2014;**23**(6):349-352. DOI: 10.1053/j.sempedsurg.2014.06.006 [Epub Jun 4, 2014]

[155] Kim JH, Choi TY, Han JH, Yoo BM, Kim JH, Hong J, et al. Risk factors of postoperative anastomotic stricture after excision of choledochal cysts with hepaticojejunostomy. Journal of Gastrointestinal Surgery. May 2008;**12**(5):822-828. [Epub Dec 6 2007]

[156] Yamataka A, Kobayashi H, Shimotakahara A, Okada Y, Yanai T, Lane GJ, et al. Recommendations for preventing complications related to Roux-en-Y hepatico-jejunostomy performed during excision of choledochal cyst in children. Journal of Pediatric Surgery. 2003;**38**(12):1830-1832

[157] Ono S, Fumino S, Shimadera S, Iwai N. Long-term outcomes after hepaticojejunostomy for choledochal cyst: A 10- to 27-year follow-up. Journal of Pediatric Surgery. 2010;**45**(2):376-378. DOI: 10.1016/j.jpedsurg.2009.10.078

[158] Cho MJ, Hwang S, Lee YJ, Kim KH, Ahn CS, Moon DB, et al. Surgical experience of 204 cases of adult choledochal cyst disease over 14 years. World Journal of Surgery. 2011;**35**(5):1094-1102. DOI: 10.1007/s00268-011-1009-7

[159] Lee KF, Lai EC, Lai PB. Adult choledochal cyst. Asian Journal of Surgery. 2005;**28**(1):29-33

Section 4

Abdominal Wall Defects

Chapter 6

Management of Gastroschisis

Alaa Obeida and Aly Shalaby

Abstract

Gastroschisis (GS) is one of the congenital abdominal wall defects, in which the bowel has prolapsed without a covering through a defect adjacent to (and nearly always to the right of) an otherwise normal umbilicus. Proper management of such cases gives them the opportunity to survive and thrive. In this chapter, simplified flowcharts for the initial management of GS, surgical intra-operative decisions and post-operative active follow-up of such cases will be presented and discussed. The first flowchart will discuss how to deal with a GS case from birth till the operative theatre, while the second flowchart will take the lead to guide the surgeon with the available surgical options and how to choose the suitable one for the case. Finally, the post-operative active follow-up fluid management and possible complications are discussed.

Keywords: gastroschisis, AWDs, fluid management, LMIC, complications

1. Introduction

Gastroschisis (GS) or more aptly "laparoschisis" is a congenital abdominal wall defect (AWD) leading to herniation of the gut more commonly to the right of the umbilical cord (**Figure 1**). It differs from other AWDs in causality, risk factors, and associated anomalies [1–3].

GS incidence is increasing worldwide [4, 5] and is estimated around 1 in 2200 live births [6, 7]. Antenatal scans detect most cases [8], survival in developed countries is excellent [7] and apart from some gastrointestinal dysfunction, long-term problems are rare [9].

This chapter is dedicated to discuss in simplified flowchart-form the initial, operative and post-operative management of GS with emphasis on low-resource settings. In addition it aims to outline salient topics such as fluid management and complications.

2. Etiology and embryology

Though unexplained, a young maternal age and low socioeconomic status are the commonest risk factors for GS [10, 11]. Smoking, drugs, environmental toxins and poor nutrition have also been implicated [12]. A genetic link in the form of homozygous gene polymorphisms has been reported [13] and is substantiated by an increased prevalence among familial cases of birth defects and twins [14].

The embryological origin of GS is still a matter of conjecture. Several theories have been put forward attempting to expound the abdominal wall defect: failed body-wall folding [15]; a vascular insult to the omphalo-mesenteric artery [16] or to the right umbilical vein [17]; a localized disruption of the amniotic membrane [18]

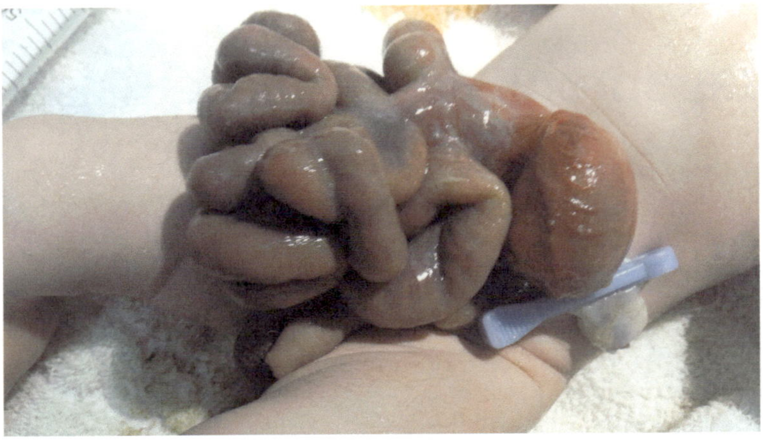

Figure 1.
Gastroschisis with prolapsed bowel to the right of the umbilicus.

or teratogen-induced mesenchymal failure [19]. None of the theories are fully satisfactory [20]. The right-sided occurrence of the defect has been linked to the position of the yolk sac [15, 21] without clear reasoning as to why. Left-sided defects have also been described [22].

3. Antenatal diagnosis

In high-income countries (HICs) routine antenatal scans may detect more than 97% of cases [23]. A diagnosis can be made as early as 10 weeks of gestation [24] and aids counseling, transfer and delivery [25, 26]. Ultrasound will typically pick up herniated bowel not covered by amnion, to the right of the umbilical cord (**Figure 2**). In contrast, an exomphalos will be covered by a membrane, lies in the

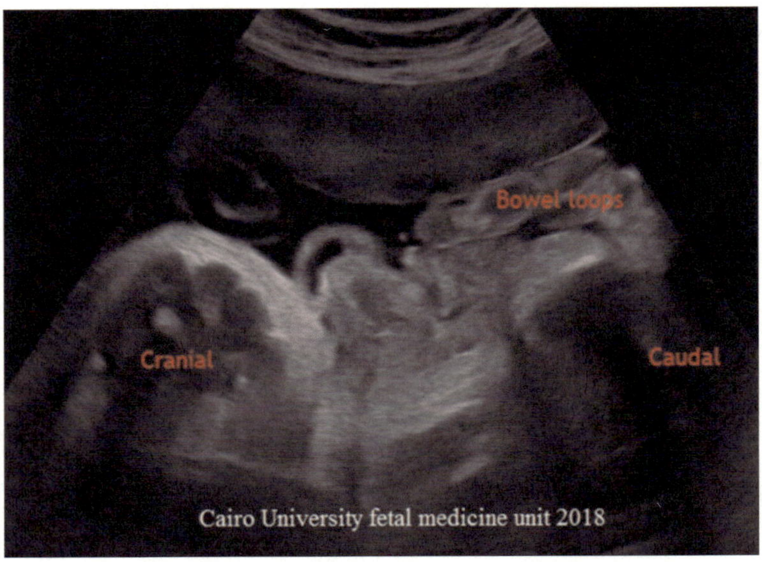

Figure 2.
Antenatal scan showing GS.

midline and may involve solid organ prolapse. Ultrasound is instrumental in picking up closing GS which is defined as a worsening ratio of intra vs. extra peritoneal bowel dilatation [27]. Further aids to diagnosis of GS are high levels of maternal serum alpha-fetoprotein (MSAFP) [28], intrauterine growth retardation with or without oligo-/an-hydramnios [7, 29, 30]. As GS is usually an isolated anomaly with very few risks to the mother or child, termination of pregnancy is not habitually offered [2, 31, 32].

4. Timing and mode of delivery

A spontaneous onset of labor will typically occur around 36 weeks gestation and the route of delivery is dependent on obstetric indications [33, 34]. There is a lack of high-level evidence to support early induction of labor in uncomplicated GS cases [35, 36] and a similar lack of evidence to support cesarean section [37]. Early (emergency) delivery is beneficial in closing GS [26].

5. GS in low to middle income countries (LMICs)

LMICs have an overall high mortality rate in neonates with correctable congenital anomalies [38, 39] and suffer from a lack of medical facilities and personnel [40]. Non-governmental and governmental organizations have been criticized for not doing enough [41, 42] though new partnerships are attempting to redress this [43, 44].

Mortality from GS in low-to-middle-income countries (LMICs) can reach up to 80–100% [45–48] which is in sharp contrast to the <10% in HICs [49]. Sepsis is a major culprit in most cases of neonatal mortality in LMICs [48]. The Gastroschisis International (GiT) network has suggested that poor resuscitation combined with sepsis and abdominal compartment syndrome is directly linked to the poor outcome [50].

Antenatal care may not be well developed [51] or mothers may engage poorly with it [52] which risks births in areas far from the reach of the pediatric surgeon. A delay in transfer of the neonate with GS remains a main concern [47, 53] however a recent study from South Africa has suggested that resuscitation at the initial point of care and throughout transfer may be the key to improving the end result [51].

6. Initial management (pre-operative management)

A GS infant is ideally delivered at or near a facility with pediatric surgical support [25]. Conversely, outborn cases have been shown to have worse outcomes such as longer days on parenteral nutrition and longer duration to achieving full feeds [54].

The accepted approach to managing GS is to cover the gut with a sterile bag (**Figure 3**), nasogastric decompression and fluid resuscitation. Hypothermia is a major risk due to the exposed gut and significant fluid losses [55]. Premature babies are particularly prone to hypothermia because of their high ratio of skin surface to weight and a lower amount of subcutaneous and brown fat. They may also have respiratory issues which impact on their oxygen consumption and heat production [55].

The authors follow the protocol outlined in **Figure 4**. At the outset doctors and nurses are reminded that the triad of hypovolemia, hypothermia and sepsis are the major threats to this neonate and that resuscitation is directed to mitigating their

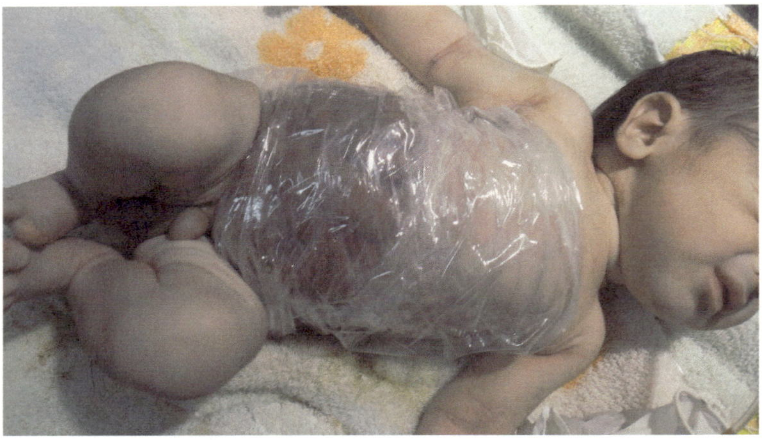

Figure 3.
Cling film covering the bowel in gastroschisis.

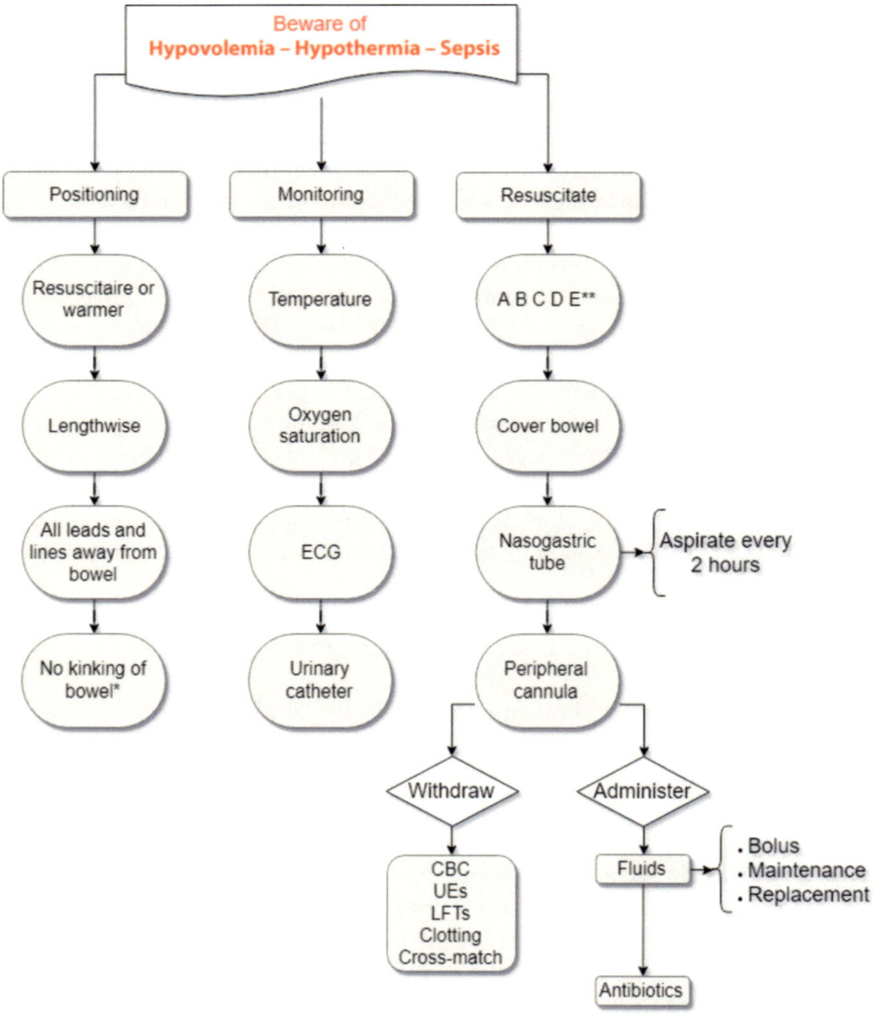

Figure 4.
*Initial management of gastroschisis. *Kinking can be avoided by laying the child on their side or by propping up the bowel with gauze rolls while the child is supine. **ABC of basic resuscitation. Do not forget blood sugar. CBC, complete blood count; UEs, urea and electrolytes; LFTs, liver function tests.*

effects. Almost simultaneously, certainly not sequentially, the baby is positioned lengthwise on a resuscitaire or warmer to facilitate access. Any wires, leads or lines are shifted away from the baby and the bowel. Kinking of the bowel is avoided by laying the child on their side or by propping up the bowel with gauze rolls in the supine position. Probes for temperature and oxygen saturation are connected. ECG leads are placed and connected to a monitor. A urinary catheter is placed with an aseptic technique. Resuscitation follows APLS guidelines of airway, breathing, circulation, rapid initial examination while the bowel is covered with cling film. An appropriately-sized nasogastric tube is placed on free drainage supplemented by 2-hourly active aspiration. Peripheral vascular access is secured and bloods are taken for blood sugar (if not done earlier), a complete blood picture, kidney and liver functions, clotting and cross-match. A fluid bolus is then administered followed by maintenance according to body weight. Broad-spectrum antibiotics are given according to the hospital protocol.

7. Intra-operative decision making

The aspired aim is to achieve full reduction of the bowel with muscle and skin closure of the abdominal wall, as cosmetically as possible. Safety of the child and the gut are paramount therefore if a complete primary closure is not possible staged reduction should be considered.

All manipulations should be done in a sterile environment. The authors routinely take all cases to theatre, however bedside procedures are also possible. Central vascular access is secured and a urinary catheter would have been placed during initial resuscitation in all cases.

The authors follow the guideline outlined in **Figure 5**: cases of simple GS with no obvious viscero-peritoneal disproportion (VPD) will undergo primary closure. If very straightforward, sutureless closure with steri-strip dressings is done. On occasion some cases will require division of bands or strands of omentum adherent to the defect and they go on to have formal sutured closure of the defect. Primary (sutured) closure has excellent cosmetic results (**Figures 6** and 7). Sutureless closure is associated with a higher incidence of umbilical hernia [56, 57] Guided by ventilation pressures, cases with moderate VPD will undergo a skin closure with the size of the defect determining if the umbilicus, the skin or a prosthetic patch is needed. Marked VPD and high ventilation pressures call for staged silo closure. The authors fashion surgical silos from sterile intravenous fluid bags (**Figure 8a–c**). Surgical silos can be made from a variety of materials which are summarized in **Box 1.** Spring-loaded (pre-formed) silos are ready-made and obviate the need for suturing to the abdominal wall [20, 55]. They come in various sizes to allow for the variability in the GS defect (**Figure 9**). One may rely on gravity alone, active tucking or a combination of both to reduce the contents into the abdominal cavity. There is weak evidence in favor of the routine use of pre-formed silos instead of primary closure [20, 55, 58].

Complex GS is defined as any case with associated bowel atresia, stenosis, perforation or volvulus. In the presence of atresia, the authors' preference is to plan a delayed repair but a primary resection and anastomosis at the time of abdominal closure is also acceptable if the bowel is healthy and not too edematous. Stoma formation is fraught with high-output stoma complications such as failure to thrive and peri-stoma skin breakdown—therefore is not the surgery of choice in low-resource settings. Closing GS represents a spectrum of disease where the defect has started to narrow down around the prolapsed gut. At its simplest form it can lead to intestinal stenosis but may progress to atresia, gut ischemia up to complete

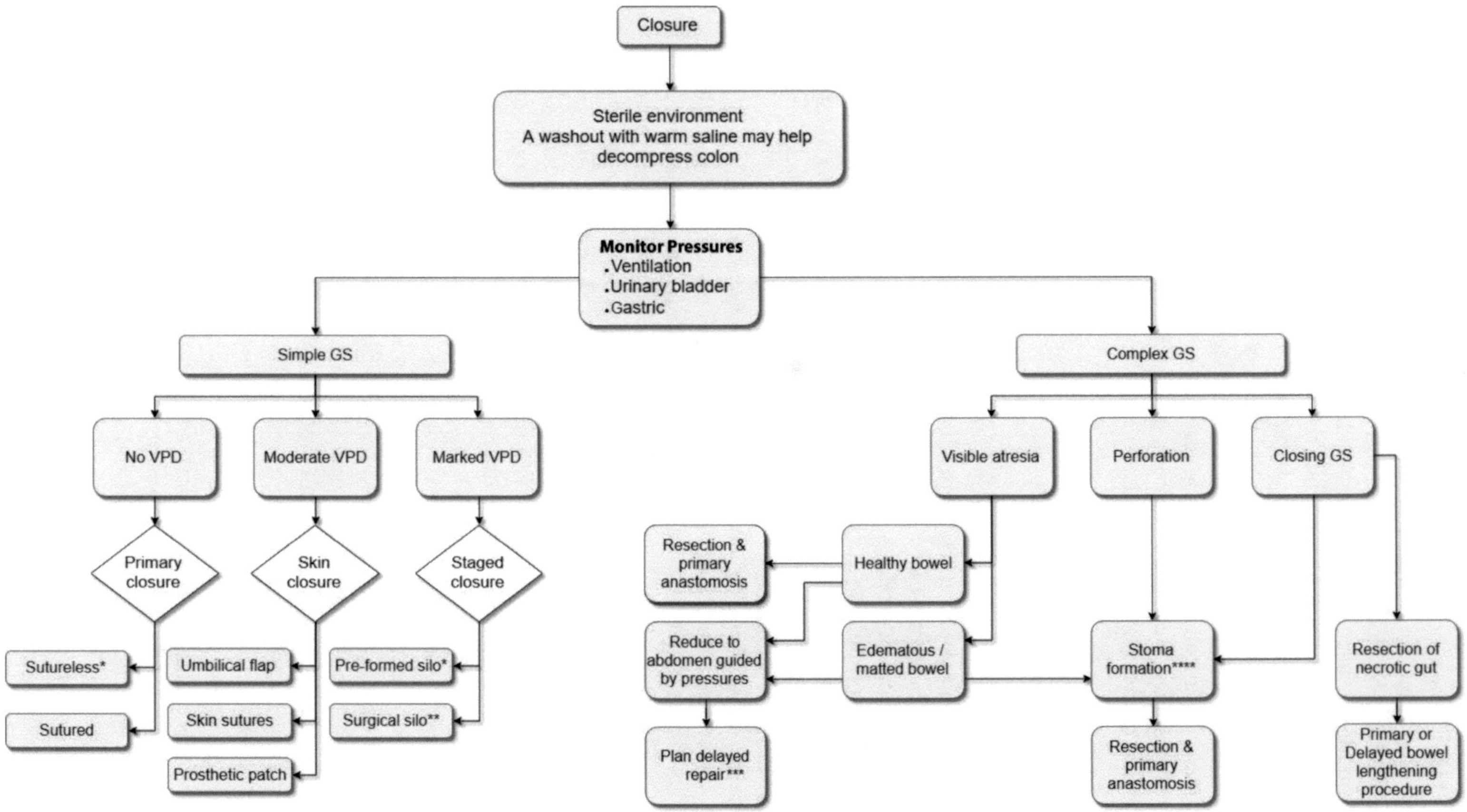

Figure 5.
Options for closure of gastroschisis. **Can be done cotside.* ***Silo material, see* **Box 2**. ****Delayed repair is around 6 weeks post-operatively.* *****Avoid stoma in a low-resource setting. GS, gastroschisis; VPD, viscero-peritoneal disproportion.*

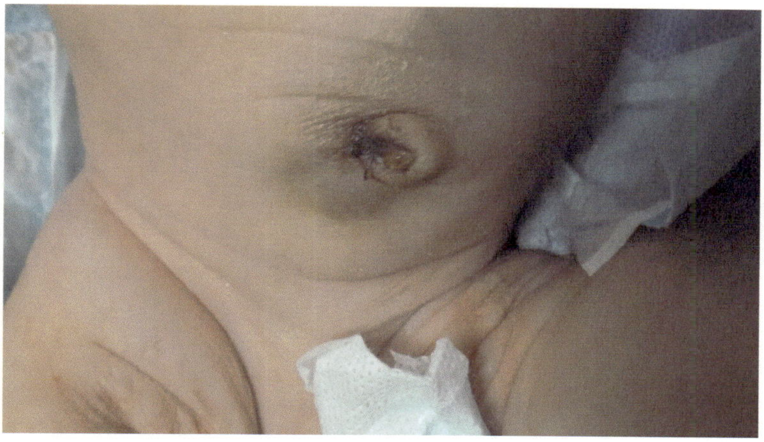

Figure 6.
Cosmetic result after primary closure.

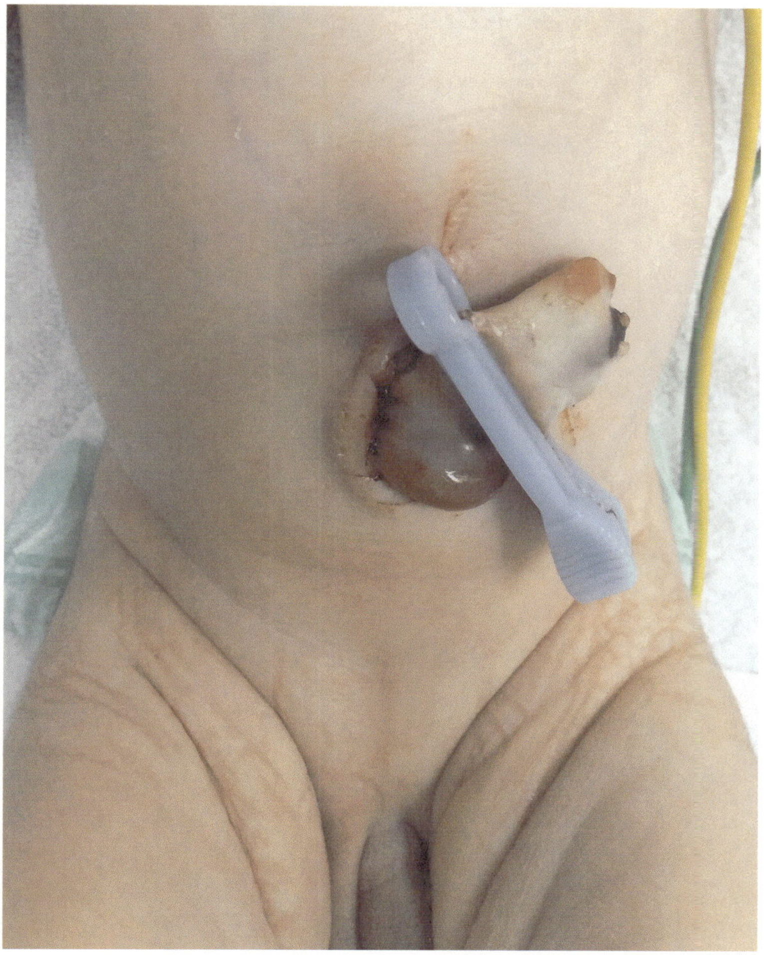

Figure 7.
Primary Closure.

disappearance of the prolapsed bowel if the defect closes completely, aka closed GS or "vanishing gut syndrome" [61]. Closing GS is challenging even in HICs and is associated with worse outcomes compared to simple GS. Narrowing or atresia may

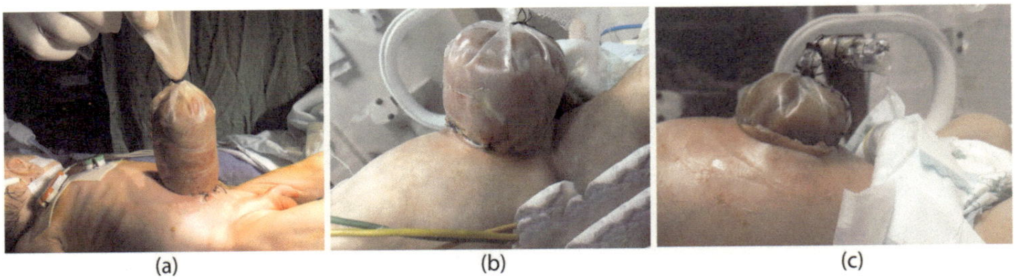

Figure 8.
(a–c) Staged silo reduction.

- Prolene mesh
- Silicone sheet
- Goretex mesh
- Sterile adhesive drapes +/− prolene mesh
- Biomaterials (Alloderm, Permacol)
- IV fluid bag
- Female condom
- Alexis wound protector

Box 1.
Available silo materials [55, 59, 60].

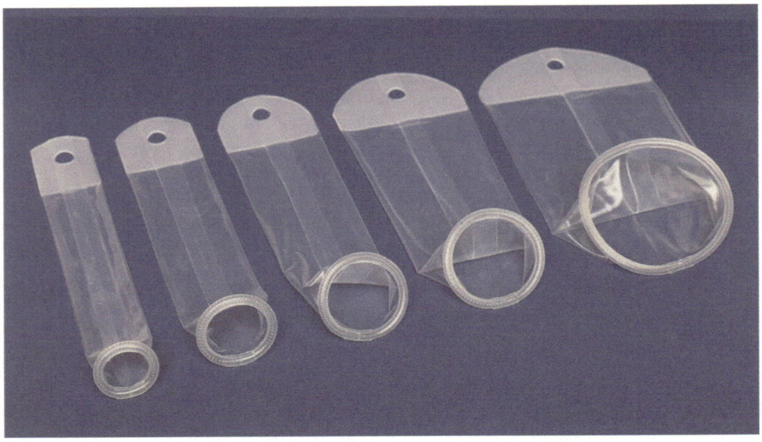

Figure 9.
Pre-formed silos http://bentecmed.com/bentec-medical-products/ventral-wall-defect-silo-bags/.

lend themselves to resection and primary anastomosis (either at the time of reduction, or delayed). Necrotic gut will require resection (**Figures 10** and **11**) and vanished gut will indicate an ultra-short intra-abdominal segment. These cases will require either primary or delayed bowel lengthening procedures [62].

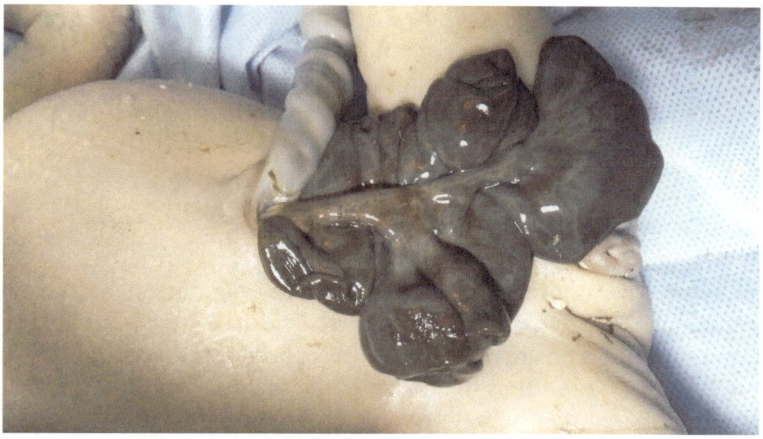

Figure 10.
Closing gastroschisis with necrotic bowel.

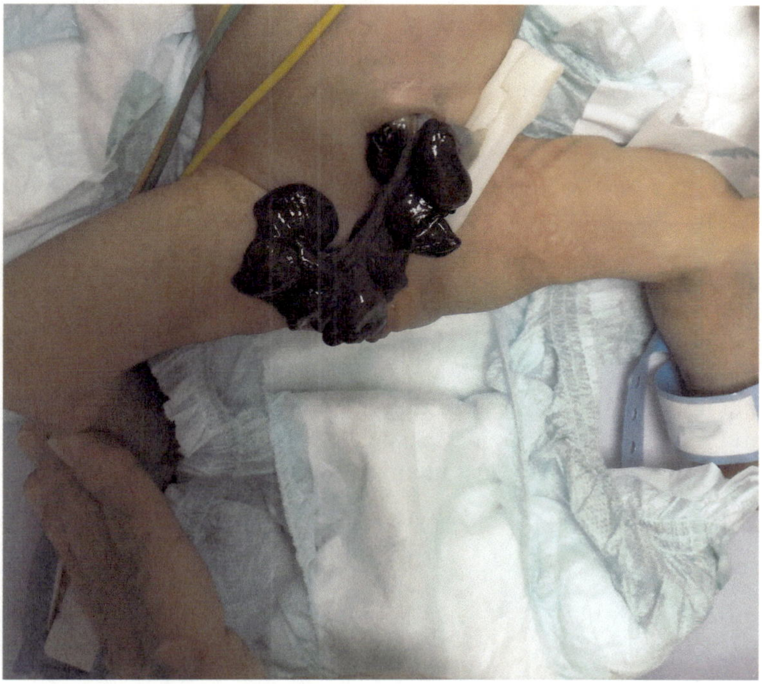

Figure 11.
Closing gastroschisis with necrotic bowel.

8. Post-operative care

The staged reduction process should take between 1 day and 2 weeks and is dependent on the degree of VPD. Enteral feeds are started once the gastro-intestinal system shows signs of resumed function: decreased nasogastric aspirates <20 ml/kg and bowel motions. Ideally expressed maternal breast milk is used [63–65], but formula feeds are acceptable. Elemental feeds may help protect against necrotizing enterocolitis. GS infants fed at around 7 days post closure seem to have the best outcome [66]. If the bowels do not open within 10–14 days a water-soluble contrast enema should be done to rule out a bowel atresia. An atresia detected at the time of initial closure of by subsequent imaging may be safely repaired after 3–6 weeks. Albeit uncommon in GS, cases with any associated malformations will require further investigations and management according to the findings.

9. Fluid management in GS

Publications frequently refer to a "consensus" among doctors on the optimal fluids required for GS. However, there is sparse evidence-based literature to guide the perioperative fluid management [65, 66]. Reports of fluid administration have varied from twice to three-times the normal maintenance volumes for neonates [67, 68] and were based on original research by Phillippart et al. in 1972 [69].

Fluid overload in the absence of hypovolemia has been proven to be deleterious in neonates [70]. It affects a patent ductus arteriosus, may cause intracranial hemorrhage, bronchopulmonary dysplasia or may even be fatal [71, 72]. Therefore the mere assumption that GS cases need vigorous volume expansion may be harmful. Preterm neonates may also benefit from fluid restriction according to a recent Cochrane review [73]. It has been suggested that the fluid overload will contribute to intestinal edema leading to a longer hospital stay and longer duration of parenteral nutrition through the increase of total body water and salt [65]. It may also play a part in development of NEC [74].

This practice of over transfusion is routinely carried out postoperatively as well [75]. While it may be of value in cases with a silo where there are ongoing losses of fluid from the base, it has no real justification in cases which undergo primary closure.

Few published sources will give an outright volume to go by. They will always be ranges and the clinician must be guided by continuous assessment of the child. Postnatal diuresis can complicate fluid-balance calculations but a useful milestone to assess the cardiovascular status is after administering 40 ml/kg of fluid. Albumin has been advocated as a volume expander in hypovolemic GS cases. It is not particularly useful in hypoalbuminemia associated with sepsis [76, 77]. An additional tool to help restore insensible water loss incurred through breathing is the humidification of incubator air.

10. Complications

10.1 Abdominal compartment syndrome (ACS)

A large degree of viscero-peritoneal disproportion and over-zealous reduction runs the risk of increased intra-abdominal pressure. The latter will result in restricting diaphragmatic movement and compression of the inferior vena cava, which will in turn result in respiratory distress, renal, liver and bowel ischemia, respectively. They manifest as metabolic acidosis, oliguria, renal and liver dysfunction [55].

Frequent monitoring of oxygen saturation/ventilation setting, serial blood gases, urine output, serial abdominal examinations, lower limb perfusion are important in early detection of ACS. Oliguria alone is not a sensitive indicator of ACS as it may be due to hypovolemia. Pressure measurements can be taken using sophisticated transducers used with anesthesia machines or by simply connecting the tubing to a CVP water manometer. Reference values are quoted in **Box 2** [78–81].

- Gastric/urinary bladder pressure < 200 cm H_2O or < 15–20 mmHg
- End-tidal CO_2 < 50 mmHg
- CVP < 4 mmHg or < 5.4 cm H_2O
- Ventilation <24 cm H_2O

Box 2.
Reference values for safe abdominal closure [78–81].

10.2 Sepsis

Sepsis is a common complication in LMICs. Most common sources are intra-abdominal, silo/wound infections, indwelling central lines or urinary catheters [50, 51].

As always, prevention is better than cure. Meticulous antisepsis protocols and timely use of antibiotics are important first tools. Early suspicion of central line-associated blood stream infection (CLABSI) or urinary tract infection (UTI) should prompt urgent cultures to be sent to the lab. The authors remove the urinary catheter once there is a stable urine output and no further risk of abdominal compartment syndrome.

10.3 Silo complications

Both pre-formed and surgical silos are prone to dislodgement and may cause bowel kinking, ischemia and perforation [58]. It is prudent to keep the silo and its contents visible at all times to allow early detection of any of these complications.

10.4 Pneumothorax

Iatrogenic pneumothorax secondary to barotrauma is an unfortunate complication in ventilated neonates and occurs in around 8.7% of the cases [82]. In GS this may be due to high intra-abdominal pressure after bowel reduction. This is best anticipated in theatre and if pressures exceed 24 cm H_2O, a staged reduction should

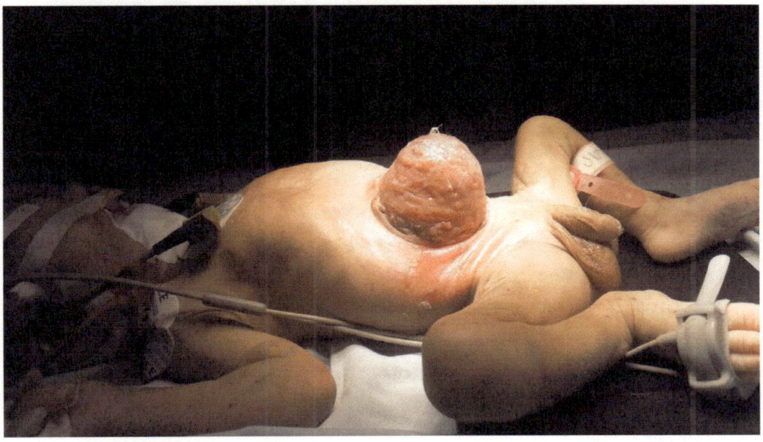

Figure 12.
Large abdominal wall defect with granulation in long-standing silo.

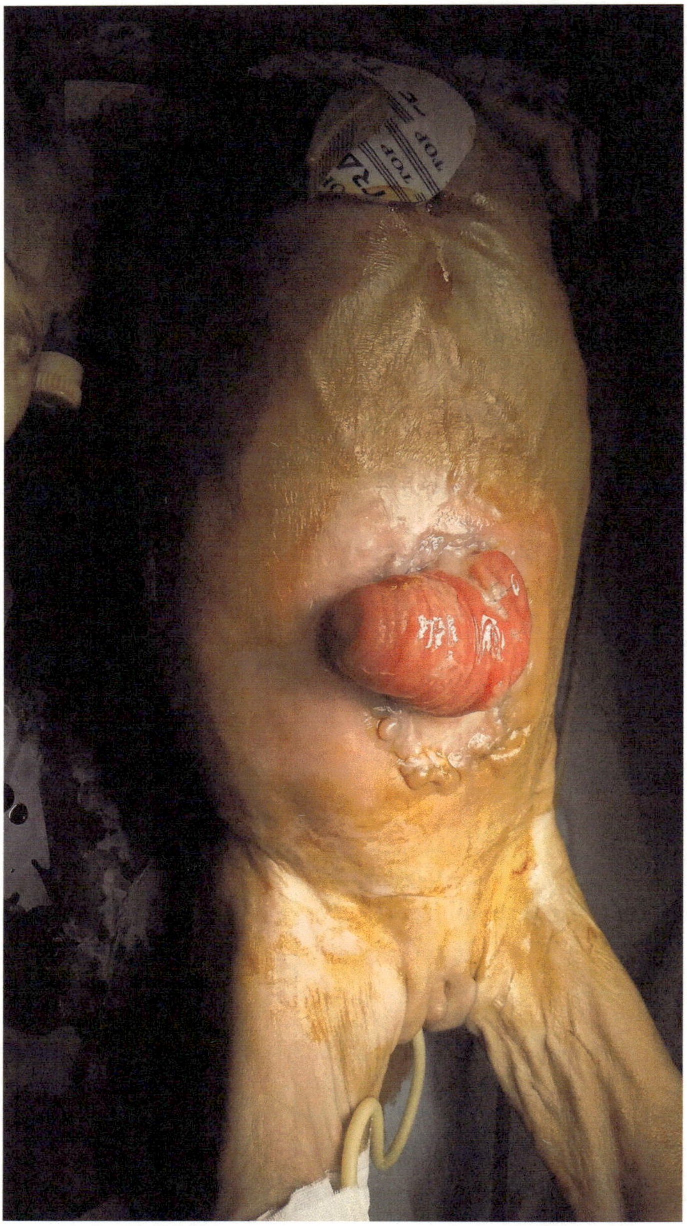

Figure 13.
Entero-cutaneous fistula.

be the surgery of choice. If post-operative ventilation is unavoidable then positive end-expiratory pressure (PEEP) or high-frequency oscillation ventilation (HFOV) is used. Neuromuscular paralysis may also help reduce ventilation pressures but is not always available in low-resource settings.

A pneumothorax is suspected when oxygen saturation drops and ventilation pressures rise sharply with absent ipsilateral air entry. An urgent plain chest x-ray will confirm this and should be followed by immediate needle decompression then a formal chest drain with an underwater seal. Bilateral asynchronous pneumothoraces are not uncommon [82].

10.5 Others

- **NEC:** It follows the same patterns and risk factors as with non-GS infants. Prematurity, formula feeds, rapid increase in feed volume—have all been implicated. Treatment is standard: nasogastric tube decompression, gut rest and antibiotics will often suffice [83, 84].

- **Large abdominal defect**: The GS defect is seldom large to start with and is occasionally enlarged by the surgeon to facilitate bowel reduction. Hence a large defect is a rare complication which may occur in long-standing cases of staged-reduction (**Figure 12**). Standard closure techniques include the use of a prosthetic material or plastic surgery techniques such as abdominal wall rotational flaps with or without lateral release incisions [85].

- **Enterocutaneous fistula:** (**Figure 13**) rare complication which may occur secondary to wound infection, NEC, or a combination of both. Vacuum dressings have been of value in treating such a complication [55, 86]. It is the authors' experience that vacuum dressings may paradoxically cause an enterocutaneous fistula if incorrectly placed or if the suction is too vigorous. Surgical closure when the infant is in a positive nitrogen balance is beneficial.

Author details

Alaa Obeida* and Aly Shalaby
Pediatric Surgery Department, Cairo University, Specialized Pediatric Hospital, Cairo, Egypt

*Address all correspondence to: alaa.obeida@gmail.com

References

[1] Wilson RD, Johnson MP. Congenital abdominal wall defects: An update. Fetal Diagnosis and Therapy. 2004;**19**(5): 385-398

[2] David AL, Tan A, Curry J. Gastroschisis: Sonographic diagnosis, associations, management and outcome. Prenatal Diagnosis: Published in Affiliation With the International Society for Prenatal Diagnosis. 2008; **28**(7):633-644

[3] Gow KW, Bhatia A, Saad DF, Wulkan ML, Heiss KF. Left-sided gastroschisis. The American Surgeon. 2006;**72**(7):637-640

[4] Tan KH, Kilby MD, Whittle MJ, Beattie BR, Booth IW, Botting BJ. Congenital anterior abdominal wall defects in England and Wales 1987–93: Retrospective analysis of OPCS data. BMJ. 1996;**313**(7062):903-906

[5] International Clearinghouse for Birth Defects Surveillance and Research (ICBDSR). ICBDSR Annual Report 2005, with data 2003. Rome: ICBDSR Centre; 2005. www.icbd.org

[6] Parker SE, Mai CT, Canfield MA, Rickard R, Wang Y, Meyer RE, et al. Updated national birth prevalence estimates for selected birth defects in the United States, 2004–2006. Birth Defects Research Part A: Clinical and Molecular Teratology. 2010;**88**(12):1008-1016

[7] Holland AJ, Walker K, Badawi N. Gastroschisis: An update. Pediatric Surgery International. 2010;**26**(9): 871-878

[8] Bond SJ, Harrison MR, Filly RA, Callen PW, Anderson RA, Golbus MS. Severity of intestinal damage in gastroschisis: Correlation with prenatal sonographic findings. Journal of Pediatric Surgery. 1988;**23**(6):520-525

[9] Langer JC, Longaker MT, Crombleholme TM, Bond SJ, Finkbeiner WE, Rudolph CA, et al. Etiology of intestinal damage in gastroschisis. I: Effects of amniotic fluid exposure and bowel constriction in a fetal lamb model. Journal of Pediatric Surgery. 1989;**24**(10):992-997

[10] Loane M, Dolk H, Bradbury I. A EUROCAT Working Group. Increasing prevalence of gastroschisis in Europ. 1980–2002: A phenomenon restricted to younger mothers? Paediatric and Perinatal Epidemiology. 2007;**21**(4):363-369

[11] Mac Bird T, Robbins JM, Druschel C, Cleves MA, Yang S, Hobbs CA, et al. Demographic and environmental risk factors for gastroschisis and omphalocele in the National Birth Defects Prevention Study. Journal of Pediatric Surgery. 2009;**44**(8): 1546-1551

[12] Forrester MB, Merz RD. Comparison of trends in gastroschisis and prenatal illicit drug use rates. Journal of Toxicology and Environmental Health, Part A. 2006; **69**(13):1253-1259

[13] Torfs CP, Christianson RE, Iovannisci DM, Shaw GM, Lammer EJ. Selected gene polymorphisms and their interaction with maternal smoking, as risk factors for gastroschisis. Birth Defects Research Part A: Clinical and Molecular Teratology. 2006;**76**(10): 723-730

[14] Hwang PJ, Kousseff BG. Omphalocele and gastroschisis: An 18-year review study. Genetics in Medicine. 2004;**6**(4):232

[15] Feldkamp ML, Carey JC, Sadler TW. Development of gastroschisis: Review of hypotheses, a novel hypothesis, and

implications for research. American Journal of Medical Genetics Part A. 2007;**143**(7):639-652

[16] Hoyme HE, Higginbottom MC, Jones KL. The vascular pathogenesis of gastroschisis: Intrauterine interruption of the omphalomesenteric artery. The Journal of Pediatrics. 1981; **98**(2):228-231

[17] Devries PA. The pathogenesis of gastroschisis and omphalocele. Journal of Pediatric Surgery. 1980;**15**(3):245

[18] Shaw A. The myth of gastroschisis. Journal of Pediatric Surgery. 1975;**10**(2): 235-244

[19] Duhamel B. Embryology of exomphalos and allied malformations. Archives of Disease in Childhood. 1963; **38**(198):142

[20] Haddock C, Skarsgard ED. Understanding Gastroschisis and its Clinical Management: Where are We? [Internet]. Expert Review of Gastroenterology & Hepatology. Vol. 12. Taylor & Francis; 2018. pp. 405-415

[21] Blechschmidt E. The Stages of Human Development before Birth: An Introduction to Human Embryology. Philadelphia: Saunders; 1961

[22] Ashburn DA, Pranikoff T, Turner CS. Unusual presentations of gastroschisis. The American Surgeon. 2002;**68**(8):724

[23] Fillingham A, Rankin J. Prevalence, prenatal diagnosis and survival of gastroschisis. Prenatal Diagnosis. 2008; **28**(13):1232-1237

[24] Nicholas SS, Stamilio DM, Dicke JM, Gray DL, Macones GA, Odibo AO. Predicting adverse neonatal outcomes in fetuses with abdominal wall defects using prenatal risk factors. American Journal of Obstetrics and Gynecology. 2009;**201**(4):383-3e1

[25] Murphy FL, Mazlan TA, Tarheen F, Corbally MT, Puri P. Gastroschisis and exomphalos in Ireland 1998–2004. Does antenatal diagnosis impact on outcome? Pediatric Surgery International. 2007; **23**(11):1059-1063

[26] Shalaby A, Davenport M. Closed gastroschisis. Pediatric Surgery International. 2011;**27**(3) 335

[27] Vegunta RK, Wallace LJ, Leonardi MR, Gross TL, Renfroe Y, Marshall JS, et al. Perinatal management of gastroschisis: Analysis of a newly established clinical pathway. Journal of Pediatric Surgery. 2005;**40**(3):528-534

[28] Palomaki GE, Hill LE, Knight GJ, Haddow JE, Carpenter M Second-trimester maternal serum alpha-fetoprotein levels in pregnancies associated with gastroschisis and omphalocele. Obstetrics and Gynecology. 1988;**71**(6 Pt 1):906-909

[29] Luton D, Guibourdenche J, Vuillard E, Bruner J. Prenatal management of gastroschisis: The place of the amnioexchange procedure. Clinics in Perinatology. 2003;**30**(3):551-572

[30] Reid KP, Dickinson JE, Doherty DA. The epidemiologic incidence of congenital gastroschisis in Western Australia. American Journal of Obstetrics and Gynecology. 2003; **189**(3):764-768

[31] Campbell KH, Copel JA. Gastroschisis. In: Obstetric Imaging: Fetal Diagnosis and Care. Second ed. 2018. pp. 78-84

[32] Hunter A, Soothill P. Gastroschisis —An overview. Prenatal Diagnosis. 2002;**22**:869-873

[33] Abdel-Latif ME, Bolisetty S, Abeywardana S, Lui K. Mode of delivery and neonatal survival of infants with gastroschisis in Australia and New

Zealand. Journal of Pediatric Surgery. 2008;**43**(9):1685-1690

[34] Lausman AY, Langer JC, Tai M, Seaward PG, Windrim RC, Kelly EN, et al. Gastroschisis: What is the average gestational age of spontaneous delivery? Journal of Pediatric Surgery. 2007; **42**(11):1816-1821

[35] Cohen-Overbeek TE, Hatzmann TR, Steegers EA, Hop WC, Wladimiroff JW, Tibboel D. The outcome of gastroschisis after a prenatal diagnosis or a diagnosis only at birth: Recommendations for prenatal surveillance. European Journal of Obstetrics & Gynecology and Reproductive Biology. 2008;**139**(1): 21-27

[36] Moir CR, Ramsey PS, Ogburn PL, Johnson RV, Ramin KD. A prospective trial of elective preterm delivery for fetal gastroschisis. American Journal of Perinatology. 2004;**21**(05):289-294

[37] Mozurkewich E, Chilimigras J, Koepke E, Keeton K, King VJ. Indications for induction of labour: A best-evidence review. BJOG: An International Journal of Obstetrics & Gynaecology. 2009;**116**(5):626-636

[38] Murray CJ, Vos T, Lozano R, Naghavi M, Flaxman AD, Michaud C, et al. Disability-adjusted life years (DALYs) for 291 diseases and injuries in 21 regions, 1990–2010: A systematic analysis for the global burden of disease study 2010. The Lancet. 2012; **380**(9859):2197-2223

[39] Black RE, Cousens S, Johnson HL, et al. Global, regional, and national causes of child mortality in 2008: A systematic analysis. Lancet. 2010;**375**: 1969-1987

[40] Rosano A, Botto LD, Botting B, Mastroiacovo P. Infant mortality and congenital anomalies from 1950 to 1994: An international perspective. Journal of Epidemiology & Community Health. 2000;**54**(9):660-666

[41] Ameh EA, Chirdan LB. Paediatric surgery in the rural setting: Prospect and feasibility. West African Journal of Medicine. 2001;**20**(1):52-55

[42] Bickler SW, Kyambi J, Rode H. Pediatric surgery in sub-Saharan Africa. Pediatric Surgery International. 2001;**17** (5–6):442-447

[43] Badrinath R, Kakembo N, Kisa P, Langer M, Ozgediz D, Sekabira J. Outcomes and unmet need for neonatal surgery in a resource-limited environment: Estimates of global health disparities from Kampala, Uganda. Journal of Pediatric Surgery. 2014; **49**(12):1825-1830

[44] Galukande M, Luboga S, Kijjambu SC. Improving recruitment of surgical trainees and training of surgeons in Uganda. East and Central African Journal of Surgery. 2006;**11**(1):17-24

[45] Arnold M. Is the incidence of gastroschisis rising in South Africa in accordance with international trends?— A retrospective analysis at Pretoria academic and Kalafong hospitals, 1981-2001. South African Journal of Surgery. 2004;**42**(3):86-88

[46] Ameh EA, Chirdan LB. Ruptured exomphalos and gastroschisis: A retrospective analysis of morbidity and mortality in Nigerian children. Pediatric Surgery International. 2000;**16**(1–2): 23-25

[47] Vilela PC, de Amorim MM, Falbo GH, Santos LC. Risk factors for adverse outcome of newborns with gastroschisis in a Brazilian hospital. Journal of Pediatric Surgery. 2001;**36**(4):559-564

[48] Askarpour S, Ostadian N, Javaherizadeh H, Chabi S. Omphalocele, gastroschisis: Epidemiology, survival, and mortality in imam Khomeini

hospital, Ahvaz-Iran. Polish Journal of Surgery. 2012;**84**(2):82-85. DOI: https://doi.org/10.2478/v10035-012-0013-4

[49] Driver CP, Bruce J, Bianchi A, Doig CM, Dickson AP, Bowen J. The contemporary outcome of gastroschisis. Journal of Pediatric Surgery. 2000; **35**(12):1719-1723

[50] Ford K, Poenaru D, Moulot O, Tavener K, Bradley S, Bankole R, et al. Gastroschisis: Bellwether for neonatal surgery capacity in low resource settings? Journal of Pediatric Surgery. 2016;**51**(8):1262-1267

[51] Stevens P, Muller E, Becker P. Gastroschisis in a developing country: Poor resuscitation is a more significant predictor of mortality than postnatal transfer time. South African Journal of Surgery. 2016;**54**(1):4-9

[52] Abou-Zahr C, Wardlaw T. Antenatal Care in Developing Countries. Promises, Achievements and Missed Opportunities: An Analysis of Trends, Levels and Differentials 1990-2001. Geneva: World Health Organization, UN Children's Fund; 2003

[53] Harrison DS. Factors associated with mortality among neonates presenting with gastroschisis in Zimbabwe. South African Journal of Surgery. 2006;**44**(4): 157

[54] Kitchanan S, Patole SK, Muller R, Whitehall JS. Neonatal outcome of gastroschisis and exomphalos: A 10-year review. Journal of Paediatrics and Child Health. 2000;**36**(5):428-430

[55] Marven S, Owen A. Contemporary postnatal surgical management strategies for congenital abdominal wall defects. Seminars in Pediatric Surgery. 2008;**17**(4):222-235

[56] Witt RG, Zobel M, Padilla B, Lee H, MacKenzie TC, Vu L. Evaluation of clinical outcomes of sutureless vs sutured closure techniques in gastroschisis repair. Journal of the American Medical Association surgery. 2019;**154**(1):33-39

[57] Tullie LG, Bough GM, Shalaby A, Kiely EM, Curry JI, Pierro A, et al. Umbilical hernia following gastroschisis closure: A common event? Pediatric Surgery International. 2016;**32**(8): 811-814

[58] Charlesworth P, Akinnola I, Hammerton C, Praveena P, Desai A, Patel S, et al. Preformed silos versus traditional abdominal wall closure in gastroschisis: 163 infants at a single institution. European Journal of Pediatric Surgery. 2014;**24**(01): 088-093

[59] Bustorff-Silva JM, Schmidt AF, Gonçalves A, Marba S, Sbragia L. The female condom as a temporary silo: A simple and inexpensive tool in the initial management of the newborn with gastroschisis. The Journal of Maternal-Fetal & Neonatal Medicine. 2008;**21**(9): 648-651

[60] Kusafuka J, Yamataka A, Okazaki T, Okawada M, Urao M, Lane GJ, et al. Gastroschisis reduction using "applied Alexis", a wound protector and retractor. Pediatric Surgery International. 2005;**21**(11):925-927

[61] Perrone EE, Olson J, Golden JM, Besner GE, Gayer CP, Islam S, et al. Closing gastroschisis: The good, the bad, and the not-so ugly. Journal of Pediatric Surgery. 1 Jan 2019;**54**(1):60-64

[62] Emil S. Surgical strategies in complex gastroschisis. Seminars in Pediatric Surgery. 2018;**27**(5):309-315

[63] Jayanthi S, Seymour P, Puntis JW, Stringer MD. Necrotizing enterocolitis after gastroschisis repair: A preventable complication?. Journal of Pediatric Surgery. 1 May 1998;**33**(5):705-707

[64] Aljahdali A, Mohajerani N, Skarsgard ED. Effect of timing of enteral feeding on outcome in gastroschisis. Journal of Pediatric Surgery. 1 May 2013;**48**(5):971-976

[65] Jansen LA, Safavi A, Lin Y, MacNab YC, Skarsgard ED. Preclosure fluid resuscitation influences outcome in gastroschisis. American Journal of Perinatology. 2012;**29**(04):307-312

[66] Gamba P, Midrio P. Abdominal wall defects: Prenatal diagnosis, newborn management, and long-term outcomes. Seminars in Pediatric Surgery. 2014; **23**(5):283-290

[67] Ledbetter DJ. Gastroschisis and omphalocele. Surgical Clinics. 2006; **86**(2):249-260

[68] Cooney DR. Defects of the abdominal wall. In: O'Neill JA, Rowe MI, Grosfeld JL, et al., editors. Pediatric Surgery. 5th ed. Vol. 1045. St Louis: Mosby; 1998

[69] Philippart AI, Canty TG, Filler RM. Acute fluid volume requirements in infants with anterior abdominal wall defects. Journal of Pediatric Surgery. 1972;**7**(5):553-558

[70] Ewer AK, Tyler W, Francis A, Drinkall D, Gardosi JO. Excessive volume expansion and neonatal death in preterm infants born at 27–28 weeks gestation. Paediatric and Perinatal Epidemiology. 2003;**17**(2):180-186

[71] Arikan AA, Zappitelli M, Goldstein SL, Naipaul A, Jefferson LS, Loftis LL. Fluid overload is associated with impaired oxygenation and morbidity in critically ill children. Pediatric Critical Care Medicine. 2012;**13**(3):253-258

[72] Willson DF, Thomas NJ, Tamburro R, Truemper E, Truwit J, Conaway M, et al. The relationship of fluid administration to outcome in the pediatric calfactant in acute respiratory distress syndrome trial. Pediatric Critical Care Medicine. 2013;**14**(7): 666-672

[73] Bell EF, Acarregui MJ. Restricted versus liberal water intake for preventing morbidity and mortality in preterm infants. Cochrane Database of Systematic Reviews. 2014;**12**. Artical ID: CD000503

[74] Oldham KT, Coran AG, Drongowski RA, Baker PJ, Wesley JR, Polley TZ. The development of necrotizing enterocolitis following repair of gastroschisis: A suprisingly high incidence. Journal of Pediatric Surgery. 1988;**23**(10):945-949

[75] Bonasso PC, Lucke-Wold B, Hobbs GR, Vaughan RA, Shorter NA, Nakayama DK. Excessive postoperative fluid administration in infants with gastroschisis. The American Surgeon. 2016;**82**(8):704-706

[76] AL-Khafaji A, Webb AR. Should albumin be used to correct hypoalbuminemia in the critically ill? No. Transfusion Alternatives in Transfusion Medicine. 2003;**5**(4): 392-396

[77] Vincent JL, Russell JA, Jacob M, Martin G, Guidet B, Wernerman J, et al. Albumin administration in the acutely ill: What is new and where next? Critical Care. 2014;**18**(4):231

[78] Puffinbarger NK, Taylor DV, Tuggle DW, Tunell WP. End-tidal carbon dioxide for monitoring primary closure of gastroschisis. Journal of Pediatric Surgery. 1996;**31**(2):280-282

[79] Olesevich M, Alexander F, Khan M, Cotman K. Gastroschisis revisited: Role of intraoperative measurement of abdominal pressure. Journal of Pediatric Surgery. 2005;**40**(5):789-792

[80] Banieghbal B, Gouws M, Davies MR. Respiratory pressure monitoring as

an indirect method of intra-abdominal pressure measurement in gastroschisis closure. European Journal of Pediatric Surgery. 2006;**16**(02):79-83

[81] Hong CM, Patel A. Novel intra-operative pulse oximetry monitoring for gastroschisis: A noninvasive monitor of intra-abdominal pressure. Pediatric Anesthesia. 2008;**18**(4):344-345

[82] Watkinson M, Tiron I. Events before the diagnosis of a pneumothorax in ventilated neonates. Archives of Disease in Childhood-Fetal and Neonatal Edition. 2001;**85**(3):F201-F203

[83] Snyder CL. Outcome analysis for gastroschisis. Journal of Pediatric Surgery. 1999;**34**(8):1253-1256

[84] Gupta R, Cabacungan ET. Outcome of neonates with gastroschisis at different gestational ages using a national database. Journal of Pediatric Surgery. 2018;**53**(4):661-665

[85] Svetanoff WJ, Zendejas B, Demehri FR, Cuenca A, Nath B, Smithers CJ. Giant gastroschisis with complete liver herniation: A case report of two patients. Case Reports in Surgery. 2019; **2019**:8. Article ID: 4136214. https://doi.org/10.1155/2019/4136214

[86] Waldhausen JH. Surgical management of gastroschisis. NeoReviews. 2005;**6**(11):e500-e507

Section 5

Minimally Invasive Surgery

Chapter 7

Single-Incision Pediatric Endosurgery (SIPES)

Enaam Raboei, Ameen Alsaggaf, Yazeed Owiwi, Syed Salahuddin, Alaa Ghallab and Mazen Zidan

Abstract

Most centers advocate laparoscopy in order to minimize the size and the number of skin incisions. Many comparative studies, systematic review, and pooled analysis demonstrate that single-incision laparoscopic surgery (SILS) is comparable to conventional laparoscopic surgery (CLS). However, this review identifies the need for randomized controlled trials to clarify the efficacy of SIPS compared with CLS. SIPES pediatric has gained significant popularity. Longer M OT with SIPES was the main concern in most published series. One study has shown that SIPES in children is safe and feasible when performed by resident doctors in comparison to the fellow. We started SIPES in 2003. It is carried out routinely by trainees and specialists. Interferences and collisions between surgical instruments are worse in SIPES than CLS. These challenges extended the OT. Although the use of flexible laparoscopic instruments instead of straight instruments may overcome these technical difficulties, only straight laparoscopic instruments are currently used in our institution. Our aim is to standardize this approach in pediatric age group. The technique can be imparted satisfactorily to trainees. However, its successful incorporation into surgical training programs will depend on the development of innovative simulation strategies.

Keywords: SILS, SIPES, single incision, laparoscopy

1. Introduction

There are many nomenclatures and abbreviations found in literatures: SILS, single-incision laparoscopic surgery; LESS, laparo-endoscopic single-site surgery; TUES, trans-umbilical endoscopic single-site surgery; SPA, single portal access; E-NOTES, embryologic natural orifice transluminal endoscopic surgery; SAS, single access surgery; S3, single-site surgery; NOTUS, natural orifice trans-umbilical surgery; SAVES, single access video endoscopic surgery; and SIPES, single-incision pediatric endoscopic surgery. Cultural changes affected the way of managing patients. It has been over 30 years since the first laparoscopic cholecystectomy. Von Ott inspected the abdominal cavity of pregnant women in 1901. Georg Kelling performed "koelioscopie." Jacobeus published his first report "Laparothorakoskopie." Lukichev in 1983 and Muhe in 1985 performed laparoscopic cholecystectomy in humans [1]. Kalloo performed trans-gastric peritoneoscopy in 2004 [2]. Multiple centers performed NOTES in humans, trans-gastric appendectomy and transvaginal cholecystectomy. Limitations of NOTES technique lead to make SILS to go in parallel with it [3]. The first published report in general surgery appeared in 1992 with appendectomies [4]. In the same year, D'Alessio described a technique for appendectomy in pediatric patients in which a special port was used at the umbilicus to allow the surgeon to bring the appendix out through the umbilicus to perform an extracorporeal appendectomy [5]. 19% of 166 patients in their series required additional trocars, and 4% required conversion to an open operation. The MOT (MOT) was 35 min with a 7-day return to normal activity, compared with 10 days for those that required additional trocars. SIPES has been introduced in our institute by 2003. Now SIPES is our standard technique for many procedures like cholecystectomy, splenectomy, appendectomy, assisted Mitrofanoff, SIPES hernia repair percutaneous internal ring suturing (PIRS), ovarian cystectomy, and fundoplication since 2011. We have performed around 400 SIPES cases up-to-date.

2. Limitations of SIPES

SIPES is not a new technique. It is actually a modification of current laparoscopic technique with some modified instruments and approach used successfully for multiple laparoscopic procedures. Almost all cases which could be done by conventional laparoscopy are amenable to be done by SIPES like splenectomy, appendectomy, cholecystectomy, colectomy, anterior resection, hernia repair, splenectomy, Nissen fundoplication, and sleeve gastrectomy. The approach failed to gain momentum for several years, due to technical limitations with conventional instrumentation. These limitations did not prevent surgeons from using SIPES in pediatric age group. Barbaros and Dinccag [6] published the first two adult cases of SILS splenectomy in 2009. Later Dutta reported the first SIPES splenectomy in 2012 [7]. Recently still few centers worldwide have advanced pediatric SIPES [7–13].

3. Advantage of SIPES

Fewer incisions, cosmesis, and non-violation of natural orifices are the most attractive reasons for the patient to choose SILS technique; as a surgeon, ease of tissue retrieval and combination procedures are the main reasons. Using standard laparoscopic equipment has facilitate the procedure for the surgeon with less cost.

4. Disadvantage of SIPES

In comparison with CLS, increased postoperative pain and violation of ergonomic principles in SIPES were not proven in the published studies. Hernia might be a problem in adults published series, but we did not encounter any in our patients. In reverse SIPES, it is an opportunity to repair the umbilical hernia when closing the wound in pediatric age group. Wound infection was not different from conventional laparoscopy. Learning curve escalates fast, and the cost-effectiveness was proven to be less costly than conventional laparoscopy [3].

5. Public opinion

Which technique the public choose if NOTES and SIPES were the only options offered to them? [14]

Most people choose SILS over NOTES when asked about this scenario.

- 208 (20.7%) choose NOTES
- 795 (79.0%) choose SILS
- 3 (0.3%) would refuse surgery

1006 individuals completed the questionnaire explained by F1 medical intern, so as not to bias anyone. All individuals were from around London. 458 (45.5%) were males and 548 (54.5%) were females. 129 were < 20 yrs. old, 460 were 20–29 yrs. old, 186 were 30–39 yrs. old, 103 were 40–49 yrs. old, 61 were 50–59 yrs. old, and 67 were ≥ 60 yrs. old. 80 were physician, 88 medical students, 39 were nurses, and 6 were NHS admin [15]. 793 were nonmedical. Taking the choices by gender, profession, and age, the preference order for the four approaches was:

- 1st—SILS
- 2nd—conventional lap
- 3rd—NOTES
- 4th—open

Summary

- SIPES is safe and feasible technique for pediatric age group.
- The disadvantages are balanced with the patient satisfaction and excellent cosmetic results.

6. Port position

The position of SIPES port may be different depending on many factors like choice of surgeon, type of surgery, and the age of the patient. The different locations commonly used are:

1. Omega-shaped incision made around the upper half of umbilicus.
2. Trans-umbilical incision.
3. Incisions are also given above and below umbilicus.
4. Incision maybe placed in the pubic hairline medially.

The author prefers trans-umbilical incision as its ideal to prevent any visible scar, easy access, and quick closure with no port site hernia. In pediatric it gives opportunity to repair the umbilical hernia.

7. Types of ports

There are many types of ports with different sizes in the market. The devices are either disposable or reusable: SILS device by Covidien© (Medtronic), GelPOINT system by Applied Medical, R-Port and TriPort by Advanced Surgical Concepts,

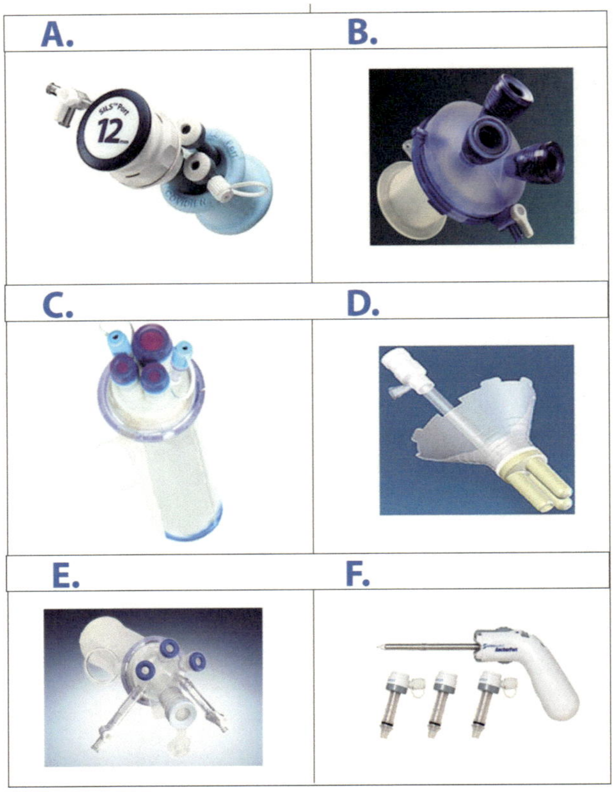

Figure 1.
Types of ports. A) Sils covidien, B) Gel point, C) Triport, D) Uni-X, E) Quadric port. F) Anchorport R by Surgiquest.

Uni-X by Pnavel, Tri or quadric port by Olympus, and AnchorPort R by SurgiQuest. (**Figure 1**) Each port has its own unique feature, so the selection of the port depends on the surgeon, availability, and cost factor. The author has found that Covidien© (Medtronic) port is the most suitable one as it is small in size and it can adopt 15 mm port for introducing GIA stapler and endobag.

8. Problems and solutions seen in SIPES

Rivas [16] has given a good list of problems and solutions in SILS. The encountered problems were clashing of instruments, lack of ideal operative ports, interference and deflection of laparoscope's light source by operating instruments, interference of wires or tubing that connect perpendicularly to instruments, difficulty with retraction of organs or structures, lack of time and patience to learn, loss of proprioception due to crossed instrument, and change of surgeon's mindset. The solutions suggested by him were the use of curved, reticulating, or flexible instruments, use of novel multichannel ports, use of an extra-long 5-mm angled laparoscope (50 cm), use of retracting sutures, continuous medical education, implementation of magnetically anchored instruments deployed though a single incision, and use of a 90° adaptor for the light source (for sharp change in its direction parallel to the laparoscope).

Collision of instruments is considered the main limiting factor for popularizing this technique. Other surgeons conquer this problem by using articulating instruments and angled tip fiber-optic camera. The use of articulating instruments was difficult and almost impossible in small age group due to narrow and small working space, so the author has replaced it by standard straight instruments. The cameraman can stand away from the operating surgeon by using a 50 cm long laparoscope. The articulating and bent instrumentation requires training and experience, and we as other SIPES surgeons are confident that they are not needed in neonates and children. Bent graspers and the 45° rigid endoscope or the deflectable tip laparoscope to minimize instrument collision, both internally and externally, might be of help in obese children and bariatric surgery.

Retraction difficulties is again one of the most important challenges in SIPES; to overcome this problem, there are many tricks being used by surgeons like placing a thin grasper (2-mm Minilap Alligator-Stryker Endoscopy, San Jose, CA), transabdominal sutures, insertion of additional trocarless instrument, and using special laparoscopic magnetic graspers which coupled with external magnets [16, 17]. Transabdominal suturing is useful in small children due to their thin abdominal wall. These sutures are used to encircle the round ligament for liver retraction and seromuscular bites through hollow organs like intestine and gallbladder [16, 19].

Coordination between the surgeon and the camera driver is essential as much or more than it's needed in CLS. In case of intraoperative complication or failure of progression, the introduction of other transabdominal conventional laparoscopic ports to aid completion of the surgical procedure is still there.

Engagement of OR staffs is essential to develop SIPES skills. In the beginning "converting an easy procedure into a harder one" is the sentence which you will hear as a SILS surgeon. Surgeons performing SIPES should have MIS skills and should attend SILS workshops.

In our institute we are providing surgical trainees with advanced laparoscopic and SILS animal workshops. The trainees are doing many SIPES procedures during their rotation, like appendectomies, cholecystectomies, and splenectomies. Although our rotating trainees did not have previous experience in SILS, as we are the only SILS center in the region, by the end of their rotation, they will be able to perform SIPES safely.

Summary

- The position of SIPES port is mainly trans-umbilical, but it might be introduced in the left upper quadrant for sleeve gastrectomy.
- Many types of ports are available, but Covidien© (Medtronic) is more suitable for pediatric patients, and Olympus is more suitable for bariatric surgery.
- Many challenges exist with SIPES, but there are always solutions as in conventional laparoscopy.
- Surgeons performing SIPES should have MIS skills and should attend SILS workshops.
- Insertion of extra port is always an option and is considered as conversion to mini laparoscopy (two ports).

9. SIPES tips and tricks

9.1 Tips & Tricks in SIPES appendectomy

SIPES appendectomy is increasing for its well-known cosmetic benefit. SIPES appendectomy is the most common procedure done in pediatric surgical units. The incision is strategically placed in the umbilicus with a perceived scarless abdomen. The technique is almost the same as in conventional procedure; it is performed through a 1.5 cm umbilical incision. Single-incision port Medtronic 5–12 mm is placed using the open technique. The mesoappendix is divided by diathermy or sealing device, endo-loops is applied to secure the base of the appendix, and the appendix is then divided and retrieved through the port. Interferences and collisions between surgical instruments are worse than they are when conventional laparoscopic appendectomy (CLA) is performed using three incisions; this may extend the MOT. However, even with these challenges, difficult appendectomy can be completed successfully and safely by SIPES.

9.2 SIPES cholecystectomy

Cholecystectomy is one of the most popular SIPES procedures. Our technique is to place a SILS port Covidien© (Medtronic) 5–12 mm in 1.5 cm trans-umbilical incision by open access. Obtaining the critical view of safety to properly visualize the cystic duct and artery is perhaps of utmost importance. The author modified the placement of straight needle for gallbladder fundus traction by transabdominal suture which is introduced percutaneously by curved needle. Once the gallbladder is properly retracted, the cystic duct and artery are identified, double clipped, and divided. The gallbladder is then dissected off the liver bed with hook cautery, and when completely detached, it is extracted from the abdomen through 12 mm port. No need for endobag.

9.3 SIPES splenectomy

SIPES splenectomy gives a good access for retrieving large-sized spleen through the umbilicus, instead of Pfannenstiel-Kerr incision used in conventional laparoscopic splenectomy CLS. Our technique is to place the patient in supine position with left side tilted 30°. Open-access trans-umbilical single-incision of 1.5 cm is used for placement of SILS port, Covidien (Medtronic) 12–15 mm SILS ports. Pneumoperitoneum is created and maintained at a constant pressure of 10–12 mm Hg. We insert 3 mm extra port in left flank for splenic retraction. We use only straight regular instruments. Dissection is performed by sealing device (LigaSure) in four stages: division of spleno-colic ligament at lower pole, dissection of vascular hilum, division of short gastric vessels, and detachment of diaphragmatic ligaments. The spleen is placed in a plastic bag and retrieved after morcellation with Péan forceps.

Insertion of portless extra 3 mm port in the left upper quadrant is necessary for elevation of the spleen to facilitate dissection of the hilum [20]. There is some argument about the use of extra port that it contradicts the concept of SIPES.

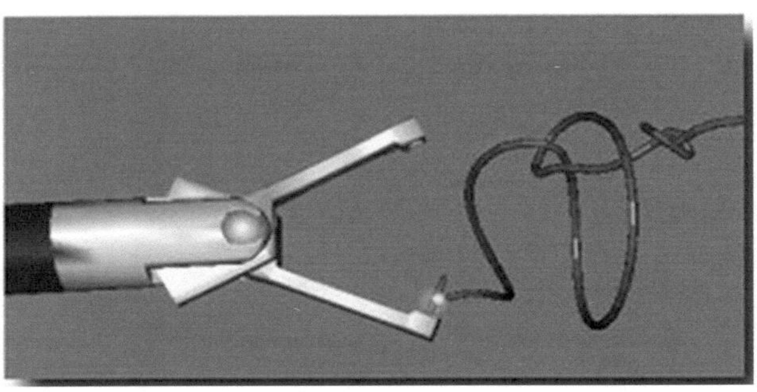

Figure 2.
Endo Stitch device.

There are some options to replace this port by using tug-exposure or suture suspension techniques [21, 22].

9.4 SIPES inguinal herniorrhaphy

Our technique for inguinal herniorrhaphy is percutaneous internal ring suturing (PIRS). The child is placed on supine position, and the surgeon stands on contralateral site of hernia. Laparoscopic camera is inserted through supra umbilical incision. Both sides of deep inguinal ring are explored. Stab wound is placed on the skin crease above deep inguinal ring. Epidural needle inserted in pre-peritoneal area with looped 4/0 nonabsorbable suture. In female the suture surrounds the sac entirely. In boy the needle enters the peritoneum adjacent to vas or vessels for exchange of the suture.

9.5 SIPES cystectomy/oopherectomy

We are using bronchoscope with foreign body retrieval forceps to retrieve the cyst and deliver it from the wound in neonate. In older children we use SIPES port and operate as in conventional laparoscopy.

9.6 SIPES fundoplication

We insert liver retractor directly through stab wound. The dissection is carried out as in conventional laparoscopy, and traction suture around the esophagus is taken out from the abdominal wall. We performed two cases with large hiatus hernia. Intracorporeal suturing is done by Endo Stitch device (**Figure 2**).

9.7 SIPES-assisted Mitrofanoff appendicovesicostomy

We ligate the base of appendix by extracorporeal sutures instead of endo-loop. The urinary bladder filled to come near the umbilical wound. The operation finished through the umbilical incision.

9.8 Obesity and SIPES

In the beginning adult surgeons were doing SILS cholecystectomy on patients with BMI less than 34. Later with improvement of instrumentations and development of disposable and reusable SILS trocars, SILS is now is recommended technique for obese, and it is used for sleeve gastrectomy.

Summary

- Many procedures have been done in our center
- We found out that appendectomy, cholecystectomy, splenectomy, cystectomy, oopherectomy, orchidectomy, Mitrofanoff, nephrectomy, herniorrhaphy, adhesiolysis, malrotation, and Morgagni hernia are easier to be performed
- Sleeve gastrectomy and fundoplication are less frequently done in our center; the reason in fundoplication is difficulty in suturing.
- This difficulty in older age group could be overcome with Endo Stitch instrument or the use of extracorporeal sliding notes.

10. Outcomes of SIPES at King Fahad Armed Forces Hospital (KFAFH)

The outcome of our retrospective study of all SIPES cases which was done from 2010 to 2016 is shown in (**Table 1** and **Figure 3**).

10.1 SIPES splenectomy

Few centers worldwide are performing SIPES pediatric splenectomy (**Table 2**). On extensive review there were only 166 SILS splenectomy cases, out of them only 61 SIPES pediatric splenectomy published in English, German, Greek, French, Italian, or Spanish literatures in all age groups (0.6–90 years) [23–28]. No publications regarding the safety of SIPES splenectomy were performed by trainees. Laparoscopic splenectomy is a demanding technique which needs high level of skills and mainly performed by the most experienced trained surgeon. Our SIPES splenectomy series is the largest one. 49 SIPES splenectomies were performed by 15 trainees. 25 (51%) were male and 24 (49%) were female. Mean age was 6.9 years (2.5–14.8 years). Six cholecystectomies were done simultaneously. 45 patients were having sickle cell disease, two with thalassemia, one spherocytosis, and one Fanconi's anemia. MOT for splenectomy was 182 min (130–190) and 251 min for splenectomy with cholecystectomy (230–270) min depending on severity of adhesions and size of the spleen

Procedures	Age	OT (min)	#	Conversion
Cholecystectomy (one with inguinal hernia repair+ 1 with appendectomy)	7–16	85 ± 40	52	2 (extra port)
Splenectomy (6 with cholecystectomy)	2.5–14.8	130–270	49	2
Appendectomy (carcinoid, adhesion, 6 perforated, 4 appendix mass)	3–12	70–160	137	0
SIPES hernia repair percutaneous internal ring suturing (PIRS)	2 months–12 years	20–45	46	22 (extra port)
Fundoplication (liver retract, Endo Stitch, 2 hiatal hernia)	18 months–7 years	90–180	8	0
Ovarian cystectomy (oophorectomy) (2 teratomas)	4 days–13 years	30–90	10	0
Intussusception	10 months	90	I	0
Malrotation (Ladd's procedure)	16 and 17 years	90 and 120	2	0
Assisted Mitrofanoff one with nephrectomy and orchidectomy	1.5–13 years	90–180	10	0
SIPES nephrectomy	18 months	100	1	0
SIPES abdominal orchidectomy	18 months	20	1	0
Morgagni hernia	3 and 5 years	90 and 120	2	0
Adhesiolysis	3 and 6 years	80 and 100	2	0
Sleeve gastrectomy	13–18 years	40–120	3	0
Total				324

Table 1.
SIPES outcome at KFAFH.

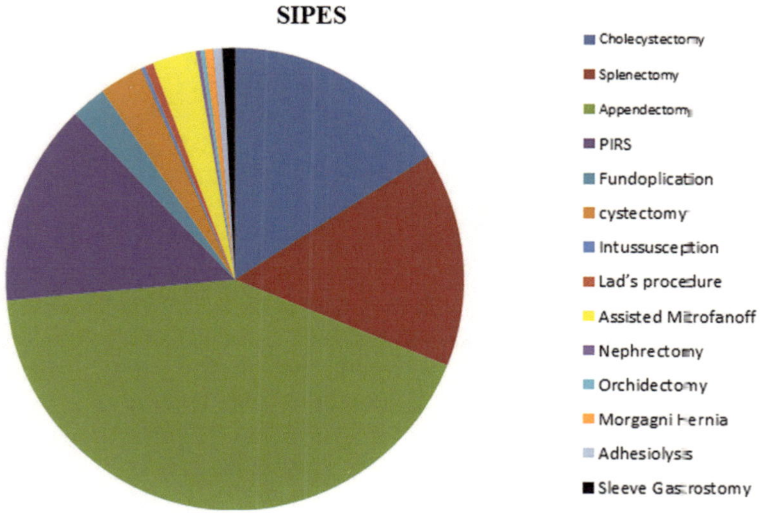

Figure 3.
KFAFH SIPES outcome.

Conversion	Time/min	Detail procedures	Age years	Number	Authors
0	90–176	4 splenectomy 2 combined splenectomy/ cholecystectomy	2–17	20 SIPES procedures 8 months	Dutta [18]
2 (excluded)	116	SIPES	7.1 (2.7–9.7)	37 patients (20 with extra port)	Seims et al. [20]
0	125 min (range, 45–420 min)	SILS and SIPES splenectomy	0.6–90	81	Gkegkeset al [23]
		SIPES splenectomy	6 months	1	Joshi et al. [24]
2	130–190	SIPES splenectomy	2.5–14.8	49	Raboei [25]

Table 2.
Comparison of SIPES splenectomy in pediatric age group.

P value <0.001 (**Figures 4** and **5**). Two were converted to open due to bleeding and were in the beginning of the series. There is neither wound infection nor incisional hernia update. SIPES splenectomy is now the standard of care in our unit, and we highly recommend it as excellent approach for splenectomy.

Summary

- This is the first series of SIPES splenectomy for hematological diseases done by trainees.

Procedures	Age	OT (min)	#	Conversion
Splenectomy (six with cholecystectomy)	2.5–14.8	130–270	49	2

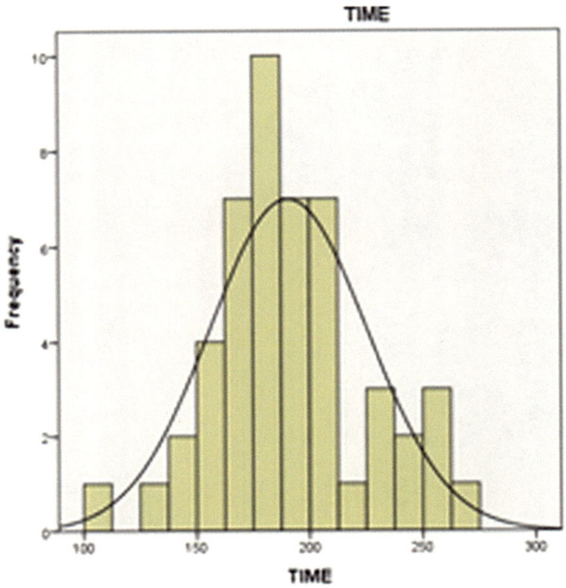

Figure 4.
MOT SIPES splenectomy.

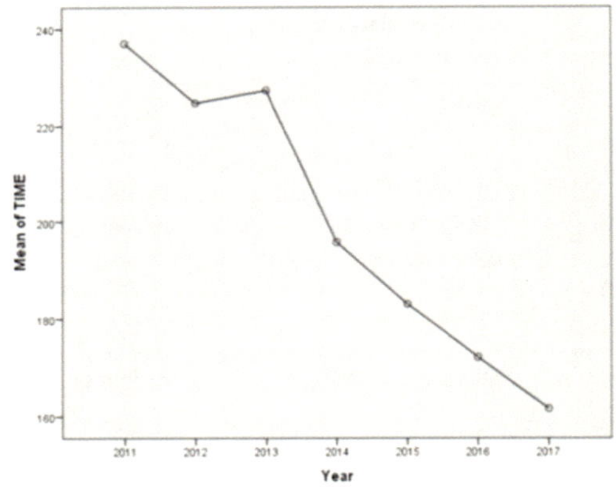

Figure 5.
SIPES MOT over years.

10.2 SIPES appendectomy

Most centers advocate laparoscopy for treating acute appendicitis in order to minimize the size and the number of skin incisions even with complicated ones [29]. SIPES pediatric appendectomy has gained significant popularity, as its main advantage is preferable cosmetic result. Previous studies have typically compared SIPES and CLA appendectomy in children and showed heterogeneous results. There was no difference in duration of hospital stay or postoperative complications. Longer MOT with SIPES appendectomy was the main concern [11, 30–41]. One study has shown that SIPES appendectomy in children is safe and feasible when performed by resident doctors and compare it when performed by fellows [42]. Chandler NM et al. studied SIPES versus conventional laparoscopic appendectomy CLA in children. 110 patients underwent appendectomy; 50 SIPES Group 1 and 14 were excluded (perforated) [30, 33]. They concluded that MOT and pain medication are the only significant values between SIPES and conventional. There was no increase in wound infection [43, 44].

Operation	Performing surgeon	MOT	NO.
SIPES appendectomy	Specialist	70.723	47
	Trainee	95.289	90
	Total	86.861	137
CLA	Specialist	64.681	141
	Trainee	88.457	46
	Total	70.529	187

Table 3.
Performing surgeon and MOT.

We started SIPES appendectomy in 2011, and it became our standard approach for acute appendicitis. It is carried out routinely by trainees and specialist. We compared SIPES appendectomy with CLA between our center and another training center. We conducted retrospective study at two training military institutes, KFAFH and Prince Sultan Medical City PSMMC. A total of 322 patients were operated. 187 patients (58%) underwent CLA, and 137 patients (42%) underwent SIPES appendectomy. 120 patients (64%) of CLA and 87 (63%) patients of SIPES appendectomy were males. 67 patients (36%) of CLA and 42 (37%) patients of SIPES appendectomy were females. The mean age of the patients in CLA and SIPES appendectomy was 10 and 9.6 years, respectively. Diagnosis at time of operation was simple appendicitis in 166 patients who underwent CLA and 126 patients who underwent SIPES appendectomy, and complicated appendicitis was in 21 and 11 patients, respectively. 143 CLA (76%) were performed by specialist, and 44 cases (24%) were performed by trainees. 47 SIPES appendectomy (34%) were performed by specialist, and 90 cases (66%) were performed by trainees (**Table 3**) (P value <0.001). The MOT was 70 min for CLA and 86 min for SIPES appendectomy (P value <0.001). The mean length of hospital stay is 2.6 days for CLA and 2.8 days for SIPES appendectomy. Bilateral percutaneous internal ring suturing (PIRS) and right PIRS were performed on 2 patients who underwent SIPES appendectomy. Three cases developed intra-abdominal collection (2.2%), one case had wound infection (0.7%), and two cases had adhesion (1.5%), treated conservatively in SIPES appendectomy. There were five cases of intra-abdominal collection (2.7%), two cases of wound infection (1.1%), and one case of adhesion (0.5%) in CLA. Negative appendectomy rate has been 10%.

Summary

- SIPES appendectomy is the commonest procedure done in our center by our trainees.

Procedures	Age	OT (min)	#	Conversion
Appendectomy (carcinoid, adhesion, six perforated, four appendix mass)	3–12	70–160	137	0

10.3 SIPES cholecystectomy

Minimally invasive techniques have revolutionized surgical treatment. Few centers worldwide have advanced SIPES for pediatric age group. Many papers that were published in English literatures proved the safety and efficacy of SIPES cholecystectomy [44–48]. Up to our knowledge, there is no study regarding MOT of SIPES

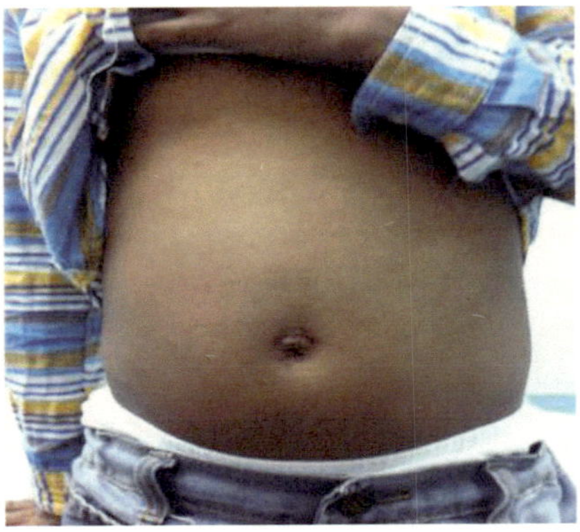

Figure 6.
SIPES cholecystectomy 6 months post-op.

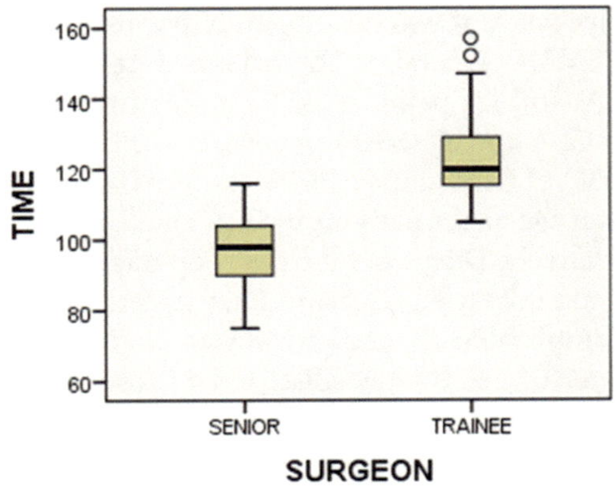

Figure 7.
SIPES cholecystectomy MOT.

cholecystectomy performed by trainees in patients with hematological disease. We conducted a retrospective study to determine the feasibility, safety, and expediency of SIPES cholecystectomy performed by trainees. 45 patients underwent SILS cholecystectomy. Age of the patients ranged from 7 to 16 years. Hematological disease were in >80% of cases. One extra port was needed in 2 patients in the beginning of the series. Eight procedures were done simultaneously, six splenectomy, one appendectomy, and one herniotomy, and were excluded from MOT. No conversion was needed. No wound infection. MOT is 85 ± 40 min. (**Figures 6** and 7). It is comparable with conventional technique.

Summary

- SIPES cholecystectomy is the second common operation in our center.
- We made a new technique for gallbladder traction by using a curved needle which visualize Calot's triangle clearly.

Procedures	Age	OT (min)	#	Conversion
Cholecystectomy (one with inguinal hernia repair + 1 with appendectomy)	7–16	85 ± 40	52	2 (extra port)

10.4 SIPES inguinal herniorrhaphy

The approach to inguinal hernia in the pediatric population has historically been via an open technique. During recent years, laparoscopic surgery has emerged as an alternative in the treatment of pediatric inguinal herniorrhaphy. Different laparoscopic technique has been used, and SIPES is a recommended approach for management of inguinal herniorrhaphy [28]. SIPES inguinal herniorrhaphy gives opportunity to explore the contralateral side. We retrospectively review all SIPES inguinal hernia cases. MOT, intra- and postoperative complications, cosmetic results, and contralateral patencies of processus vaginalis (CPPV) were recorded. Patients were followed up for 4 months postoperatively. A total of 46 patients were operated, 39 (84.8%) were male, and 7 (15.2%) were female. Right side inguinal hernias were 18 (39.1%), left were 12 (26.1%), and bilateral sides were 16 (34.8%). 56.5% were less than 1 year, 19.6% were between 1 and 5 years, and 23.9% were 6–13 years old. Mean age is 2.7 years. For unilateral procedures MOT was 27 min. For bilateral procedures MOT was 40 minutes. Seven (23%) (CPPV) was found in laparoscopic surgery. Stitch granuloma developed in one patient.

Summary

- PIRS is comparable with OH.
- It needs good ancillary services for babies below 6 months of age.

Procedures	Age	OT (min)	#	Conversion
SIPES hernia repair percutaneous internal ring suturing (PIRS)	2 months–12 years	20–45	46	22 (extra port)

11. Conclusion

SIPES has excellent cosmesis and almost invisible scar.

We can do more than one procedure at the same time with SIPES technique.

SIPES splenectomy is safe and feasible when performed by surgical trainees without adding any morbidity to the patients even those with hematological diseases.

SIPES appendectomy is feasible and safe in complicated appendicitis.

SIPES cholecystectomy MOT is comparable with conventional technique.

SIPES PIRS for inguinal herniorrhaphy is safe and efficient with good learning curve and best cosmetic result.

SIPES technique can be imparted satisfactorily to trainees. However, its successful incorporation into surgical training programs will depend on the development of innovative simulation strategies.

Our aim is to standardize this approach and to reassure our colleagues regarding the safety, feasibility, and technical challenges of SIPES.

Acknowledgements

We would like to acknowledge Dr Mohamed Al Onazi and his team from PSMC in Riyadh Saudi Arabia for their contribution.

Conflict of interest

None.

Author details

Enaam Raboei[1*], Ameen Alsaggaf[2], Yazeed Owiwi[2], Syed Salahuddin[3], Alaa Ghallab[2] and Mazen Zidan[2]

1 Pediatric Surgery Department, King Fahd Armed Forces Hospital, Jeddah, Saudi Arabia

2 King Fahd Armed Forces Hospital, Jeddah, Saudi Arabia

3 Leeds, UK

*Address all correspondence to: enaamraboei@kfafh.med.sa

References

[1] Vecchio R, MacFayden BV, Palazzo F. History of laparoscopic surgery. Panminerva Medica. 2000;**42**(1):87-90

[2] Kalloo AN, Singh VK, Jagannath SB, Niiyama H, Hill SL, Vaughn CA, et al. Flexible transgastric peritoneoscopy: A novel approach to diagnostic and therapeutic interventions in the peritoneal cavity. Gastrointestinal Endoscopy. 2004;**60**(1):114-117

[3] Li P, Chen Z-H, Li Q-G, Qiao T, Tian Y-Y, Wang D-R. Safety and efficacy of single-incision laparoscopic surgery for appendectomies: A meta-analysis. World Journal of Gastroenterology. 2013;**19**(25):4072-4082

[4] Pelosi MA, Pelosi MA 3rd. Laparoscopic appendectomy using a single umbilical puncture (minilaparoscopy). The Journal of Reproductive Medicine. 1992;**37**(7):588-594

[5] Saidy MN, Tessier M, Tessier D. Single-incision laparoscopic surgery—Hype or reality: A historical control study. The Permanente Journal. 2012;**16**(1):47-50

[6] Barbaros U, Dinççağ A. Single incision laparoscopic splenectomy: The first two cases. Journal of Gastrointestinal Surgery. 2009;**13**(8):1520-1523

[7] Dutta S. Early experience with single incision laparoscopic surgery: Eliminating the scar from abdominal operations. Journal of Pediatric Surgery. 2009;**44**(9):1741-1745

[8] Hansen EN, Muensterer OJ, Georgeson KE, Harmon CM. Single-incision pediatric endosurgery: Lessons learned from our first 224 laparoendoscopic single-site procedures in children. Pediatric Surgery International. 2011;**27**(6):643-648

[9] De Armas IA, Garcia I, Pimpalwar A. Laparoscopic single port surgery in children using Triport: Our early experience. Pediatric Surgery International. 2011;**27**(9):985-989

[10] Kocherov S, Lev G, Shenfeld OZ, Chertin B. Laparoscopic single site surgery: Initial experience and description of techniques in the pediatric population. The Journal of Urology. 2011;**186**(4 Suppl):1653-1657

[11] Oltmann SC, Garcia NM, Ventura B, Mitchell I, Fischer AC. Single-incision laparoscopic surgery: Feasibility for pediatric appendectomies. Journal of Pediatric Surgery. 2010;**45**(6):1208-1212

[12] Gasior AC, Knott EM, Holcomb GW, Ostlie DJ, St Peter SD. Patient and parental scar assessment after single incision versus standard 3-port laparoscopic appendectomy: Longterm follow-up from a prospective randomized trial. Journal of Pediatric Surgery. 2014;**49**:120-122. discussion 122

[13] Jayashingh SC. Comparison of advantages and disadvantages between SILS and NOTES. World Journal of Laparoscopic Surgery. 2011;**4**(1):67-72

[14] Fransen SA, Broeders E, Stassen L, Bouvy N. The voice of Holland: Dutch public and patient's opinion favours single-port laparoscopy. Journal of Minimal Access Surgery. 2014;**10**:119-125

[15] Chow A, Purkayastha S, Dosanjh D, Sarvanandan R, Ahmed I, Paraskeva P. Patient reported outcomes and their importance in the development of novel surgical techniques. Surgical Innovation. 2012;**19**(3):327-334. DOI: 10.1177/1553350611426011. Epub 2011 Dec 7

[16] Rivas H, Varela E, Scott D. Single-incision laparoscopic cholecystectomy:

Initial evaluation of a large series of patients. Surgical Endoscopy. 2010;**24**(6):1403-1412

[17] Padilla BE, Dominguez G, Millan C, Martinez-Ferro M. The use of magnets with single-site umbilical laparoscopic surgery. Seminars in Pediatric Surgery. 2011;**20**:224-231

[18] Dutta S. Early experience with single incision laparoscopic surgery: Eliminating the scar from abdominal operations. Journal of Pediatric Surgery. Sep 2009;**44**(9):1741-1745

[19] Blanco FC, Kane TD. Single-port laparoscopic surgery in children: Concept and controversies of the new technique. Minimally Invasive Surgery. 2012;**2012**:232347. Published Online 2012 Jun 12

[20] Seims AD, Russell RT, Beierle EA, Chen MK, Scott AA, Martin CA, et al. Single-incision pediatric endosurgery (SIPES) splenectomy: What dictates the need for additional ports? Surgical Endoscopy. 2015;**29**(1):30-33

[21] Misawa T, Sakamoto T, Ito R, Shiba H, Gocho T, Wakiyama S, et al. Single-incision laparoscopic splenectomy using the "tug-exposure technique" in adults: Results of ten initial cases. Surgical Endoscopy. 2011;**25**(10):3222-3227

[22] Li S, Li M, Xu W, Sun C, Liu L. Single-incision laparoscopic splenectomy using the suture suspension technique for splenomegaly in children with hereditary spherocytosis. Journal of Laparoendoscopic & Advanced Surgical Techniques. Part A. 2015;**25**(9):770-774

[23] Gkegkes D, Mourtarakos S, Iavazzo C. Single-incision laparoscopic splenectomy. JSLS. 2014;**18**(3):e2014.00350

[24] Joshi M, Kurhade S, Peethambaram M, Kalghatgi S, Narsimhan M, Ardhanari R. Single-incision laparoscopic splenectomy. Journal of Minimal Access Surgery. 2011;7(1):65-67

[25] Raboei E, Owiwi Y, Ghallab A, Zeinelabdeen A, Alsaggaf A, et al. Is It Safe for Trainees to Perform Single-Incision Pediatric Endosurgery Splenectomy?. Journal of Laparoendoscopic & Advanced Surgical Techniques. Mar 2019;**29**(3):420-423

[26] Hansen EN, Muensterer OJ. Single incision laparoscopic splenectomy in a 5-year-old with hereditary spherocytosis. JSLS. 2010;**14**(2):286-288

[27] Garrett D, Emami C, Anselmo DM, Torres MB, Nguyen N. Single-incision laparoscopic approach to management of splenic pathology in children: An early experience. Journal of Laparoendoscopic & Advanced Surgical Techniques. Part A. 2011;**21**:965-967

[28] Saldana LJ, Targarona EM. Single-incision pediatric endosurgery: A systematic review. Journal of Laparoendoscopic & Advanced Surgical Techniques. Part A. 2013;**23**:467-480

[29] Muensterer O, Puga Nougues C, Adibe O, Amin S, Georgeson K, Harmon C. Appendectomy using single-incision pediatric endosurgery for acute and perforated appendicitis. Surgical Endoscopy. 2010;**24**(12):3201-3204

[30] Chandler NM, Danielson PD. Single-incision laparoscopic appendectomy vs multiport laparoscopic appendectomy in children: A retrospective comparison. Journal of Pediatric Surgery. 2010;**45**(11):2186-2190

[31] Chow A1, Aziz O, Purkayastha S, Darzi A, Paraskeva P. Single incision laparoscopic surgery for acute appendicitis: Feasibility in pediatric patients. Diagnostic and Therapeutic Endoscopy. 2010;**2010**:294958

[32] Lacher M, Muensterer OJ, Yannam GR, Aprahamian CJ, Perger L, Megison M, et al. Feasibility of single-incision pediatric endosurgery for treatment of appendicitis in 415 children. Journal of Laparoendoscopic & Advanced Surgical Techniques. Part A. 2012;**22**(6):604-608

[33] Chandler NM, Danielson PD. SILS versus conventional laparoscopic appendectomy CLA in children. Journal of Pediatric Surgery. 2010;**45**(11):2186-2190

[34] Perez EA, Piper H, Burkhalter LS, Fischer AC. Single-incision laparoscopic surgery in children: A randomized control trial of acute appendicitis. Surgical Endoscopy. 2013;**27**:1367-1371

[35] Salö M, Järbur E, Hambraeus M, Ohlsson B, Stenström P, Arnbjörnsson E. Two-trocar appendectomy in children—Description of technique and comparison with conventional laparoscopic appendectomy. BMC Surgery. 2016;**16**:521-525

[36] Wu K, Yang L, Wu A, et al. Single-site laparoscopic appendectomy in children using conventional instruments: A prospective, randomized, control trial. Pediatric Surgery International. 2015;**31**:167-171

[37] Duza G, Palermo M, Khiangte E, Azfar M, Rizvi SAA, Trelles N, et al. Single port laparoscopic appendectomy vs conventional laparoscopic appendectomy: Outcomes after multicenter randomized control trial. Journal of American College of Surgeons. 2015;**221**(4 Suppl 2):e17

[38] St. Peter S, Adibe O, Juang D, Sharp S, Garey C, Laituri C, et al. Single incision versus standard 3-port laparoscopic appendectomy. Annals of Surgery. 2011;**254**(4):586-590

[39] Feng J, Cui N, Wang Z, Duan J. Bayesian network meta-analysis of the effects of single-incision laparoscopic surgery, conventional laparoscopic appendectomy and open appendectomy for the treatment of acute appendicitis. Experimental and Therapeutic Medicine. Dec 2017;**14**(6):5908-5916

[40] Park J, Kwak H, Kim SG, Lee S. Single-port laparoscopic appendectomy: Comparison with conventional laparoscopic appendectomy. Journal of Laparoendoscopic & Advanced Surgical Techniques. Part A. 2012;**22**:142-145

[41] Yannam G, Griffin R, Anderson S, Beierle E, Chen M, Harmon C. Single incision pediatric endosurgery (SIPES) appendectomy—Is obesity a contraindication? Journal of Pediatric Surgery. 2013;**48**(6):1399-1404

[42] Wakasugi M, Tsujimura N, Nakahara Y, Matsumoto T, Takemoto H, Takachi K, et al. Single-incision laparoscopically assisted appendectomy performed by residents is safe and feasible: A single institution, retrospective case series. Annals of Medicine and Surgery. 2017;**15**:43-46

[43] Sesia S, Haecker F, Kubiak R, Mayr J. Laparoscopy-assisted single-port appendectomy in children: Is the postoperative infectious complication rate different? Journal of Laparoendoscopic & Advanced Surgical Techniques. 2010;**20**(10):867-871

[44] Stringe G, Zitsman JL, Shehadi I, Kithir S. Laparoscopic Appendectomy in Children. JSLS. 1997;**1**(1):37-39

[45] Navarra G, Pozza E, Occhionorelli S, Carcoforo P, Donini I. One-wound laparoscopic cholecystectomy. The British Journal of Surgery. 1997;**84**(5):695

[46] Podolsky ER, Rottman SJ, Poblete H, King SA, Curcillo PG. Single port access (SPA) cholecystectomy: A completely transumbilical approach.

Journal of Laparoendoscopic & Advanced Surgical Techniques. Part A. 2009;**19**(4):495-499. DOI: 10.1089/lap.2008.0424

[47] Podolsky ER, Curcillo PG 2nd. Reduced-port surgery: Preservation of the critical view in single-port-access cholecystectomy. Surgical Endoscopy. 2010;**24**(12):3038-3043

[48] Podolsky ER, Rottman SJ, Curcillo PG 2nd. Single port access (SPA) cholecystectomy: Two year follow-up. JSLS. 2009;**13**(4):528-535

Frontiers and New Trends in the Science of Fermented Food and Beverages

Edited by Rosa Lidia Solís-Oviedo and Ángel de la Cruz Pech-Canul

Published in London, United Kingdom

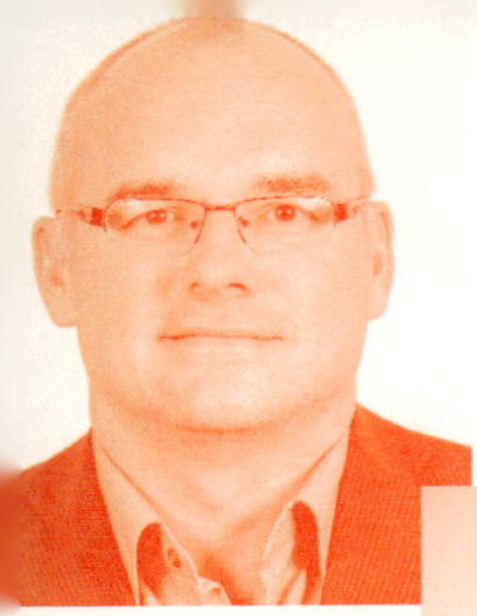
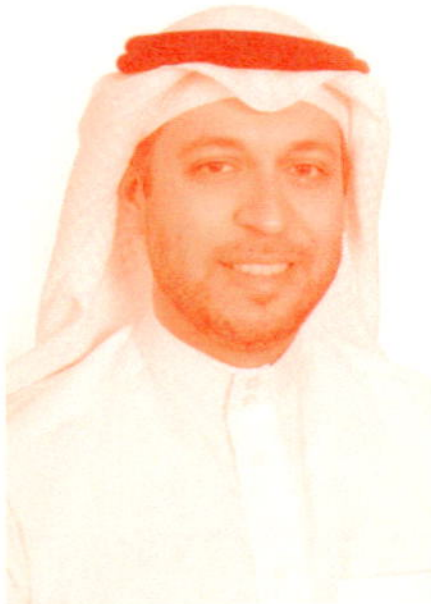
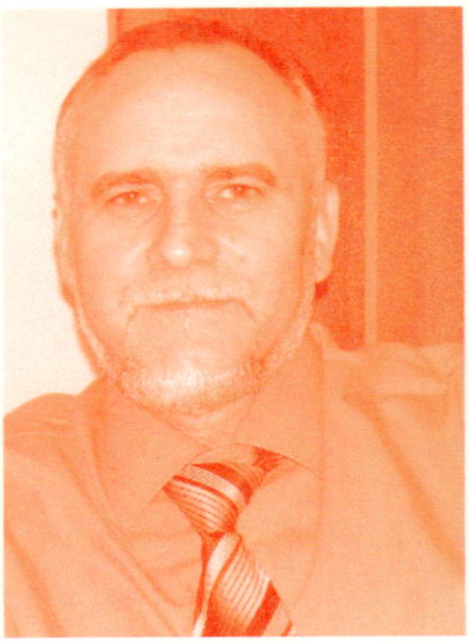
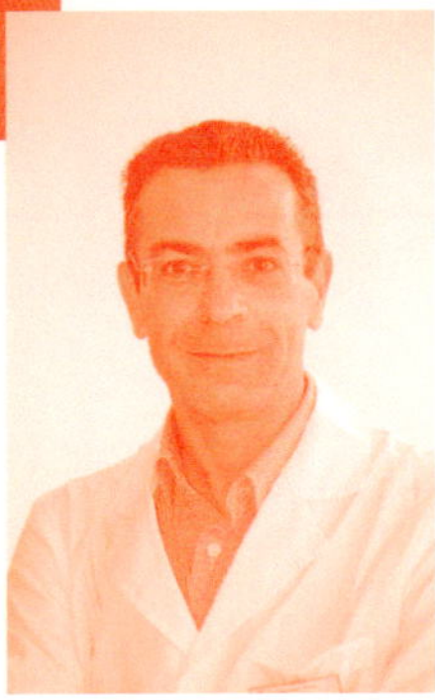
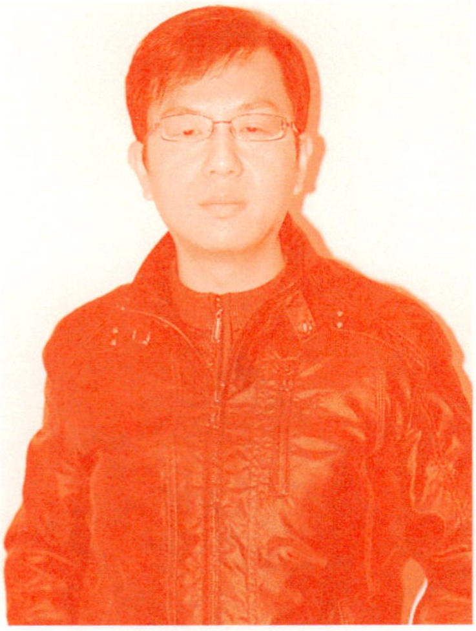
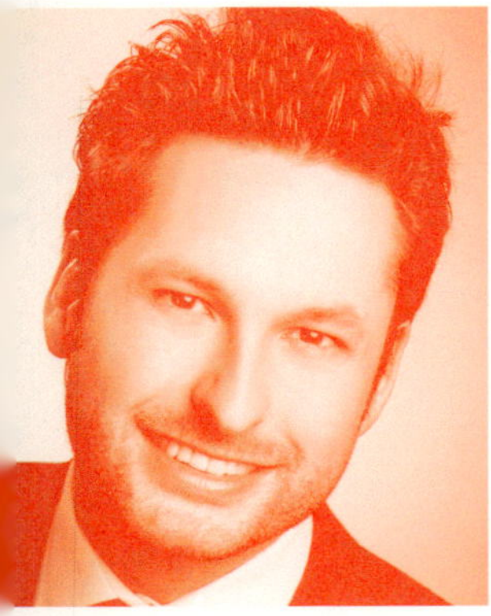
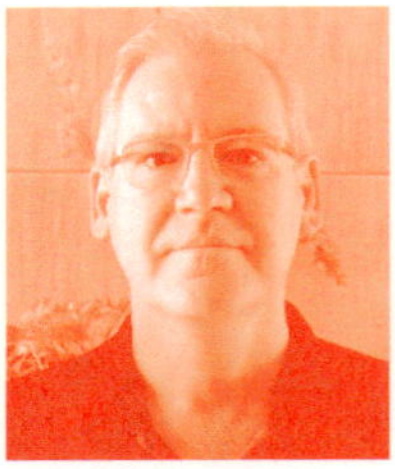

IntechOpen

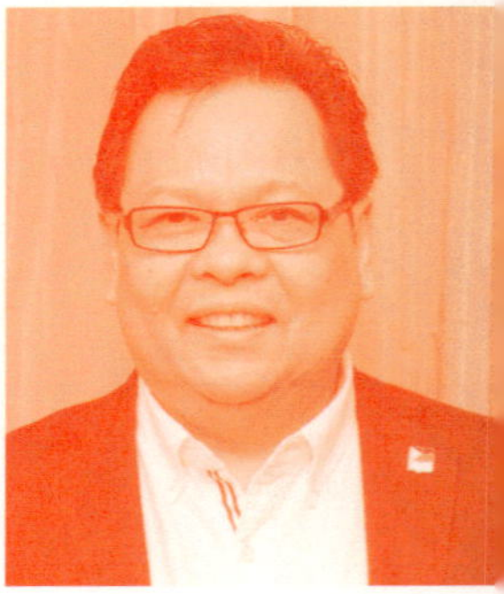
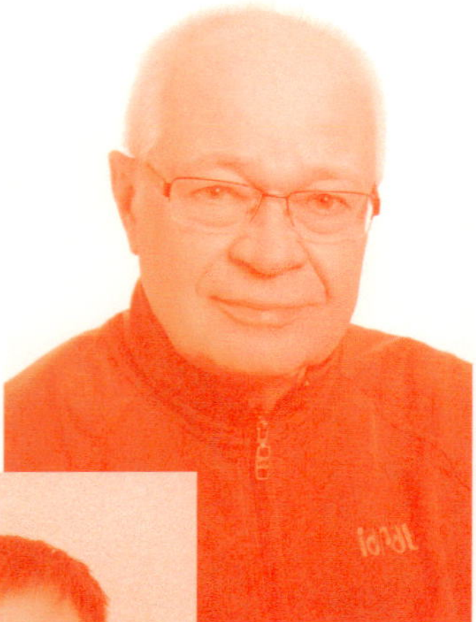
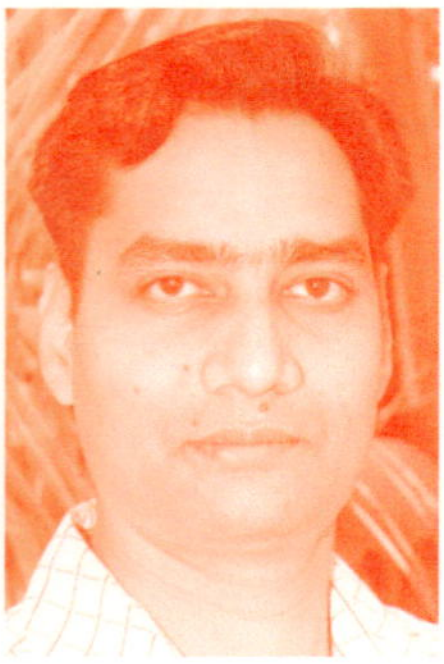
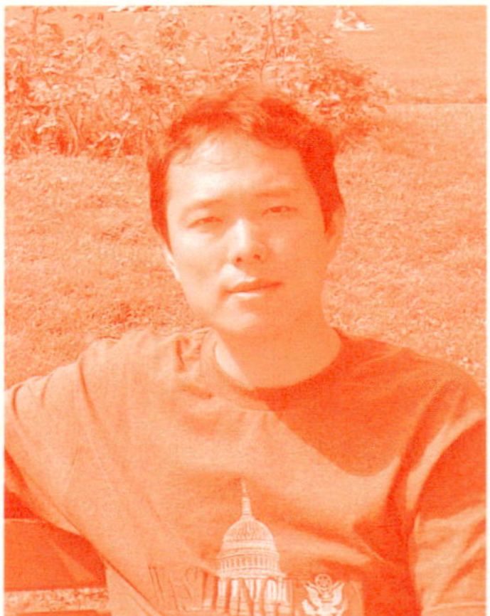
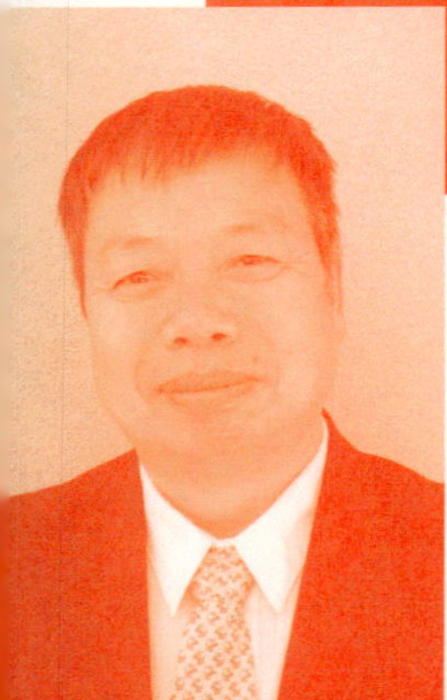
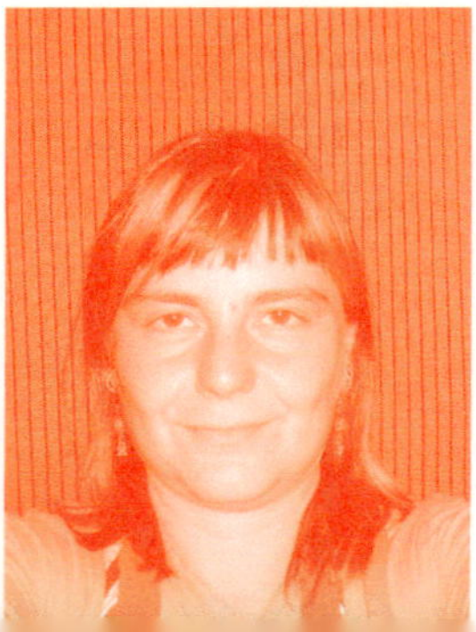

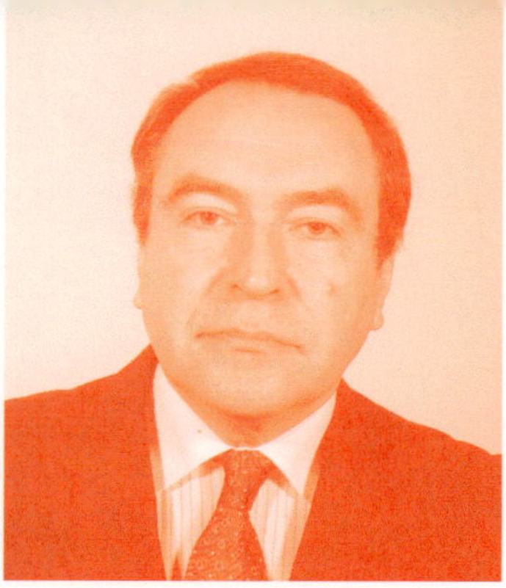
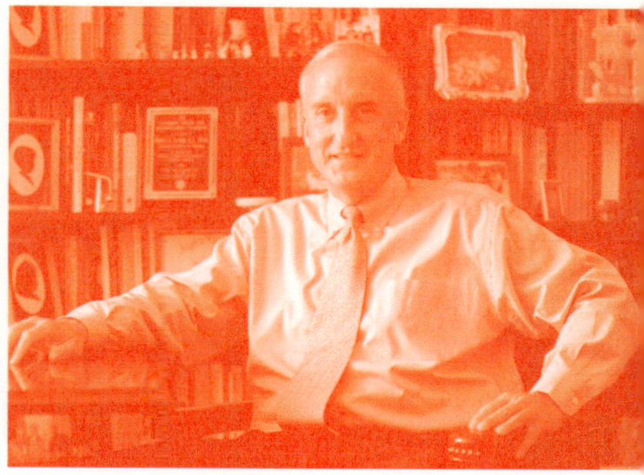
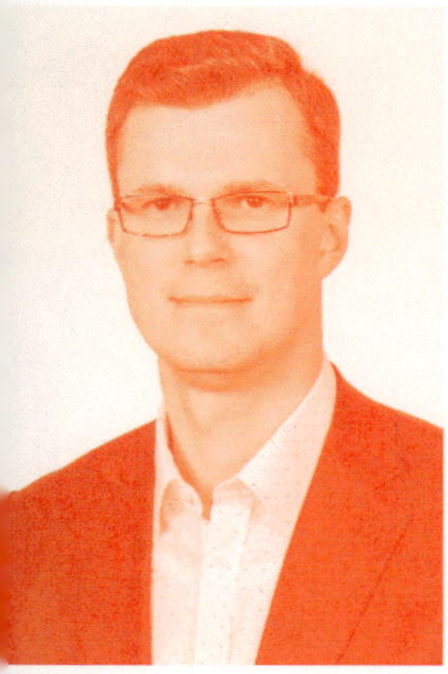
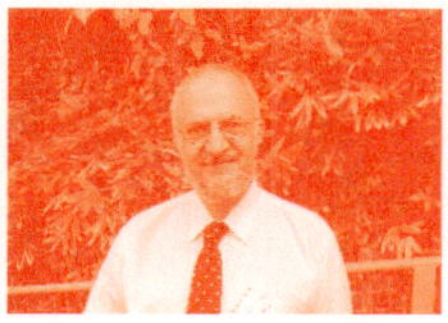
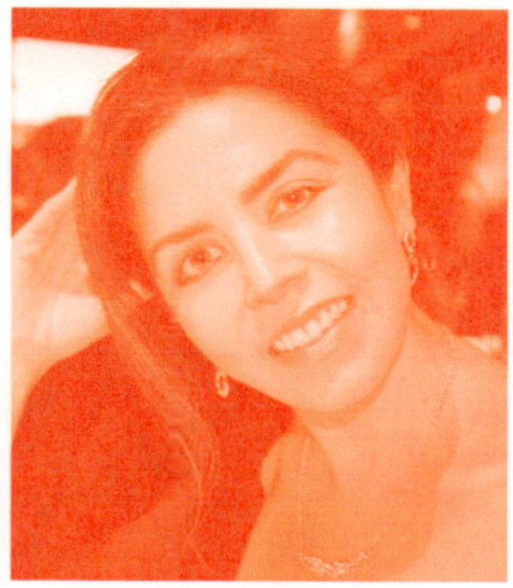

Supporting open minds since 2005

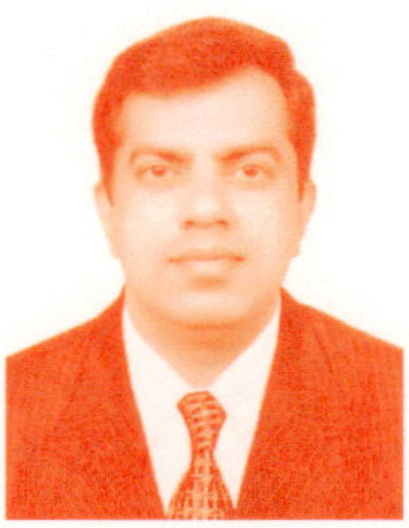
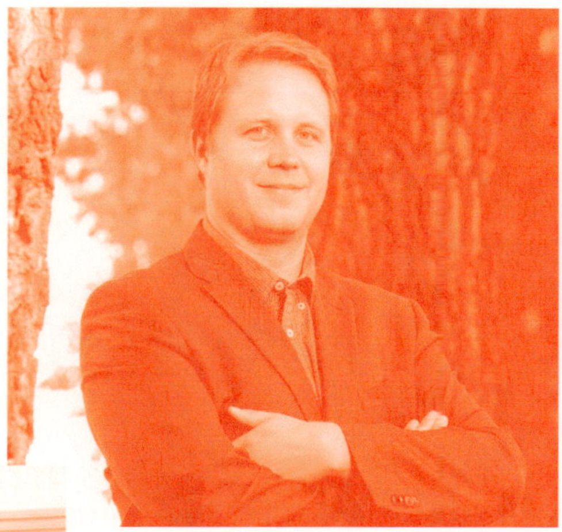
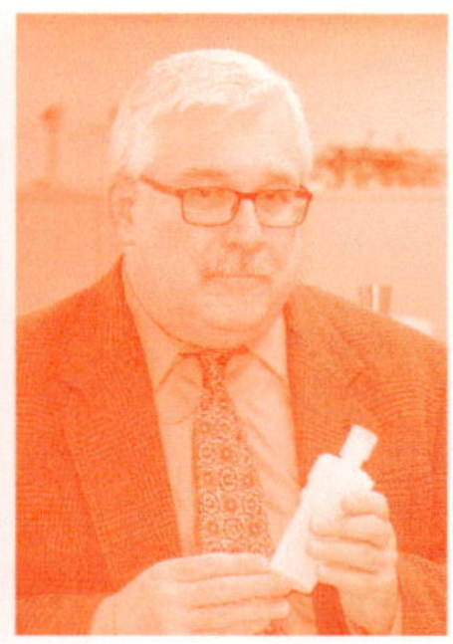
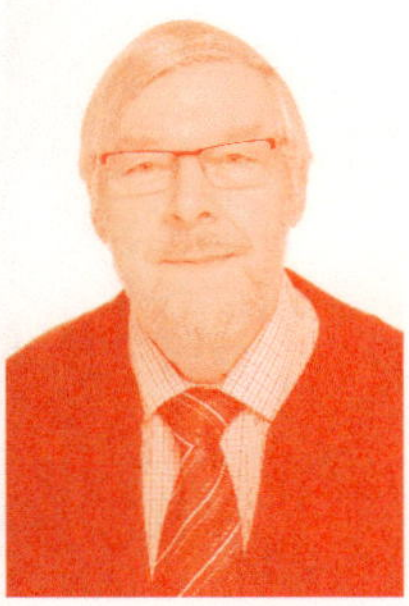
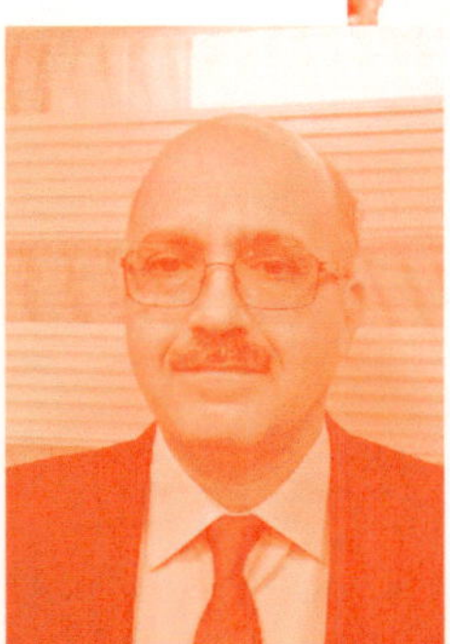
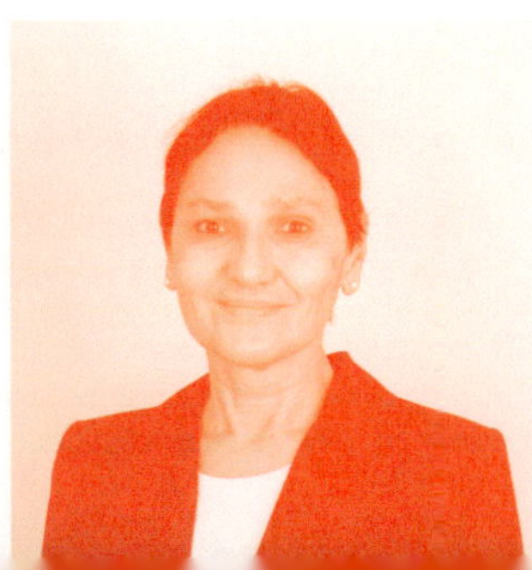
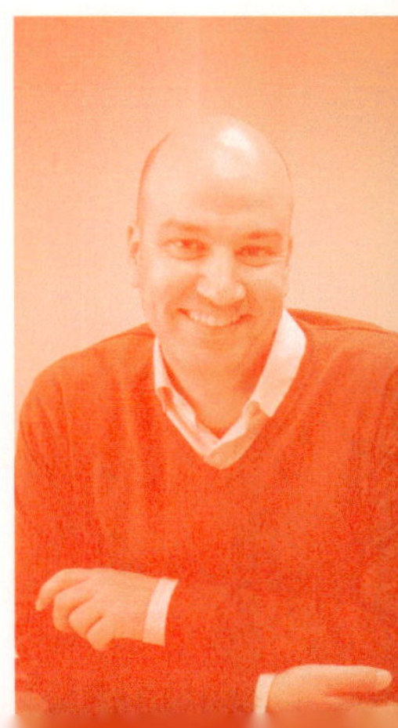

Frontiers and New Trends in the Science of Fermented Food and Beverages
http://dx.doi.org/10.5772/intechopen.73404
Edited by Rosa Lidia Solís-Oviedo and Ángel de la Cruz Pech-Canul

Contributors
Jose Luis Aleixandre-Tudo, Wessel Du Toit, Viduranga Waisundara, Nicoleta-Maricica Maftei, Waldir D. Estela-Escalante, Rosa Lidia Solís-Oviedo, David Ortega, Ángel De La Cruz Pech-Canul, Antonio Garcia-Triana, Iyabo Oladipo, Montserrat H. Iturriaga, Ramón Martínez-Peniche, Sofía M. Arvizu Medrano, Dalia E. Miranda Castilleja, Alejandro Aldrete Tapia, Lourdes Soto Muñoz, Nurudeen Olasupo, Chimezie Okorie

First published in London, United Kingdom, 2019 by IntechOpen
IntechOpen is the global imprint of INTECHOPEN LIMITED, registered in England and Wales, registration number: 11086078, The Shard, 25th floor, 32 London Bridge Street
London, SE19SG – United Kingdom
Printed in Croatia

British Library Cataloguing-in-Publication Data
A catalogue record for this book is available from the British Library

Additional hard copies can be obtained from orders@intechopen.com

Frontiers and New Trends in the Science of Fermented Food and Beverages
Edited by Rosa Lidia Solís-Oviedo and Ángel de la Cruz Pech-Canul
p. cm.
Print ISBN 978-1-78985-495-4
Online ISBN 978-1-78985-496-1

For EU product safety concerns:
IN TECH d.o.o., Prolaz Marije Krucifikse Kozulić 3, 51000 Rijeka, Croatia, info@intechopen.com or visit our website at intechopen.com.

Meet the editors

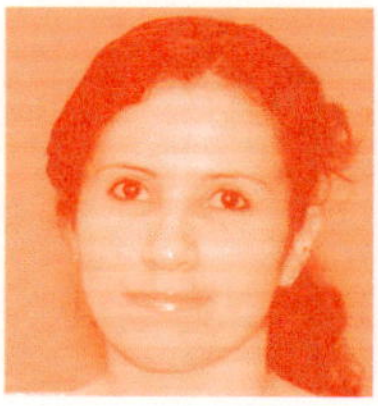

Dr. Solís-Oviedo is a researcher belonging to the National System of Researchers (SNI) from the Mexican National Council for Sciences and Technology (CONACyT). She is a member of the National Registry of Accredited Science Reviewers (RCEA-CONACyT) at the Biology/Chemistry Division. Her current interests are the exploitation of industrial properties of beneficial strains, specifically in food fermentations, and the production of chemical commodities from renewable resources. Dr. Solís-Oviedo holds a PhD in Biomedical Sciences and a BSc in Biochemical Engineering. She held a postdoctoral position at the University of Nottingham, where she gained experience working with modern genetic tools and microbial biotechnology aspects for the production of metabolites of industrial interest from industrial wastes, as well as on the training of human resources.

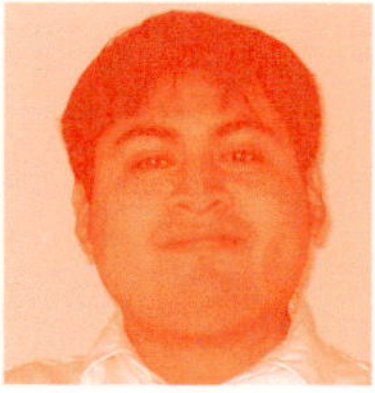

Dr. Pech-Canul is a research officer at the Mexican National Council for Sciences and Technology (CONACyT). He has extensive experience in bacterial genetics/physiology, fermentation, analytics (HPLC, GC-MS), and modern genetic tools. He is currently supported by the "Cátedras CONACyT para Jóvenes Investigadores" Programme for the identification of microorganisms with exploitable potential for industrial processes. Dr. Pech-Canul holds a PhD in Biomedical Sciences and a BSc in Biochemical Engineering. He was awarded with a CONACyT fellowship for postdoctoral training at the University of Nottingham, where he worked in modern genetic tools and microbial biotechnology aspects for the production of metabolites of industrial interest from industrial wastes. He is happy to participate in the formation of young scientists or science educators.

Contents

Preface

From time immemorial fermented foods have undoubtedly contributed to human health and well-being, and consequently to the progress of modern societies. The earliest archaeological evidence for the preparation of recipes was found in the Middle East. However, archaeological evidence, such as dedicated utensils for fermentation, are even older than these recipes. Among many fermented foods, both beer and bread flourished in the ancient Egyptian civilization and were considered as basic food items for their citizens. Historically, the preparation of bread, beer, and wine has been popular across Europe for centuries. Nevertheless, natives from many ancient cultures worldwide still conduct a wide variety of food fermentations using deep-rooted recipes and processes.

For centuries, the art of fermented foods was mastered by pure empirical observation, for example, through the domestication of yeast strains. Within the last four centuries, scientific research has started to unravel many aspects of the biological process. Hence, it has contributed to the improvement of many industrial processes. Nowadays, it is well known that fermentations are conducted by microorganisms. Therefore, fermented foods can be categorized according to either the primary metabolic product or the microorganism involved in the biological process. The food used as substrate in the fermentation process can also be used to describe fermented foods.

The modern food industry allows massive production of fermented products. However, somehow it has limited the diversification of fermented foods available in the market. Fortunately, several traditional fermented foods have recently regained attention mainly due to their nutritional values. Through our journey in the research field, we have always been attracted to the development of scientific research around autochthonous fermented foods and their cultural roots. These unique ferments are a wide-open window for new biodiversity. Furthermore, they are a natural repository of novel biological processes and biomolecules that will positively impact on many application fields from health, to food, to materials. Despite this, we find that many of these exciting results are regularly scattered and hard to find, because they are regularly spread in conference reports or in local journals. Furthermore, many of these reports remain in their original language and consequently are out of sight. Thus, most of the research progresses in this area are being hampered by the lack of publications in internationally recognized journals or books. Unfortunately, this has been a common issue, especially in developing countries where scientific research is consciously considered as a basis for economic growth.

The main purpose of this book is to provide useful and novel information for readers regarding fermented foods. The content aims to expand the knowledge of fermented foods emphasizing their research progresses, new trends, and diversity. The book also aims to promote the interest of readers in this particular area of research. Chapters focus on many different research disciplines. For example, ethanol from fermentations is presented, including its social implications. Research progresses on tea-derived beverages are also presented along with advances in prebiotic and symbiotic products. The book also includes exciting examples of African fermented foods. On the other hand, two divergent approaches to improve fermentation by the controlled inoculation of microorganisms are discussed, contrasting their strengths and weaknesses. Finally, research on genetics is presented as a valuable tool to deeply understand the basics of fermentation and its perspectives for the progress of the modern food industry. We were honoured and privileged by the valuable participation of researchers worldwide, such as from many African countries, Australia, Singapore, Romania, Argentina, Peru, and Mexico. The eclectic participation allowed us to enrich the outlook on the diversity of fermented foods and their potential impacts on human well-being.

Rosa Lidia Solís-Oviedo, PhD
Associate Research,
Faculty of Chemical Sciences, Autonomous University of Chihuahua,
Chihuahua, México

Ángel de la Cruz Pech-Canul, PhD
Research Professor,
Mexican National Council for Sciences and Technology (CONACyT),
Commissioned at the Faculty of Chemical Sciences,
Autonomous University of Chihuahua, Chihuahua, México

Chapter 1

Alcoholic Beverages and Human Health: An Overview

Oladipo Iyabo Christianah

Abstract

Production of alcohol is by fermentation of yeast, sugar, and starches. The consumption of which may be associated with some underlining risk factor depending on the quantity consumed per time. Alcohol can be consumed raw or by mixing in beverages, and whenever an alcoholic beverage is consumed, it can take about an hour for the body to metabolize one-eight of an imperial gallon. The level of the blood alcohol is increased when the quantity of alcohol consumed exceeds the normal dose which the body could metabolize, and then intoxication sets it. The higher the blood alcohol concentration, the higher the risk of diseases associated with the liver, kidney, and pancreas and the abundance of free radicals in the body system. Excessive use of alcohol can lead to alcoholism or alcohol dependence. Withdrawal from which can be life-threatening. Disulfiram, naltrexone, and acamprosate are the three approved oral medications for the treatment of alcoholism or alcohol dependence. On the other hand, moderate consumption of alcohol or red wines has been confirmed to be beneficial to human health particularly because of the antioxidant properties it confers.

Keywords: alcoholism, alcohol dependence, alcohol addiction, alcohol withdrawal, signs and symptoms

1. Introduction

Alcohol are organic compounds identified by one or more hydroxyl (^-OH) groups attached to a carbon atom of an alkyl group [1]. Alcohol is often considered as organic derivatives of water in which one of the hydrogen atoms has been replaced by an alkyl group, typically represented by R in organic structures. There are different types of alcohol: propyl, methyl, ethyl, and butyl alcohol, but for the production of alcoholic beverages, ethyl alcohol (ethanol) is the type used, while death or blindness could result if the other three are consumed at all [2]. Ethanol is normally produced from the fermentation of yeast, sugar, and starches [3]. It can also be consumed mixed in beverages or in its raw form, but the end product after digestion by the body is formaldehyde, which is deleterious to the body and also the cause of alcohol poisoning. Liver cirrhosis, gastric ulcers, gastritis, fatty liver, alcoholic hepatitis, and pancreatitis are examples of some disorders resulting from alcohol intoxication. Moderate consumption of alcohol may have some health benefits that could prolong life, but when taken in excess or as an escape route from problems, then abuse or alcoholism is inevitable.

Abuse of alcohol usually leads to alcohol use disorder also known as alcoholism or alcohol addiction which can lead to a violent behavior. Addiction to alcohol refers

IntechOpen

to physical and psychological dependency on alcohol to the point that tolerance is built up to alcohol [4]. Furthermore, once the body becomes adapted to excessive consumption of alcohol, an abrupt discontinuation leads to withdrawal symptoms which can be a threat to life and the symptoms normally includes hallucination, tremors, convulsions, anxiety, etc. Alcohol addiction may also result in the following: restlessness, depression, erratic behavior, decreased involvement in extracurricular activities, loss of interest in work or school, lack of interest in relationships, preoccupation with drinking, inability to control drinking, and violent behavior. While, nonalcoholic beverage refers to any drink that contains no alcohol or which contains less than 0.5% alcohol by volume and examples are fruit juices, mineral water, hot drinks etc.

2. Alcohol and alcoholic beverages

There are different types of alcohol based on their uses; some are used as solvents, antifreeze solutions, e.g., isopropyl and methyl alcohol, paint removers in chemistry laboratories and chemical factories, and as nail polish remover and cleansing solvent, for example, methylated spirit for domestic use [5]. There are different types of alcohol depending on the number of carbon atoms present and the position of the OH bond in the formula, but the most common alcohol is ethanol (CH_3CH_2OH or C_2H_5OH). During the process called fermentation, alcohol is produced. Fermentation of yeast usually results into sugar breaking down into carbon dioxide and alcohol. But carbon dioxide is taking off the process through gas bubbles leaving a mixture of water and ethanol. Sugar fermentation to alcohol can be used in different applications especially in the production of alcoholic beverages, for example, the extracts of grapes and barley are fermented in the wine and beer industry to produce alcoholic beverages. Any drink or beverage that contains ethanol is normally referred to as alcoholic beverage and are either produced by fermentation or distillation. There are different types of alcoholic and nonalcoholic beverages. Alcoholic drinks can be classified into five categories: (i) Wine, i.e., still, sparkling, fortified, or aromatized; (ii) beer, i.e., ales, lagers, and stouts; (iii) cider and perry; (iv) distilled spirits, i.e., vodka, gin, rum, whiskey, brandy, and others; and (v) liqueurs, i.e., flavored with fruit, citrus, herb, kernel, flower, cream, and berry. And nonalcoholic drinks can be classified into four categories: (i) Hot drinks, i.e., tea, coffee, and chocolate; (ii) fruit juices; (iii) mineral waters; and (iv) cordials/syrups.

3. Alcohol and human health

Alcohol has a complex mode of action and is majorly a depressant on the central nervous system, and the brain is affected in the process. It activates the release of the chief inhibitory neurotransmitter in the central nervous system by binding to GABA (gamma-aminobutyric acid) receptors in the brain. Absorption of alcohol which takes place from the intestine is reduced by fatty foods, and alcohol is distributed into body water. Alcoholic beverages contain ethyl alcohol, and research has shown that utilization of alcohol has here and now mental and physiological impacts on the consumer [6, 7]. Diverse absorption of alcohol in the human body affects a man, and the impacts of alcohol rely upon the quantity an individual has consumed, the level of alcohol in the mixed drinks and the time length that the utilization occurred, the measure of sustenance eaten and whether an individual has taken other remedies, and over-the-counter or road drugs, among different elements. Alcohol in carbonated drinks is absorbed faster than alcohol in noncarbonated drinks [6, 7].

Blood alcohol concentration (BAC) is dependent on amount and time range of alcohol utilization, muscle to fat ratio and weight, and nourishment impacts. Overabundance utilization of alcohol on an unfilled stomach over a brief timeframe range as a rule results to higher BAC. Drinking enough to cause a blood alcohol concentration (BAC) of 0.03–0.12% ordinarily causes a general perking up and conceivable happiness; expanded self-assurance and amiability; diminished nervousness; a flushed, red appearance in the face; impeded judgment; and fine muscle coordination. A BAC from 0.09 to 0.25% causes torpidity, sedation, adjust issues, and obscured vision. A BAC from 0.18 to 0.30% causes significant disarray, hindered discourse (e.g., slurred discourse), unsteadiness, and spewing [6, 7]. A BAC from 0.25 to 0.40% causes trance, obviousness, anterograde amnesia, retching (passing may happen because of inward breath of regurgitation (pneumonic goal) while oblivious), and respiratory melancholy (possibly dangerous). A BAC from 0.35 to 0.80% causes a state of unconsciousness (obliviousness), hazardous respiratory misery, and potentially deadly alcohol harming. Likewise with every mixed drink, drinking while at the same time driving, working an airship, or substantial hardware builds the danger of a mishap; numerous nations have punishments against driving while intoxicated [8].

Metabolization of 90% of consumed alcohol takes place in the liver; alcohol is converted to acetaldehyde by dehydrogenase (which is a sympathomimetic toxin responsible for "hangover"). Then, acetaldehyde is metabolized to acetic acid by aldehyde dehydrogenase and finally to carbon dioxide and water. Alcohol can then be excreted from the body through the sweat, lungs, and urine.

The regular consumption of alcohol, despite the bad effects it has on human's life, is called addiction or alcoholism. The causes of alcoholism usually include one or more of the following: peer pressure, usage of alcohol as remedy for mental ill health, alcoholism gene, influence of an alcoholic parent, etc. The abuse of alcohol results in over a million deaths in teenagers and young adults due to accidents every year all over the world [9]. Alcohol abuse occurs when all or one of the following happens: (i) Excess alcohol consumption in a social gathering, (ii) drinking and driving, (iii) alcohol consumption throughout the day, (iv) alcohol consumption to feel high, and (v) the need to drink alcohol every day.

Cognitive ability is impaired due to alcohol consumption, for example, in occasional and moderate drinkers the following occurs: memory impairment, blackout, recklessness, and impaired decision-making. While the following results in heavy and/or chronic drinkers: diminished brain size, inability to think abstractly, loss of visuospatial abilities, Wernicke-Korsakoff syndrome, loss of memory, and poor attention span. There are five different types of alcoholics which are (i) young adult subtype which includes young adults whose family have no history of alcoholism or mental ill health; (ii) young antisocial subtype, also includes young adult with a family history of alcoholism, mental ill health, and other addictions; (iii) functional subtype, this includes gainfully employed and successful middle-aged with a supportive family; they have a family history of alcoholism while some of them may have a history of depression (iv) intermediate familial subtype, these are middle-aged people with prior episode of depression and a family history of alcoholism, (v) chronic severe subtype are the middle-aged people with family histories of alcoholism, mental ill health, and other addictions [10].

3.1 Toxicity of alcohol

The toxic metabolic effects of alcohol are due both to its direct action when few percent of it enter the bloodstream from the stomach and that of its first metabolite called acetaldehyde (belongs to the same chemical family with formaldehyde) which is highly toxic to man [11]. Alcohol increases the rate of generation of free radicals in the body system and also inhibits the antioxidant levels thus inducing oxidative stress [6]. The excessive consumption of alcohol can also result in immunodeficiency and immunosuppressant thus exposing such individual to different kinds of infections. Research has shown that the consumption of alcohol is one of the causes of acute illness and chronic diseases throughout the world today [7].

3.2 Alcohol and pregnancy

Consumption of alcohol during pregnancy can have deleterious effects on the fetus not only in the first trimester but also throughout pregnancy as alcohol can move by the umbilical cord and placenta from the mother's bloodstream to the fetus. Alcohol consumption can cause havoc on the pregnancy before a woman is aware of the pregnancy. The havoc that can be caused on pregnancy includes miscarriage, birth deformities, retarded growth, and mental defects [2]. Excessive consumption of alcohol in pregnant women results in fetal alcohol syndrome (FAS) or fetal alcohol spectrum disorders (FASD) characterized with irreversible mental and physical changes to the baby. Fetal alcohol syndrome (FAS) may cause skeletal and facial abnormalities, growth retardation, mental disorders, and heart defects, while in fetal alcohol spectrum disorders (FASD), hyperactivity, life-long learning disabilities, poor attention span, speech or language delays, poor memory, and other disorders may result [12–14]. It is generally advised that drinking should be completely avoided by pregnant women.

3.3 Alcohol's effects on the body

Frequent alcohol consumption can be deleterious to human's health by affecting the following: (i) Brain: the communicative pathways of the brain are disrupted which may result in mood swing, lack of coordination, and coherence. (ii) Heart: it may also affect the heart by causing cardiomyopathy, arrhythmias, stroke, and high blood pressure. (iii) Liver: different types of problems may occur in the liver including liver inflammations, cirrhosis, alcoholic hepatitis, fibrosis and steatosis, or fatty liver [15]. (iv) Pancreas: heavy consumption of alcohol may cause the blood vessels in the pancreas to be swollen and inflamed thereby preventing proper digestion [16]. (v) Skin: abuse and consumption of alcohol can cause a variety of skin disorders [17]. Thermoregulation of the body also results in skin vasodilation and sweating [18]. (vi) Cancer: heavy drinkers stand the chance of developing cancers like cancer of the mouth, esophagus, throat, liver, and breast [16, 19]. Alcohol meddles with folate assimilation and function in the body, which may be one way alcohol can build danger of causing specific cancers. (vii) Immune system: alcoholism results in immune system being compromised, and the body is easily prone to diseases like pneumonia and tuberculosis.

4. Signs and symptoms of alcohol abuse and addiction

Some of the signs and symptoms of alcoholism includes the following in most adults: stomach pains, vomiting or nausea, redness of the face during or after periods of consumption, delayed reflexes, loss of consciousness or blacking out, slurred or incoherent speech, poor balance, and clumsiness. Alcoholics reach a level that the breathing is affected due to depression of the respiratory system which sometimes results into death. Some alcoholics become dependent on alcohol up to a point that their health, work, and relationship are neglected [20]. Signs of alcohol abuse include the following: insomnia, anger, loss of control and attention, etc. Alcoholism if untreated results in addiction identified by dependency. Signs of alcohol dependence are tolerance to increase in alcohol consumption, hangover, unsuccessful attempt to reduce consumption, alcohol withdrawal symptoms when alcohol is not consumed, etc. Seizures, extreme agitation or anxiety, hallucinations, nausea or vomiting, tremors, convulsions, uncontrolled shaking of the hands, persistent insomnia, and profuse sweating are some of the symptoms of withdrawal from alcohol indicative of advanced stage of addiction and should not be handled lightly [11]. Medical detoxification is usually the treatment given to alcoholism.

5. Side effects of alcohol withdrawal

Withdrawal from alcohol normally kicks off between 6 and 24 hours after the last drink, and withdrawal has been categorized into three stages according to their severity: (i) stage one which is the mild stage involves tremors, abdominal pain and/or vomiting, foggy thinking, anxiety, insomnia, nausea, loss of appetite, fatigue, depression, mood swings, and heart palpitations; (ii) stage two which is the moderate stage also involves mental confusion; irregular heart rate; profuse sweating; irritability; increased blood pressure, body temperature, and respiration; and heightened mood disturbances; and (iii) stage three which is the severe stage is often called the delirium tremens. It is characterized by fever, agitation, severe confusion, hallucination, and seizures. Delirium tremens often occur in about 3–5% alcohol withdrawal individuals. It normally kicks off without warning at 24 or 48 hours after alcohol leaves the bloodstream. Withdrawal from alcohol is influenced by factors such as stress level, family history of addiction, co-occurring mental ill health, childhood trauma, drinking duration, and quantity consumed. It can also be influenced by combined use of alcohol and other drugs thereby increasing the potential for dangers and other side effects. Withdrawal from alcohol can in some cases cause the death of an addict as the central nervous system and the brain are normally affected by continuous suppression by alcohol for a long period of time.

Withdrawal from alcohol has no definite timeline, but a general timeline has been detailed as follows: the first stage normally begins 8 hours after the first drink, while the second and third stages occur rapidly, and symptoms peak between 24 and 72 hours. Symptoms may then start to wear off 5–7 days later, but psychological symptoms may be prolonged for several weeks [21].

Physical symptoms are monitored and controlled up to a stable point during detoxification which is often achieved by medications. Restoration of the natural order to the overactivity of the central nervous system can be accomplished by using benzodiazepines during alcohol detoxification. Dangerous side effects of alcohol withdrawal can be avoided by gradual and controlled weaning of alcohol out of the body.

5.1 Managing withdrawal symptoms

Thought of suicide, anxiety, and depression can be controlled with medications alongside therapy and counseling. Disulfiram, naltrexone, and acamprosate are the three approved medications used to control alcohol cravings in the treatment of alcohol withdrawal. Naltrexone operates by blocking the opioid receptors in the brain, thereby reducing cravings for drinking, while long-term withdrawal symptoms are taken care of by acamprosate. Disulfiram makes drinking undesirable by making people sick if they drink. Another promising medication in the treatment of alcohol use disorders is topiramate [2].

6. Beneficial effects of alcohol

Red wines have been known to have antioxidant properties because they contain substances like resveratrol (polyphenol) and flavonoids which confer cardioprotective effects to the heart. Antioxidants also protect against artery damage by increasing levels of high density lipoprotein (HDL). So, moderate consumption of alcohol or red wines has been confirmed to be beneficial to human health. But it should not be used as an excuse to start drinking as it can be addictive or cause other health problems [2].

Also, it is generally known that red wine contains the most resveratrol, the antioxidant found in grape skin that may improve the health of the heart by counteracting blood vessel harm and also diminishing LDL cholesterol. Additionally, the flavonoids contained in red wine are another vital cancer prevention agent. It must then be noted that most research carried out have been on animals, and the measure of wine to be taken by an individual to level with a similar sum given to mice would neutralize any of the assumed advantages. Likewise, the 129 calories contained in a glass can accumulate, regardless of whether an individual is just drinking one daily [22]. Red wine also contains histamine that can cause headache assaults or different kinds of manifestations that happen from a histamine prejudice.

7. Treatment of alcohol abuse and alcoholism

Alcoholism treatment involves serious medical, family, and social support, while interventions like group support, individual counseling, stepped therapy, and medications are usually advocated for alcohol dependence. Three approved medications for medical treatments of alcohol dependence are naltrexone (Depade, ReVia), disulfiram (Antabuse), and acamprosate (Campral) and an injectable long-acting form of naltrexone (Vivitrol). The medication may reduce relapses and drinking and may result to total recovery and abstinence from alcohol. Naltrexone and acamprosate have been recommended as treatment alternative for alcohol dependence together with behavioral therapy in a review, but disulfiram has not been recommended for routine use in primary care as proof of its ability to increase abstinence rates or decrease relapse rates or cravings compared with placebo as not been shown [4].

8. Alcohol detoxification

Alcohol detoxification is the process by which the system of a heavy drinker is returned to normal after prolonged period of alcohol abuse. It normally involves medical treatment and counseling. The detoxification process involves three steps: (i) Step one (intake) involves a comprehensive review of drug, psychiatric, and medical histories of patients to fully understand the situation, (ii) step two (stabilization) which involves medical and psychological therapies to help a patient reach a balance of mind and body, and (iii) step three (medication) which involves medications that mimic the effects of alcohol to mitigate withdrawal symptoms. Some of the unpleasant side effects of detoxification may include nausea, insomnia, mood swing, muscle weakness, and nervousness, while kidney or liver dysfunction, seizures, extreme nausea, aspiration pneumonia, heart arrhythmias, fever, and hallucinations are examples of some of the severe side effects of alcohol detoxification. Medications are used to avoid physiological upsets and system imbalance during detoxification. Benzodiazepines are used to reduce alcohol withdrawal symptoms and also prevent alcohol withdrawal seizures which are the most common causes of fatality in alcohol withdrawal [23].

9. Nonalcoholic drink

Beverage without an alcohol is usually referred to as a nonalcoholic drink. There are different varieties of nonalcoholic beverages; examples are soft drinks, nonalcoholic beers like root beer, mineral water, aerated/carbonated, hot and cold drinks, mocktails, etc. These nonalcoholic beverages perform one or more of the following functions: (i) supply vitamins and nutrient required by the body, (ii) provide energy, (iii) hydrate, (iv) supply of the necessary calories and sugar required by the body, and (iv) some can be used as aperitif or palate stimulant.

Some beverages like soft drink, juice, and apple cider naturally may contain little amounts of alcohol. Distillation of ethanol is often to separate alcoholic drinks into what are commercially called spirit and nonalcoholic drinks. Purification of alcoholic drinks to 0.00% alcohol by volume by distillation is impossible. Furthermore, most drinks with the label nonalcoholic contain 0.5% ABV as it brings more profit than distilling it to 0.05% ABV normally found in products sold by companies specialized in nonalcoholic drinks [24]. It is said by some people that the sign nonalcoholic on drinks is misleading and therefore a threat to recovering alcoholics due to the psychoactive nature of alcohol.

Nonalcoholic beer may be beneficial to other people, but it is not advised to be consumed by a recovering alcoholic. According to a study which was conducted on some Spanish nuns who drank nonalcoholic beer for 45 days and had an increased antioxidant levels in their bloodstream, nonalcoholic beer could have positive impacts on the cardiovascular system. Among the disadvantages are (i) the perception of most people is that nonalcoholic beer does not have the rich flavor of normal alcoholic beer; (ii) most nonalcoholic beer contains a small amount of alcohol, which could result into relapse for recovering alcoholics; (iii) research has made it clear that the smell of any kind of beer may trigger cravings in the alcoholic's mind, and the level of dopamine in the brain may be raised; and (iv) there is a fear of being stigmatized as the only one not drinking alcohol in a social gathering.

10. Conclusions

Conclusively, drinks that contain ethanol are regularly alluded to as mixed refreshment and are either produced by fermentation or distillation. The utilization of which might be related with some underlining hazard factor contingent upon the amount devoured per time. The consistent utilization of alcohol, regardless of the terrible impacts it has on human's life, dependence, alcohol addiction, and withdrawal from which can be dangerous. Alcohol expands the rate of production of free radicals in the body framework and furthermore represses the antioxidant levels along these lines instigating oxidative stress. The unnecessary utilization of alcohol can likewise result in immunodeficiency and immunosuppressant subsequently presenting such individual to various types of infections. The causes of alcoholism range from alcoholism gene, peer pressure, to influence of an alcoholic parent, among others. The three affirmed oral pharmaceuticals for the treatment of alcohol addiction or dependence are disulfiram, naltrexone, and acamprosate. While, nonalcoholic beverages alludes to any drink that contains no alcohol or which contains under 0.5% alcohol by volume. Moderate consumption of alcohol or red wines has been affirmed to be gainful to human well-being especially on account of the cancer prevention agent properties it gives. Some other positive effects like reduction of diabetes, stroke, and coronary heart disease have been associated with moderate consumption of alcohol particularly among middle-aged and older men and women.

Conflict of interest

The authors hereby declare that there is no conflict of interest.

Author details

Oladipo Iyabo Christianah
Department of Science Laboratory Technology, Ladoke Akintola University of Technology, Ogbomoso, Oyo State, Nigeria

*Address all correspondence to: xtiecoker@gmail.com

References

[1] Leroy GW. Alcohol Encyclopædia Britannica [Internet]. 2018. Available from: https://www.britannica.com/science/alcohol [Accessed: 27-5-2018]

[2] Drugs.com. Alcohol. [Internet]. Available from: https://www.drugs.com/alcohol.html [Accessed: 26-5-2018]

[3] National Institutes of Health (NIH). National Institute on Drug Abuse (NIDA). Drugs of Abuse: Alcohol. [Internet]. Available from: http://www.drugabuse.gov/drugsabus e/alcohol [Accessed: 24-5-2018]

[4] Drugabuse.com. Alcohol Abuse. [Internet]. Available from: https://drugabuse.com/library/alcohol-abuse/ [Accessed: 2-6-2018]

[5] Tarek IK. A round in alcohols world between: Production, properties, uses, applications, fuel, and compounds chemistry. Chemical Science and Engineering. 2009;**14**:25. Available from: http://tarek.kakhia.org/books_eng/Alcohol.Tarek_Kakhia.pdf

[6] Nordmann R, Riviere C, Rouach H. Implication of free radical mechanisms in ethanol-induced cellular injury. Free Radical Biology & Medicine. 1992;**12**:219-240

[7] Kevin DS, Charles P, Jürgen R. Chronic diseases and conditions related to alcohol use. Alcohol Research: Current Reviews. 2014;**35**(2):155-171

[8] Horowitz M, Maddox A, Bochner M. Relationships between gastric emptying of solid and caloric liquid meals and alcohol absorption. American Journal of Physiology. 1989;**257**(92 Pt 1): G291-G298. PMID 2764113

[9] National Institute of Alcohol Abuse and Alcoholism. Overview of Alcohol Consumption; Alcohol Facts and Statistics [Internet]. Available from: https://www.niaaa.nih.gov/alcohol-health/overview-alcohol-consumption/alcohol-facts-and-statistics [Accessed: 2-6-2018]

[10] American Addiction centers. Alcoholism Addiction Treatment. [Internet]. Available from: https://Americanaddictioncenters.org/alcoholism-treatment/ [Accessed: 2-6-2018]

[11] Vaillant GE, Keller M. Alcoholism [Internet]. 2018. Available from: www.britannica.com/science/alcoholism [Accessed: 2-6-2018]

[12] Office of the Surgeon General. U.S. Department of Health and Human Services. News release. U.S. Surgeon General Releases Advisory on Alcohol Use in Pregnancy. Available from: http://www.surgeongeneral.gov/pressreleases/sg02222005.html [Accessed: 24-5-2018]

[13] Centers for Disease Control and Prevention. Fetal Alcohol Spectrum Disorders (FASDs) Alcohol Use in Pregnancy [Internet]. Available from: http://www.cdc.gov/n cbdd/fasd/alcohol-use.html [Accessed: 24-5-2018]

[14] Mayo Clinic. Heart Disease; Red Wine and Resveratrol: Good for your heart? [Internet]. March 4, 2011. Available from: http://www.mayoclinic.com/health/red-wine/HB00089 [Accessed: 24-5-2018]

[15] Naimi TS, Brewer RD, Mokdad A, Denny C, Serdula MK, Marks JS. Binge drinking among US adults. JAMA. 2003;**289**:70-75

[16] Buckman JF, Eddie D, Vaschillo EG, Vaschillo B, Garcia A, Bates ME. Immediate and complex cardiovascular adaptation to an

acute alcohol dose. Alcoholism: Clinical and Experimental Research. 2015;**39**(12):2334-2344. DOI: 10.1111/acer.12912

[17] Smith KE, Fenske NA. Cutaneous manifestations of alcohol abuse. Journal of the American Academy of Dermatology. 2000;**43**:1-16

[18] Yoda T, Crawshaw LI, Nakamura M, Saito K, Konishi A, Nagashima K, et al. Effects of alcohol on thermoregulation during mild heat exposure in humans. Alcohol. 2005;**36**:195-200

[19] Shi P, Chen Y, Guo M, Yu H. Acute effects of alcohol on heart rate variability: Time-related changes and gender difference. Biomedical Engineering Applications, Basis and Communications. 2014;(26, 3). DOI: 10.4015/S1016237214500483

[20] Timberline Knolls Residential Treatment Center. Alcohol Addiction Treatment. Alcohol Addiction Signs, Symptoms and Effects [Internet]. Available from: http://www.timberlineknolls.com/alcohol-addiction/signs-effects/ [Accessed: 12-6-2018]

[21] American Addiction Centers. Alcohol Withdrawal Treatment, Symptoms, and Time- line. [Internet]. Available from: https://americanaddictioncenters.org/withdrawal-timelines-treatments/alcohol/ [Accessed: 15-6-2018]

[22] Popsugar. Fitness. [Internet]. Available from: https://www.popsugar.com/fitness/Pros-ConsDrinking-Red-Wine-White-Wine-Champagne-14656661/ [Accessed: 18-8-2018]

[23] Addiction Centers. Alcohol Detoxification. [Internet]. Available from: https://www.addictioncenter.com/alcohol/detox/ [Accessed: 13-6-2018]

[24] Wikipedia Non Alcoholic Drinks [Internet]. Available from: https://en.wikipedia.org/wiki/Non-alcoholic_drink. [Accessed: 12-6-2018]

Chapter 2

Usage of Kombucha 'Tea Fungus' for Enhancement of Functional Properties of Herbal Beverages

Viduranga Yashasvi Waisundara

Abstract

The following herbal teas were fermented with the Kombucha "tea fungus" for 7 days: *Acacia arabica*, *Aegle marmelos* root bark, *Aerva lanata*, *Asteracantha longifolia*, *Cassia auriculata*, *Hemidesmus indicus*, *Hordeum vulgare*, *Phyllanthus emblica*, *Tinospora cordifolia*. Microbial enumerations of the bacteria and fungi present in the broth and the tea fungal mats were carried out. At the end of the period of fermentation, the pH values ranged from 4.0 to 6.0, while the titratable acidity (TA) ranging from 2.5 to 5.0 g/mL. The TA was within the acceptable limits of consumption for all beverages. The Oxygen radical absorbance capacity (ORAC) assay indicated 5 of the fermented beverages to have statistically significant increases ($P < 0.05$) by the end of the period of fermentation. By day 7, the IC_{50} values of the α-amylase inhibitory activities ranged from 52.5 to 67.2 μg/mL, while the α-glucosidase inhibitory activity values ranged from 95.2 to 196.1 μg/mL by this time point. Overall, an enhancement of the antioxidant and starch hydrolase inhibitory potential of the seven herbal teas was observed as a result of the fermentation by addition of the tea fungus. Thus, this fermentation process could be highlighted as a novel and versatile methodology to obtain functional beverages.

Keywords: antioxidant activity, ORAC, Kombucha, starch hydrolase inhibitory activity, total phenolic content

1. Introduction

Kombucha or "tea fungus" is a fermented beverage which is believed to have its origins in northeast China, and has recently gained rapid popularity among the rest of the world [1]. The beverage is produced through the symbiotic growth of bacteria and osmophilic yeast strains in a thick jelly-like membrane which is cultured in sugared black tea (**Figure 1**) [2]. While the term "Kombucha" is the most commonly used name for the beverage on a commercial basis, it is also known by other names such as Chainii grib, Chainii kvass Champignon de longue vie, Ling zhi, kocha kinoko and red tea fungus [3]. For the production of the beverage, the substrate is incubated with the tea fungal mat statically under aerobic conditions, usually for a minimum of 7 days at 20–28°C [4]. However, to obtain a pleasantly sour beverage with palatability and acceptable sensory properties, the fermentation should terminate when the titratable acidity (TA) reaches 4.0–4.5 g/L—a level which has been confirmed as acceptable by longtime consumers of the Kombucha beverage and is known as the optimal consumable acidity [5].

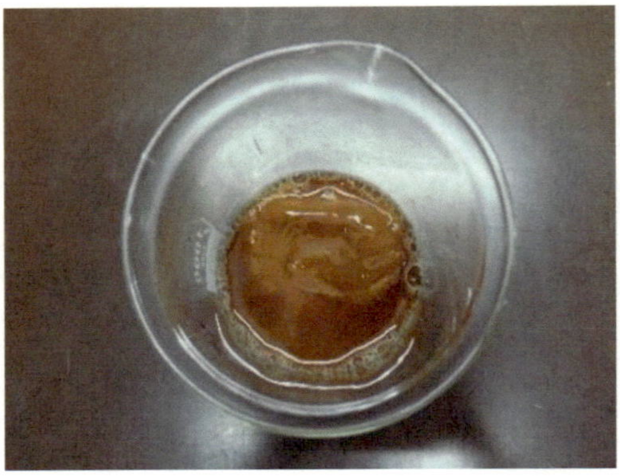

Figure 1.
Fermented black tea using the Kombucha tea fungal mat after 7 days of fermentation.

There are several types of fermentation processes which take place in the production of the beverage and obtained by-products depending on the various metabolic pathways followed by the microorganisms [6]. Kombucha fermentation is a combination of three such pathways: Alcoholic, lactic, and acetic acid production [6]. These pathways take place primarily because of the presence of several yeasts and bacteria coexisting in the medium, where the fermentation is initiated by osmotolerant microorganisms and ultimately dominated by acid-tolerant species [6].

There are many yeast genus and species in the Kombucha culture, where a broad spectrum has been reported by many researchers including *Zygosaccharomyces*, *Candida*, *Kloeckera*/*Hanseniaspora*, *Torulaspora*, *Pichia*, *Brettanomyces*/*Dekkera*, *Saccharomyces*, *Lachancea*, *Saccharomycodes*, *Schizosaccharomyces*, and *Kluyveromyces* [7–10]. The dominant bacteria of the Kombucha tea culture are acetic acid bacteria, which are aerobic and thus, are able to use alcohol as a substrate to form acetic acid [6]. However, in contrast to yeast, these bacteria require large amounts of oxygen for their growth and activity [6]. Tea provides the necessary nitrogen sources for the bacteria and yeast cultures present in the tea fungal mat [11]. Black tea is the traditional and most dominant substrate used for the Kombucha fermentation, which is independent of its comparatively lower caffeine content (2%) as compared with green tea (5%) [12]. This could be because of the comparatively more acceptable sensory qualities and flavor characteristics generated in black tea as a result of the fermentation process.

Some studies have been able to successfully demonstrate the preparation of fermented beverages through the addition of the tea fungus to various types of plant-based products which are essentially not of *Camellia sinensis* origin [13, 14]. Additionally, Watawana et al. [15] has successfully demonstrated the substitution of sugar with other types of sweetening agents for carrying out the fermentation process of the Kombucha beverage. Considering the therapeutic properties of many of the other herbal teas available in the marketplace, whether their antioxidant potential can be enhanced by natural or artificial means is a reasonable query since value-addition to existing beverages for the purpose of novelty and meeting consumer demands is a matter requiring urgent attention in the functional beverage industry.

In this study, the following plant-based herbal teas were fermented by addition of a locally available tea fungal mat: *Acacia arabica* (AA), *Aegle marmelos* root bark (AM-RB), *Aerva lanata* (Ala), *Asteracantha longifolia* (Alo), *Cassia auriculata* (CA), *Hemidesmus indicus* (HI), *Hordeum vulgare* (HV), *Phyllanthus emblica* (PE), *Tinospora cordifolia* (TC). All these herbs which are commonly consumed in Sri Lanka for health and wellness purposes have almost similar taste and color as black tea. This somewhat reassures that the fermented product does not essentially result in any adverse sensory properties which may discourage consumer acceptability.

The selection of herbs was also based with the intention of widening the application of the tea fungus to other types of herbal teas which maybe more readily available depending on the vegetation of various regions and countries. Jayawardena et al. [16] has investigated the antioxidant and starch hydrolase inhibitory potential of these herbs, further justifying their selection as a fermentation medium for preparation of the novel beverages. Identification of the dominant bacteria and yeast species were carried out as well as the changes to the overall population of bacteria and yeast in the broth and pellicle. Other than pH and TA, the enhancement of the antioxidant potential was evaluated. Another aspect of this study was the investigation of the starch hydrolase inhibitory activities, namely α-amylase and α-glucosidase enzyme activities, of the fermented beverages. Starch hydrolase inhibitors retard the absorption of glucose by curbing the action of α-amylase and α-glucosidase [17]. Compounds which are able to impede these enzymes and thereby, delay starch digestion, resulting in a reduction in the rate of glucose absorption, which in turn blunts the postprandial plasma glucose increase in diabetic patients. The enhancement of the starch hydrolase inhibitory potential of the herbal teas through addition of the tea fungal mat was also investigated in this study.

2. Materials and methods

Acetobacter aceti was found to be the dominant bacterial strain present in the tea fungal mat which was used for the study. The dominant yeast components were identified as *Zygosaccharomyces bailii* and *Brettanomyces claussenii*. These aspects were confirmed through DNA sequencing as per the method by Marsh et al. [14]. Dried powders of the plants were obtained from the Ayurveda Medicinal Hall in Kandy, Sri Lanka during the months of June–July 2014.

2.1 Preparation of the fermented beverages and determination of pH, TA and overall population of bacteria and yeast in the broth and pellicle

One gram each of the plant powders were added to 100 mL of boiling water and infused for 5 min followed by filtration through a sterile sieve. Sucrose (10%) was dissolved in each beverage and the preparation was left to cool to room temperature at 24 ± 3°C. The cooled teas were aseptically inoculated with 10 mL of the freshly grown tea fungal broth which was originated from black tea for 7 days at 24 ± 3°C. Sampling was performed on a daily basis in order to avoid contamination. Broths of the fermented beverages were centrifuged at 7240 g for 10 min prior to the assays to remove any particulate matter present as a result of microbial action and coalescence of proteins, which might interfere with the measurements. An electronic pH meter (Orion model 290A) was used to measure the pH of the broths, while the TA was measured according to the method by Chen and Liu [12] using acid-based titration. Fermented broth (10 mL) was titrated with 0.1 M NaOH and the end-point was determined by measuring the pH using the electronic pH meter (Orion model 290A), where pH = 7.0 was taken as the end-point. The final TA of the fermented broths was expressed in g/mL.

Changes to the overall population of bacteria and yeast in the fermented broth and pellicle was determined according to the method by Chen and Liu [12]. Glucose-yeast extract-calcium carbonate agar (GYCA) and potato dextrose agar (PDA) media, were used for the growth of bacteria and yeast, respectively. As per the method by Chen and Liu [12], the GYCA medium was composed of 30 g of glucose, 5 g of yeast extract, 3 g of peptone, 10 g of calcium carbonate, 30 mL of 95% ethanol, 20 g of agar, and distilled water added to make a final volume of 1 L. Aliquots of 1 mL were taken from both the broth and the tea fungal mat, while the upper pellicle portion was filtered with a sterile cheesecloth before sampling to remove the cellulose fibers. Both bacterial and yeast counts were expressed as colony-forming units per mL (cfu/mL).

2.2 Determination of the total phenolic content (TPC) and antioxidant activity

The method by Huang et al. [18] was used for determining the TPC. The results were expressed as milligrams of gallic acid equivalents (GAE) per milliliters (mg GAE/mL), using a gallic acid standard curve. The assay was carried out in 96-well format where the following constituent volumes were added in this particular order to a single well to add up to a total volume of 200 μL per well: Sample / blank (deionized water) / gallic acid standard—20 μL, Folin-Ciocalteu reagent—100 μL, Na_2CO_3 (30 g/L)—80 μL. The microplate was incubated at room temperature for 15 min following which the absorbance was read at 540 nm using a Thermo Scientific Multiskan GO Microplate Reader. The TPC value was back-calculated using the gallic acid standard curve.

The Oxygen Radical Absorbance Capacity (ORAC) assay was carried out according to the methodology by Prior et al. [19]. The final values for this assay were expressed as micromoles of trolox equivalents (TE) per milliliters (μmol TE/mL) using a trolox standard curve. Trolox is a vitamin E analogue and is ideal for the calculation of the ORAC value. This assay was carried out in 96-well format as well [19]. The following components were added to a single well in this particular order, adding up to a total volume of 200 μL per well: (1) Blank (phosphate buffered saline)/ trolox standard/sample—20 μL, (2) fluorescein working solution—160 μL, (3) 2,2′-azobis(2-amidinopropane) dihydrochloride (AAPH)—20 μL. AAPH was added in last since it is a radical initiator and for the reaction kinetics to occur in all wells at the same time point. The reaction kinetics were monitored for two hours as a fluorecence decay [485 nm (ex)/525 nm (em)], following which the area under the curve was used to calculate the ORAC value compared with those of the trolox standards.

As for the di(phenyl)-(2,4,6-trinitrophenyl)iminoazanium (DPPH) radical scavenging activity assay, 100 μL of each of the broths of the fermented beverages were mixed with 1 mL of 0.1 mM DPPH in ethanol along with 450 L of 50 mM Tris-HCl buffer at pH 7.4. The solution was incubated at room temperature for 30 min and reduction of DPPH radicals was measured by reading the absorbance of the resulting solution at 517 nm. The antioxidant activity was calculated as % DPPH radical scavenging activity. Scavenging ability of superoxide radical (O_2^-) was assessed by the method described by Lee et al. [20], and was carried out in 96-well format using the Thermo Scientific Multiskan GO Microplate Reader similar to the TPC and ORAC assays.

2.3 Determination of the α-amylase and α-glucosidase inhibitory activities

The α-amylase inhibitory activity was evaluated according to the method by Liu et al., where acarbose was used as the positive control [17]. The reduction of turbidity at 660 nm was monitored over time using the Thermo Scientific Multiskan GO Microplate Reader, and the area under the curve was used to calculate the overall inhibitory activity. The α-glucosidase inhibitory activity was carried out according to the method by Koh et al., and the same positive control was used in this instance as well [21]. A reaction substrate consisting of 4-nitrophenyl R-D-glucopyranoside (PNPG), (30 mM) and α-glucosidase (16.65 mg/mL) were prepared in phosphate buffer saline (PBS). A volume of 340 μL of inhibitor solutions of different concentrations was pipetted into separate reaction vials. Then, 20 μL of the α-glucosidase solution was added into each vial, and incubated at 37°C for 10 min. The PNPG solution (40 μL) was added to initiate the digestion. After 15 min, 200 μL of 1 M Na_2CO_3 solution was added to terminate the reaction. Aliquots of 300 μL from the reacted solutions were withdrawn and added each well of a 96-well microplate. Absorbance at 400 nm was read using the Thermo Scientific Multiskan GO Microplate Reader.

For both assays, experiments were performed in triplicate, and a curve of percentage inhibition against inhibitor concentration was plotted with the averaged values to back-calculate to the enzyme inhibitory values in the samples. Although for both assays, acarbose equivalence could also be used to express the final enzyme inhibitory data, in this instance, for ease of reference and comparison, the results were expressed as IC_{50} (mg/mL).

2.4 Statistical analysis

For the statistical evaluations, IBM SPSS Statistics version 21.0 released in 2012 (IBM Corp., Armonk, NY, USA) for Windows was used. Three or more independent analyses were utilized to calculate and express the results as mean ± standard error mean (SEM). *P* values of >0.05 were considered to be significant.

3. Results and discussion

As per **Figure 2**, all the beverages had a statistically significant decrease ($P < 0.05$) in the pH values by the end of the fermentation process on day 7. Out of the nine fermented beverages, HI and TC had statistically significant decreases ($P < 0.05$) in the pH from day 1 itself, whereas changes took place slightly later in the rest of the beverages. The decrease in pH of all the Kombucha samples as a whole would have been due to the increased concentration of organic acids (typically in the form of acetic acid) produced during the fermentation process. As per **Figure 1**, all unfermented teas had an initial pH value of between 6.0 and 8.0 prior to fermentation, while the pH values were between 4.0 and 6.0 on day 7 at the end of the fermentation period.

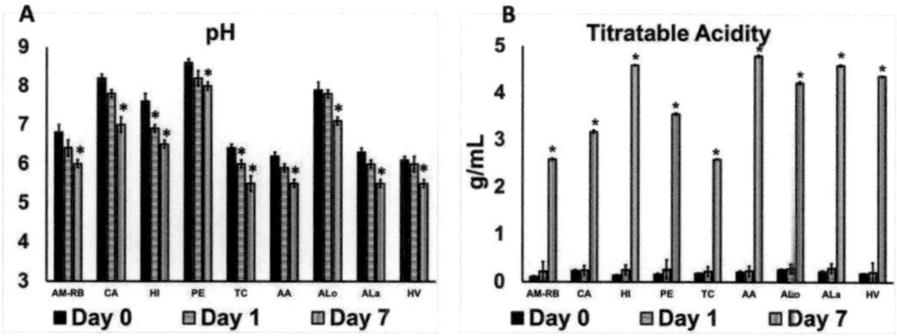

Figure 2.
*The (A) pH and (B) titratable acidity (TA) of the beverages prior to addition of the tea fungal mat (day 0), followed by day 1 and day 7 of fermentation. Values are expressed as mean ± SEM. * P < 0.05 versus the value of each tea at day 0. Abbreviations: Acacia arabica (AA), Aegle marmelos root bark (AM-RB), Aerva lanata (Ala), Asteracantha longifolia (Alo), Cassia auriculata (CA), Hemidesmus indicus (HI), Hordeum vulgare (HV), Phyllanthus emblica (PE), Tinospora cordifolia (TC).*

As per **Figure 2**, the TA of all the unfermented beverages had initial values ranging from 0.1 to 0.5 g/mL. Once the fermentation was complete by day 7, the TA values ranged between 2.5 and 5.0 g/mL, where all beverages had statistically significant increases in this particular parameter ($P < 0.05$). Given that the optimum consumable acidity level is 4.0–4.5 g/L for Kombucha beverages, only AA and HI did not have TA levels falling within this range by the end of the period of fermentation. Nevertheless, on a comparative basis, according to the TA reference levels as indicated by Reiss [5], it may be assumed that all of the Kombucha beverages were acceptable for consumption in terms of acidity.

The TPC and ORAC values are shown in **Figure 3**. AM-RB had the highest TPC prior to fermentation with HV being the lowest. By day 7, statistically significant increases ($P < 0.05$) in the TPC were observed in AM-RB, CA, HI and TC. Correlating with the TPC values, AM-RB had the highest ORAC values with HV being the lowest. The DPPH EC_{50} values appear to have complemented the ORAC values with the exceptions of AM-RB, TC, AA and ALa, where their values were observed to have statistically significant increases ($P < 0.05$) by day 7 (**Figure 3**).

As for the antioxidant assay of superoxide scavenging activity, the trends of increase or decrease whether it be statistically significant or not, were not as clear as the ORAC and DPPH EC_{50} values (**Figure 4**). A better correlation between the TPC and the ORAC values rather than the DPPH EC_{50} and superoxide scavenging values of all beverages on all days of analysis ($R^2 = 0.985$ for ORAC versus $R^2 = 0.745$ DPPH EC_{50} and $R^2 = 0.632$ for superoxide scavenging potential). This showed that the phenolic compounds present in the fermented beverages were better scavengers of the peroxyl radical which is generated through the AAPH.

The starch hydrolase inhibitory activities of α-amylase and α-glucosidase enzymes are shown in **Figure 5**. On the first day of fermentation, only CE, HI, PE and AA had statistically significant increases ($P < 0.05$) in the α-amylase inhibitory activities. However, by day 7 at the end of the fermentation period, all the beverages had statistically significant increases ($P < 0.05$) as compared with day 0. As for the α-glucosidase inhibitory activities, AM-RB, CA, HI, PE, AA, ALa and HV had statistically significant increases ($P < 0.05$) during both day 1 and 7 as compared with day 0. The fermentation process was able to enhance the

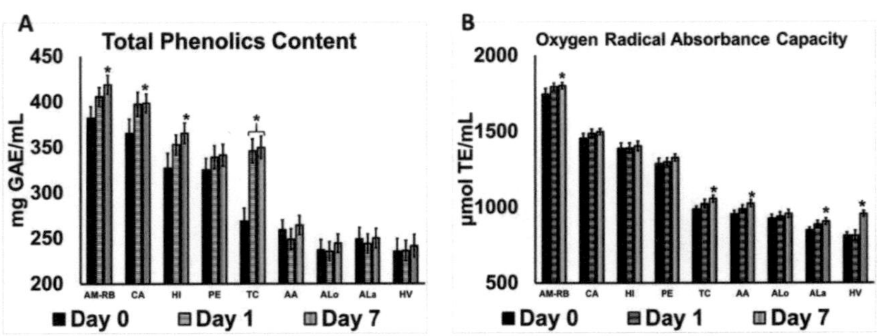

Figure 3.
*The (A) Total phenolic content (TPC) and (B) ORAC values of the herbs prior to addition of the tea fungal mat (day 0), followed by day 1 and day 7 of fermentation. Values are expressed as mean ± SEM. * P < 0.05 versus the value of each tea at day 0. Abbreviations: Acacia arabica (AA), Aegle marmelos root bark (AM-RB), Aerva lanata (Ala), Asteracantha longifolia (Alo), Cassia auriculata (CA), Hemidesmus indicus (HI), Hordeum vulgare (HV), Phyllanthus emblica (PE), Tinospora cordifolia (TC).*

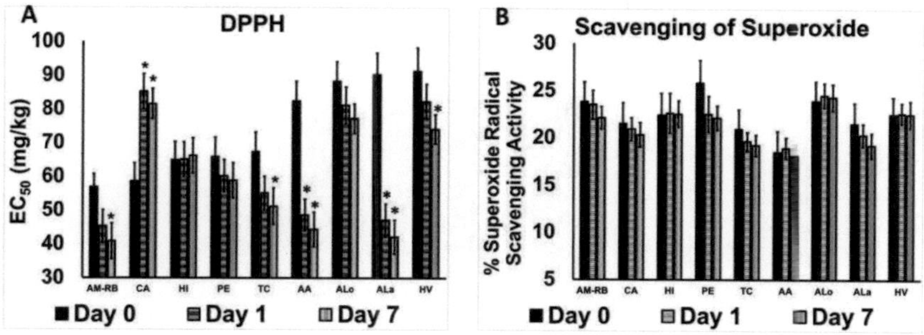

Figure 4.
*The (A) DPPH and (B) superoxide radical scavenging values of the herbs prior to addition of the tea fungal mat (day 0), followed by day 1 and day 7 of fermentation. Values are expressed as mean ± SEM. * P < 0.05 versus the value of each tea at day 0. Abbreviations: Acacia arabica (AA), Aegle marmelos root bark (AM-RB), Aerva lanata (Ala), Asteracantha longifolia (Alo), Cassia auriculata (CA), Hemidesmus indicus (HI), Hordeum vulgare (HV), Phyllanthus emblica (PE), Tinospora cordifolia (TC).*

α-amylase inhibitory activity better than the α-glucosidase inhibitory activity. This is an important aspect, given that α-amylase is required for the subsequent reactions of α-glucosidase, and therefore, curbing the reactivity of α-amylase is important from the perspective of reducing the release of simple sugars into physiological system [22].

Changes to the composition of the overall population of bacteria and yeast present in the broth and pellicle on days 1 and 7 are shown in **Tables 1** and **2**, respectively. As per the measurements from day 0, the inoculum of 10 mL which was added to initiate the fermentation process contained various numbers of bacteria and yeast. However, overall, an increase in the bacteria and yeast population in all of the fermented beverages was observed by the end of the period of fermentation. The increase in these numbers was indicative of the microbes' viability and successful livelihood in the beverages, thus, confirming their ability of thrive in the environments in similar fashion to black tea. An aspect which remains to be investigated concerning this parameter is whether some of the microbes have entered a viable but nonculturable (VBNC) state. Since the origins of the bacteria and yeast are from black tea itself, it is possible that some of the microbes have entered a state of low metabolic activity, and thus were not accounted for during the measurement of this parameter.

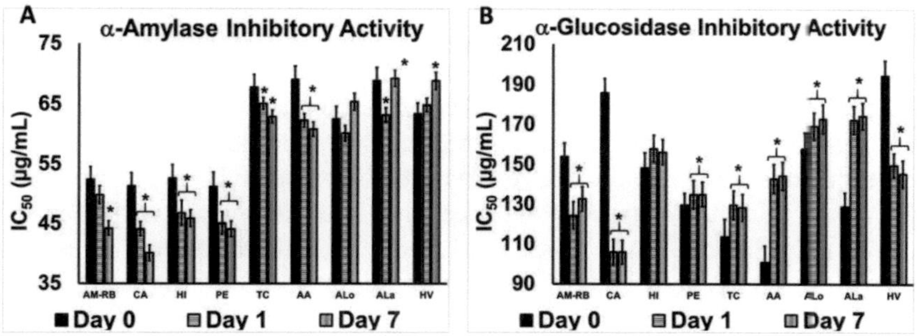

Figure 5.
*α-amylase and α-glucosidase inhibitory activity values of the herbs prior to addition of the tea fungal mat (day 0), followed by day 1 and day 7 of fermentation. Values are expressed as mean ± SEM. * P < 0.05 versus the value of each tea at day 0. Abbreviations: Acacia arabica (AA), Aegle marmelos root bark (AM-RB), Aerva lanata (Ala), Asteracantha longifolia (Alo), Cassia auriculata (CA), Hemidesmus indicus (HI), Hordeum vulgare (HV), Phyllanthus emblica (PE), Tinospora cordifolia (TC).*

Herb	Microbes	Days		
		0 (cfu/mL)	1 (cfu/mL)	7 (cfu/mL)
AA	Bacteria	$2.9 \pm 0.1 \times 10^6$	$8.6 \pm 0.2 \times 10^6$	$3.9 \pm 0.3 \times 10^9$
	Yeast	$1.5 \pm 0.2 \times 10^6$	$8.9 \pm 0.1 \times 10^6$	$9.2 \pm 0.1 \times 10^9$
AM-RB	Bacteria	$3.9 \pm 0.1 \times 10^6$	$6.5 \pm 0.3 \times 10^6$	$9.1 \pm 0.1 \times 10^{10}$
	Yeast	$6.9 \pm 0.2 \times 10^6$	$6.6 \pm 0.2 \times 10^7$	$9.5 \pm 0.1 \times 10^{10}$
ALa	Bacteria	$3.5 \pm 0.1 \times 10^6$	$6.6 \pm 0.2 \times 10^7$	$7.5 \pm 0.2 \times 10^9$
	Yeast	$5.3 \pm 0.1 \times 10^6$	$9.3 \pm 0.2 \times 10^5$	$9.6 \pm 0.1 \times 10^{10}$
ALo	Bacteria	$3.4 \pm 0.2 \times 10^6$	$6.6 \pm 0.2 \times 10^6$	$9.8 \pm 0.1 \times 10^{10}$
	Yeast	$5.1 \pm 0.2 \times 10^6$	$5.5 \pm 0.1 \times 10^7$	$1.8 \pm 0.1 \times 10^{10}$
CA	Bacteria	$1.9 \pm 0.2 \times 10^6$	$2.5 \pm 0.1 \times 10^6$	$3.6 \pm 0.1 \times 10^{10}$
	Yeast	$1.2 \pm 0.2 \times 10^6$	$8.8 \pm 0.2 \times 10^6$	$9.2 \pm 0.1 \times 10^{10}$
HI	Bacteria	$3.6 \pm 0.2 \times 10^6$	$5.9 \pm 0.1 \times 10^6$	$3.9 \pm 0.1 \times 10^{10}$
	Yeast	$5.3 \pm 0.1 \times 10^6$	$6.5 \pm 0.2 \times 10^7$	$9.0 \pm 0.1 \times 10^{10}$
HV	Bacteria	$4.1 \pm 0.1 \times 10^6$	$3.5 \pm 0.3 \times 10^6$	$4.8 \pm 0.1 \times 10^{10}$
	Yeast	$2.5 \pm 0.1 \times 10^6$	$4.4 \pm 0.3 \times 10^5$	$8.0 \pm 0.2 \times 10^{10}$
PE	Bacteria	$1.2 \pm 0.2 \times 10^6$	$3.9 \pm 0.2 \times 10^6$	$7.1 \pm 0.1 \times 10^9$
	Yeast	$3.2 \pm 0.1 \times 10^6$	$5.0 \pm 0.1 \times 10^7$	$8.0 \pm 0.2 \times 10^9$
TC	Bacteria	$1.9 \pm 0.2 \times 10^6$	$3.2 \pm 0.1 \times 10^6$	$2.3 \pm 0.2 \times 10^9$
	Yeast	$4.1 \pm 0.1 \times 10^6$	$8.3 \pm 0.2 \times 10^6$	$1.9 \pm 0.1 \times 10^{10}$

Abbreviations: AA, Acacia arabica; AM-RB, Aegle marmelos root bark; Ala, Aerva lanata; Alo, Asteracantha longifolia; CA, Cassia auriculata; HI, Hemidesmus indicus; HV, Hordeum vulgare; PE, Phyllanthus emblica; TC, Tinospora cordifolia.

Table 1.
Changes to the composition of the overall population of bacteria and yeast present in the broth prior to fermentation (day 0) as well as on day 1 and day 7.

The hypothesis for the increase in the TPC was explained by Blanc [23], where phytases liberated by bacteria and yeast in the tea fungus consortium were identified as capable of liberating polyphenol compounds from the cellulosic backbone of the fermentation medium. This metabolic reaction would have resulted in an increase in the polyphenols in the soluble fraction of the fermented beverages produced in this study. Phytases liberated by bacteria and yeast during Kombucha fermentation are also able of causing degradation of complex polyphenols to smaller molecules which would also result in the increase of TPC. The therapeutic effect of the Kombucha fermentation process has been associated with the increased presence of polyphenols, compounds produced during the fermentation period, and synergistic action between different compounds which are liberated at various stages of the fermentation process [24–26].

The opportunities and challenges for the food and beverage industry in the area of evidence-based functional foods with a low glycemic index which are able to curb the starch digestion rates are on the rise, given the increasing incidence of diabetes throughout the world [27]. Given the noteworthy starch hydrolase inhibitory activities of the fermented herbal beverages generated in this study, their importance in

Herb	Microbes	Days	
		1 (cfu/mL)	7 (cfu/mL)
AA	Bacteria	$3.7 \pm 0.2 \times 10^6$	$2.2 \pm 0.1 \times 10^8$
	Yeast	$1.1 \pm 0.2 \times 10^5$	$1.5 \pm 0.2 \times 10^7$
AM-RB	Bacteria	$1.1 \pm 0.1 \times 10^6$	$1.5 \pm 0.1 \times 10^8$
	Yeast	$1.5 \pm 0.2 \times 10^5$	$5.5 \pm 0.2 \times 10^7$
ALa	Bacteria	$6.6 \pm 0.2 \times 10^6$	$7.5 \pm 0.1 \times 10^8$
	Yeast	$1.5 \pm 0.1 \times 10^5$	$9.2 \pm 0.1 \times 10^7$
ALo	Bacteria	$2.1 \pm 0.2 \times 10^6$	$9.5 \pm 0.1 \times 10^8$
	Yeast	$1.6 \pm 0.2 \times 10^5$	$1.9 \pm 0.1 \times 10^7$
CA	Bacteria	$2.8 \pm 0.1 \times 10^6$	$2.8 \pm 0.1 \times 10^8$
	Yeast	$5.5 \pm 0.1 \times 10^5$	$4.8 \pm 0.2 \times 10^7$
HI	Bacteria	$3.9 \pm 0.1 \times 10^6$	$3.9 \pm 0.1 \times 10^8$
	Yeast	$4.9 \pm 0.1 \times 10^5$	$5.9 \pm 0.3 \times 10^7$
HV	Bacteria	$4.4 \pm 0.2 \times 10^6$	$7.5 \pm 0.1 \times 10^8$
	Yeast	$4.7 \pm 0.1 \times 10^5$	$5.5 \pm 0.1 \times 10^7$
PE	Bacteria	$3.5 \pm 0.1 \times 10^6$	$6.6 \pm 0.2 \times 10^8$
	Yeast	$2.2 \pm 0.1 \times 10^5$	$2.9 \pm 0.1 \times 10^7$
TC	Bacteria	$3.1 \pm 0.1 \times 10^6$	$2.5 \pm 0.1 \times 10^8$
	Yeast	$6.6 \pm 0.1 \times 10^5$	$1.9 \pm 0.2 \times 10^7$

Abbreviations: AA, Acacia arabica; AM-RB, Aegle marmelos root bark; Ala, Aerva lanata; Alo, Asteracantha longifolia; CA, Cassia auriculata; HI, Hemidesmus indicus; HV, Hordeum vulgare; PE, Phyllanthus emblica; TC, Tinospora cordifolia.

Table 2.
Changes to the composition of the overall population of bacteria and yeast present in the pellicle on day 1 and day 7.

support of preventing metabolic diseases such as diabetes could be highlighted in this aspect. Recently, there have been many warnings on the side effects of anti-diabetic drugs such as Rosiglitazone and Pioglitazone which highlight the urgent need of alternative and safer means of blood glucose control—a prospect which could be ideally achieved through functional foods which contain bioactive ingredients with the ability to regulate blood glucose concentration toward the normal range [28].

Last but not least, the selection of a particular fermentation period for this study requires justification. The beverages and their analytical parameters were monitored for 7 days. This was the minimum duration by which the fermented beverages could be consumed without the presence of metabolic artifacts resulting from prolonged fermentation according to literature [25, 29, 30]. In particular, according to the study by Amarasinghe et al. [30] where the study was conducted for monitoring the fermentation for a period of 8 weeks, the Kombucha samples displayed a decrease in the antioxidant activity during the 2 months of fermentation. This was suggestive that suggestive the functional properties of the beverage had decreased. It was also implied in this study that it is possible through prolonged fermentation to result in the accumulation of organic acids, which might reach harmful levels for direct consumption [30].

4. Conclusions

Given the ease of preparation of the beverages which were investigated in this study, as well as the economic viability, the products could be promoted as functional beverages which could be consumed as means of supportive therapy. In particular, they could be used for the prevention and containment of disease conditions in association with their demonstrated antioxidant and starch hydrolase inhibitory properties. Although the therapeutic mechanisms of action of these beverages in the human physiology is yet to be elucidated. However, this study serves as a platform for the identification and promotion of some novel beverages as functional food which can be easily prepared in households using edible plants. Nevertheless, having mentioned as such, during the selection of plant material for fermentation with the Kombucha tea fungal mats, care needs to be taken to identify plant-based material which carry similar sensory perceptions as black tea, thus, reducing the chances of the fermented products possessing adverse sensory perceptions.

During this study, the sensory evaluations of the novel fermented beverages was not carried out. This is one aspect which needs to be explored in future studies. It is only hypothesized in this instance that the organoleptic properties would be acceptable, since the teas are similar in physical properties to *Camellia sinensis*-based tea. However, for a proper verification, sensory evaluation needs to be carried out.

The microbial interactions taking place during the fermentation needs to be investigated further as well. For instance, as mentioned previously, whether the microbes undergo a state of VBNC needs to be elucidated. Additionally, whether microorganisms which have probiotic effects such as *Lactobacillus* spp., and *Bifidobacterium* are able to thrive in the fermented beverage and thus be incorporated, is an aspect worth exploring as well. Should this be successful, the consumer value of the beverages would increase and have a superior marketability due to its combined functional properties of comprising of phenolic compounds as well as probiotics.

Acknowledgements

Dr. Waisundara would like to express her gratitude to Miss Mindani I. Watawana and Miss Nilakshi Jayawardena—former Research Assistants at the National Institute of Fundamental Studies and Miss Candy Choo of Temasek School of Applied Sciences, Temasek Polytechnic, Singapore, for their assistance rendered toward the experimental work.

Conflict of interest

The author has no conflicts of interest to declare, financial or otherwise.

Author details

Viduranga Yashasvi Waisundara
Department of Food Technology, Faculty of Technology, Rajarata University of Sri Lanka, Mihintale, Sri Lanka

*Address all correspondence to: viduranga@gmail.com

References

[1] Jayabalan R, Malbaša RV, Lončar ES, Vitas JS, Sathishkumar M. A review on Kombucha tea—Microbiology, composition, fermentation, beneficial effects, toxicity, and tea fungus. Comprehensive Reviews in Food Science and Food Safety. 2014;**13**:538-550. DOI: 10.1111/1541-4337.12073

[2] Jayabalan R, Malini K, Muthuswamy S, Swaminathan K, Yun SE. Biochemical characteristics of tea fungus produced during Kombucha fermentation. Food Science and Biotechnology. 2010;**19**:843-847

[3] Malbaša RV, Lončar ES, Vitas JS, Čanadanović-Brunet JM. Influence of starter cultures on the antioxidant activity of kombucha beverage. Food Chemistry. 2011;**127**:1727-1731

[4] Jayabalan R, Marimuthu S, Swaminathan K. Changes in content of organic acids and tea polyphenols during kombucha tea fermentation. Food Chemistry. 2007;**102**:392-398

[5] Reiss J. Influence of different sugars on the metabolism of the tea fungus. Zeitschrift fur Lebensmittel-Untersuchung und-For-schung. 1994;**198**:258-261

[6] Villarreal-Soto VA, Beaufort S, Bouajila J, Souchard JP, Taillandier P. Understanding Kombucha tea fermentation: A review. Journal of Food Science. 2018;**83**(3):580-588. DOI: 10.1111/1750-3841.14068

[7] Chakravorty S, Bhattacharya S, Chatzinotas A, Chakraborty W, Bhattacharya D, Gachhui R. Kombucha tea fermentation: Microbial and biochemical dynamics. International Journal of Food Microbiology. 2016;**220**:63-72. DOI: 10.1016/j.ijfoodmicro.2015.12.015

[8] Coton M, Pawtowski A, Taminiau B, Burgaud G, Deniel F, Coulloumme-Labarthe L, et al. Unraveling microbial ecology of industrial-scale Kombucha fermentations by metabarcoding and culture-based methods. FEMS Microbiology Ecology. 2017;**93**(5):1-16. DOI: 10.1093/femsec/fix048

[9] Marsh AJ, Hill C, Ross RP, Cotter PD. Fermented beverages with healthpromoting potential: Past and future perspectives. Trends in Food Science and Technology. 2014;**38**(2):113-124. DOI: 10.1016/j.tifs.2014.05.002

[10] Marsh AJ, O'Sullivan O, Hill C, Ross RP, Cotter PD. Sequence-based analysis of the bacterial and fungal compositions of multiple Kombucha (tea fungus) samples. Food Microbiology. 2014;**38**:171-178. DOI: 10.1016/j.fm.2013.09.003

[11] Sreeramulu G, Zhu Y, Knol W. Kombucha fermentation and its antimicrobial activity. Journal of Agricultural and Food Chemistry. 2000;**48**:2589-2594

[12] Chen C, Liu BY. Changes in major components of tea fungus metabolites during prolonged fermentation. Journal of Applied Microbiology. 2000;**89**:834-839

[13] Watawana MI, Jayawardena N, Waisundara VY. Enhancement of the functional properties of coffee through fermentation by "tea fungus" (Kombucha). Journal of Food Processing and Preservation. 2015;**39**(6):2596-2603. DOI: 10.1111/jfpp.12509

[14] Watawana MI, Jayawardena N, Gunawardhana CB, Waisundara VY. Enhancement of the antioxidant and starch hydrolase inhibitory activities of king coconut water (*Cocos nucifera* var. *aurantiaca*) by fermentation with Kombucha "tea fungus".

International Journal of Food Science and Technology. 2016;**51**(2):490-498. DOI: 10.1111/ijfs.13006

[15] Watawana MI, Jayawardena N, Ranasinghe SJ, Waisundara VY. Evaluation of the effect of different sweetening agents on the polyphenol contents and antioxidant and starch hydrolase inhibitory properties of Kombucha. Journal of Food Processing and Preservation. 2017;(1):41. DOI: 10.1111/jfpp.12752

[16] Jayawardena N, Watawana MI, Waisundara VY. Evaluation of the total antioxidant capacity, polyphenol contents and starch hydrolase inhibitory activity of ten edible plants in an *in vitro* model of digestion. Plant Foods for Human Nutrition. 2015;**70**:71-76. DOI: 10.1007/s11130-014-0463-4

[17] Liu T, Song L, Wang H, Huang DJ. A high-throughput assay for quantification of starch hydrolase inhibition based on turbidity measurement. Journal of Agricultural and Food Chemistry. 2011;**59**:9756-9762

[18] Huang D, Ou BX, Hampsch-Woodill M, Flanagan JA, Deemer EK. Development and validation of oxygen radical absorbance capacity assay for lipophilic antioxidants using randomly methylated b-cyclodextrin as the solubility enhancer. Journal of Agricultural and Food Chemistry. 2002;**50**:1815-1821

[19] Prior RL, Hoang H, Gu LW, Wu XL, Bacchiocca M, Howard L, et al. Assays for hydrophilic and lipophilic antioxidant capacity [oxygen radical absorbance capacity ($ORAC_{FL}$)] of plasma and other biological food samples. Journal of Agricultural and Food Chemistry. 2003;**51**:3273-3279

[20] Lee JC, Kim HR, Jim K, Jang YS. Antioxidant property of an ethanol extract of the stem of *Opuntia ficus indica* var. saboten. Journal of Agricultural and Food Chemistry. 2002;**50**:6490-6496

[21] Koh LW, Wong LL, Loo YY, Kasapis S, Huang DJ. Evaluation of different teas against starch digestibility by mammalian glycosidases. Journal of Agricultural and Food Chemistry. 2009;**58**:148-154

[22] Waisundara VY. Assessment of bioaccessibility: A vital aspect for determining the efficacy of superfoods. In: Superfoods. Croatia: InTech Open; 2018. pp. 67-80. DOI: 10.5772/intechopen.73152

[23] Blanc PJ. Characterization of the tea fungus metabolites. Biotechnology Letters. 1996;**8**:139-142

[24] Jayabalan R, Marimuthu S, Thangaraj P, Sathishkumar M, Binupriya AR, Swaminathan K, et al. Preservation of Kombucha tea: Effect of temperature on tea components and free radical scavenging properties. Journal of Agricultural and Food Chemistry. 2008;**56**:9064-9071

[25] Jayabalan R, Subathradevi P, Marimuthu S, Sathishkumar M, Swaminathan K. Changes in free-radical scavenging ability of kombucha tea during fermentation. Food Chemistry. 2008;**109**:227-234

[26] Watawana MI, Jayawardena N, Gunawardhana CB, Waisundara VY. Health, wellness, and safety aspects of the consumption of Kombucha. Journal of Chemistry. 2015:1-11. DOI: 10.1155/2015/591869

[27] Stumvoll M, Goldstein BJ, van Haeften TW. Type 2 diabetes: Pathogenesis and treatment. Lancet. 2006;**371**:2153-2156

[28] Graham DJ, Ouellet-Hellstrom R, McCurdy TE, Ali F, Sholley C, Worrall C, et al. Risk of acute myocardial infarction, stroke, heart

failure and death in elderly medicare patients treated with rosiglitazone or pioglitazone. Journal of the American Medical Association. 2010;**304**:411-418

[29] Chu SC, Chen CH. Effects of origins and fermentation time on the antioxidant activities of kombucha. Food Chemistry. 2006;**98**:502-507

[30] Amarasinghe H, Weerakkody NS, Waisundara VY. Evaluation of physicochemical properties and antioxidant activities of kombucha "tea fungus" during extended periods of fermentation. Food Science & Nutrition. 2018;**6**:659-665. DOI: 10.1002/fsn3.605

Chapter 3

The Role of UV-Visible Spectroscopy for Phenolic Compounds Quantification in Winemaking

Jose Luis Aleixandre-Tudo and Wessel du Toit

Abstract

Phenolic compounds are bioactive substances present in a large number of food products including wine. The importance of these compounds in wine is due to their large effect on the organoleptic attributes of wine. Phenolic compounds play a crucial role in the colour as well as mouthfeel properties of wines. UV-visible spectroscopy appears as a suitable technique for the evaluation of phenolic compounds' properties and content. The ability of the phenolic ring to absorb UV light and the fact that some of the phenolic substances are coloured compounds, i.e. show absorption features in the visible region, make UV-visible spectroscopy a suitable technique to investigate and quantify grape and wine phenolic compounds. A number of analytical techniques are currently used for phenolic quantification. These include both simpler approaches (spectrophotometric determinations) as well as more complex methodologies such liquid chromatography analysis. Moreover, a number of spectroscopy applications have also been recently reported and are becoming popular within the wine industry. This chapter reviews information on the UV-visible spectral properties of phenolic compounds, changes occurring during wine ageing and also discusses the current UV-visible based analytical techniques used for the quantification of phenolic compounds in grapes and wine.

Keywords: UV-visible, spectrophotometry, phenolic compounds, anthocyanins, tannins, liquid chromatography, spectroscopy, chemometrics, fluorescence

1. Introduction

Phenolic compounds are bioactive molecules that are involved in some of the most relevant wine organoleptic attributes. Phenolic substances have been reported as being responsible for wine colour, mouthfeel perception and flavour. The appropriate management of the phenolic accumulation in the berry, extraction during the skin contact phase as well as the evolution during ageing in barrels or bottles will ensure a desired phenolic content and composition that will lead to a good quality wine [1]. Furthermore, the ability of phenolic molecules to act as antioxidant has placed this group of compounds in the spotlight of a considerable amount of research. Phenolic compounds have been reported as effective antioxidants and their preventive role against inflammatory, neurodegenerative, cardiovascular diseases or even against cancer has been widely acknowledged [2]. The quantification of phenolic compounds is thus of high importance and UV-visible spectroscopy has proven to be one of the most suitable and reliable techniques to quantify these substances during the winemaking process.

The accumulation of the amino acid phenylalanine is the first step towards the biosynthesis of phenolic compounds. Phenolic substances or polyphenols are thus secondary metabolites that contain at least one aromatic ring and one or several hydroxyl groups. Two main families of phenolic compounds are generally classified as the non-flavonoids and the flavonoids. Phenolic acids, including hydroxycinnamic and hydroxybenzoic acids and stilbens are part of the structurally less complex non-flavonoid group (**Figure 1**). Flavonoids share a common C3-C6-C3 structure and contain flavonols, anthocyanins and flavanols, with the latter also known as proanthocyanidins or more widely as tannins [3]. The biosynthesis and accumulation of these key substances is due to a number of plant biological functions which include growth, plant reproduction and plant protection roles against environmental signals as well as biotic and abiotic stresses [4].

Phenolic compounds are released from the solid parts of the berries into the must during the winemaking process. The contact period refers to the period of time that the must is in contact with the skins and seeds and generally coincides with the alcoholic fermentation. The presence or absence of the solid parts during the winemaking process will determine the phenolic content and composition. In white winemaking the skin contact period is limited to a minimum and the levels of phenolic compounds found in wines are thus lower than in red wines (where the fermentation takes place in the presence of skins and seeds). Due to its location in the flesh, hydroxycinnamic acids are therefore the main phenolic compounds found in white wines. On the contrary, red wines contain high levels of tannins, anthocyanins and flavonol compounds that are extracted from the solid parts of the berries during the aforementioned skin contact phase [5].

Among the subclasses of phenolic compounds found in grapes, two of the subfamilies are mostly of importance to wine production. Anthocyanins are coloured compounds responsible for the red wine colour attributes. The state of the anthocyanins and the wine medium conditions have a major impact on the final wine colour. Anthocyanins are found in red grapes and wines in five mono-glucoside forms. The 3-glucoside forms of delphinidin, cyanidin, petunidin, peonidin and malvidin are present in *Vitis vinifera* cultivars (**Figure 2**). Monomeric anthocyanins are highly reactive substances involved in a large number of reactions and interactions. Simple anthocyanins are acylated with a number of grape components such as acetic acid, *p*-coumaric or caffeic acid, they are also able to combine with themselves through intra- and intermolecular copigmentation interactions [6]. During the winemaking and ageing processes further reactions to form pyranoanthocyanins have also been documented, in combination with several associations with tannins, some of them through acetaldehyde mediated reactions. Anthocyanin interactions and reactions lead to a number of complex pigments with increased

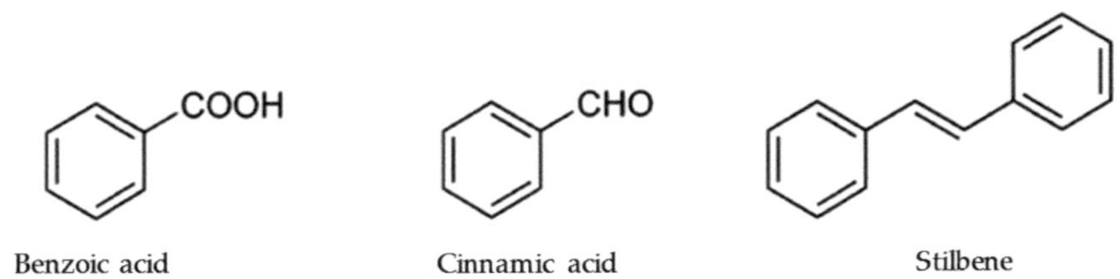

Figure 1.
Chemical structure of the non-flavonoid group of phenolic compounds found in grapes and wines.

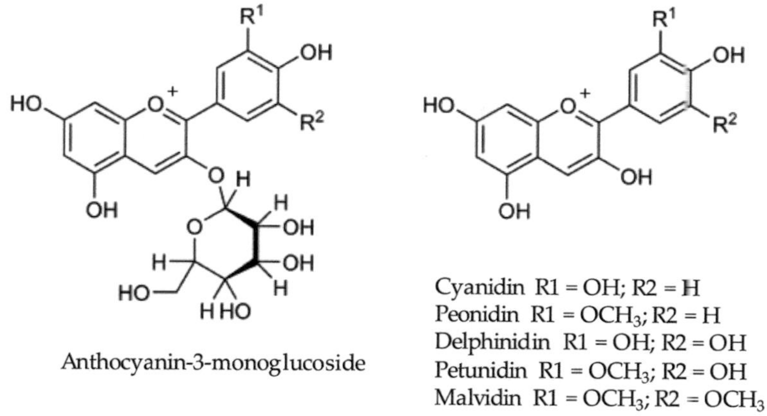

Figure 2.
Chemical structure of the main anthocyanins found in grapes and wines.

stability during wine ageing. These combinations also entail a modification of the anthocyanin coloration, phenomena that gives rise to the large variety of red and brown based colours found in red wines [7]. Additionally, tannin-anthocyanin interactions give rise to a decrease in the ability of tannins to elicit astringency [8].

Proanthocyanidins or tannins are the most abundant class of phenolic compounds. Tannins are polymeric compounds of varying size and structure, containing a combination of five flavanol monomers. The polymerisation of catechin, epicatechin, gallocatechin, epigallocatechin and catechin gallate subunits gives rise to larger and more polymerised tannin compounds (**Figure 3**) with varying ability to elicit astringency and bitterness [3, 9]. The reactivity of the hydroxyl groups towards salivary proteins creates a macromolecular complex that precipitates from solution and leads to a puckering and drying sensation, also known as astringency. Small molecular weight tannins are initially bitter and they became more astringent as the molecular size increases [9]. Young wines, initially more astringent, contain tannins that have been polymerising and have therefore and increased ability to react with salivary proteins. During the ageing process several phenomena explain why the wines become softer (less astringent). When a certain molecular size is reached the tannin molecule may become insoluble, thus precipitating from solution and lowering the tannin content of the wines. Moreover, as molecules grow in size, its conformation might hinder the tannin protein interactions which will also lead to decreased astringency intensity. It is also possible that large tannin molecules cleavages give rise to smaller and less astringent tannins. Finally, the tannin-anthocyanin combinations that take place during the ageing process may also be involved in the decrease of the astringency intensity experienced in older wines [1, 10].

The use of UV and visible light for the quantification of chemical compounds is a widely used technique [1]. Due to their biochemical and molecular properties, phenolic compounds are highly suitable to be quantified with UV-visible light. The ability of the phenolic ring to absorb UV light is exploited to quantify these compounds [11]. In addition to this, visible light can also provide valuable information due to the coloured nature of some of the phenolic compounds (e.g. red anthocyanins or yellow flavonols). The UV-visible spectra of a wine is thus attributed to the electronic transitions occurring within the hydroxyl groups of the phenolic molecules, with different transitions corresponding to the different phenolic subclasses [12]. A number of UV-visible applications have been exploited to quantify phenolic compounds. Among these the use of UV-visible spectrophotometry to estimate the content of phenolic compounds stands out as the most widely used approach. A number of methods have been optimised for the different phenolic subclasses, making nowadays the efficient estimation of

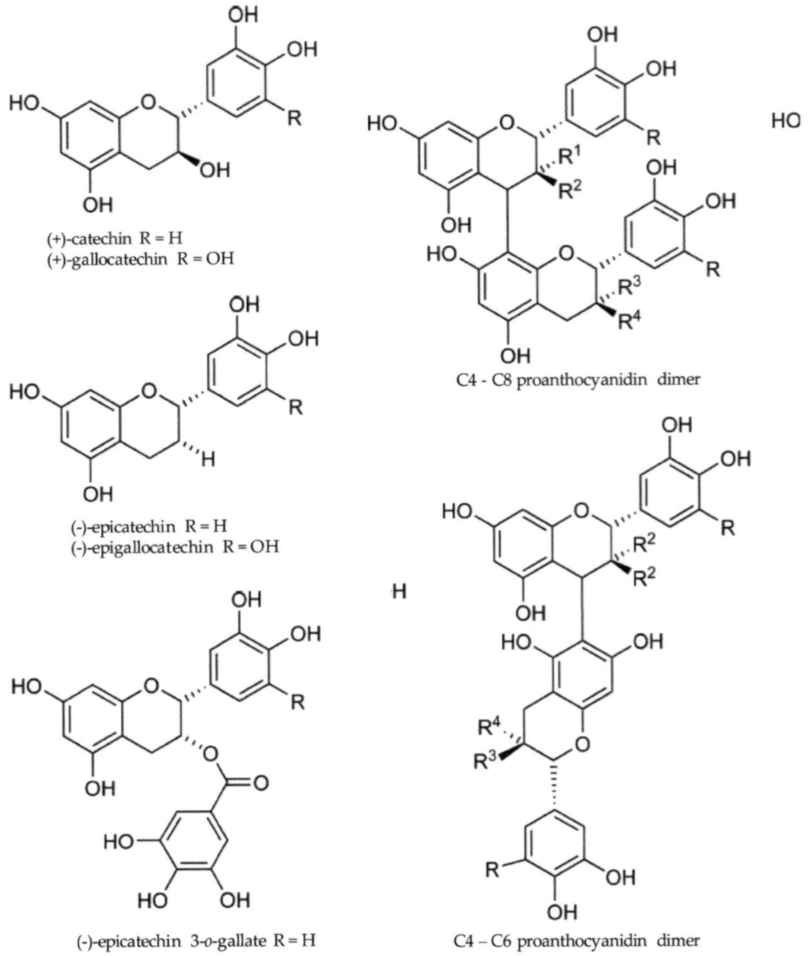

Figure 3.
Chemical structure of flavan-3-ol compounds found in grapes and wines.

phenolic content using a simple UV-visible spectrophotometer possible [1]. However, UV-visible spectroscopy is also used in more advanced separation techniques, such as liquid chromatography, that allows for the quantification of individual phenolic compounds [13]. The quantification of phenolic compounds is thus achieved through the UV-visible signal given by the individually separated phenolic compounds. On the other hand, fluorescence spectroscopy also makes use of the UV-visible spectral features of the excited substances. After the excitation process a coloured fluorophore is quantified based on its absorption intensity projected in the visible region [14]. Finally, UV-visible spectroscopy combined with chemometrics is also included in the techniques used for phenolic compounds' quantification [15]. In this case the spectral properties are used to predict the phenolic content of a given grape phenolic extract or wine [16]. This approach makes use of partial least squares regression analysis to correlate spectral information with reference data (phenolic levels). If successfully performed, a validated calibration can provide accurate predictions of phenolic content by only measuring the UV-visible spectral properties of wines.

This manuscript, in its different sections, reports therefore the current status of the different analytical techniques available for the quantification of phenolic content in grapes and wines. Moreover, the UV-visible spectral features observed in wines during the winemaking process, from the early stages of fermentation and through the ageing process are also reported and discussed.

DOI: http://dx.doi.org/10.5772/intechopen.79550

2. UV-visible features of wines during winemaking and ageing

Among other analytical techniques, UV-visible spectroscopy appears to be suitable for the quantification of phenolic compounds. This is due to two main reasons. First of all, phenolic substances have the ability to strongly absorb UV light [11] and secondly, certain compounds due to the coloured nature can lead to absorption features in the visible range [17]. Polyphenols are biological compounds containing π conjugated systems with hydroxyl-phenolic groups. The π type molecular orbitals electronic transitions provide the UV-visible spectrum of this group of compounds. UV-visible spectroscopy is used in winemaking to quantify different sub-groups within the phenolic family [18]. The most common procedures for phenolic analysis are reported to quantify anthocyanins, phenolic acids (including hydroxycinnamates and hydroxybenzoates), stilbenes, flavonols and flavanols or tannins.

The main absorption feature of the flavanol monomers is a strong absorption band around 280 nm (**Figure 4c**). These colourless compounds do not show absorption features in the visible region of the electromagnetic spectrum. The flavanol monomers may contain a galloyl molecule attached to the flavan-3-ol structure. A galloylated flavanol has been reported to have higher absorption intensity, when compared to its non-galloylated form, it also shows a shoulder at 310 nm, characteristic of the galloyl group (see gallic acid as example in **Figure 4d**) [11]. For flavanol polymers or tannins the absorption features remain the same despite the degree of polymerisation (number of monomers) of the proanthocyanidin structure with a predominant absorption band at 280 nm.

Anthocyanin compounds co-exist under different forms and its colour intensity and tonality depends on the proportion of the different molecular structures

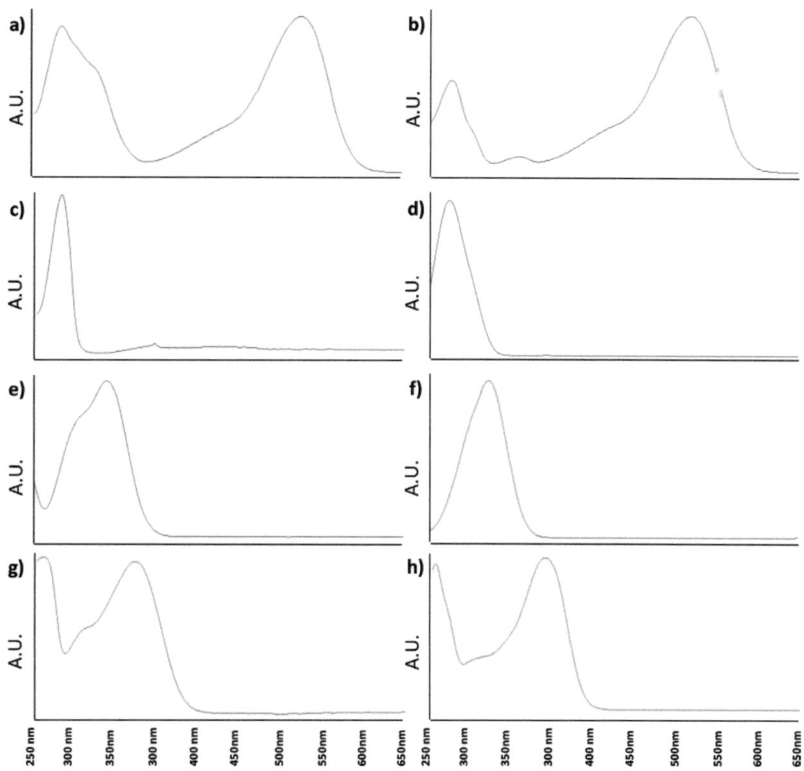

Figure 4.
UV-vis spectral properties of individual phenolic compounds. (a) Malvidin-3-glucoside, (b) malvidin-3-p-coumarylglucoside, (c) catechin, (d) gallic acid, (e) caftaric acid, (f) coutaric acid, (g) rutin, (h) quercetin.

present at the time of evaluation. The main absorption features of this phenolic subfamily are given by an intense absorption band at 280 nm, common to all phenolic substances, and by a characteristic absorption intensity around 520 nm characteristic of red colouring substances (**Figure 4a**). In addition, the anthocyanins are found in grapes and wines acylated with a number of other wine components, including some phenolic acids such as caffeic or *p*-coumaric acids [3]. In this case the anthocyanin molecule will also show a characteristic broad band around 320 nm (see malvidin-3-*p*-coumarylglucoside in **Figure 4b**). Anthocyanins are highly reactive phenolic compounds strongly influenced by the pH conditions and by the presence of SO_2 [19]. Lower pH values increase the proportion of anthocyanins present in the red flavylium form, leading to increased colour intensity, through an hyperchromic effect in the visible region. The opposite behaviour is thus observed if the wine's pH increases to higher values, leading to a decrease of the absorption intensity at 520 nm (hypochromic effect). On the other hand, the ability of anthocyanins to exist in its red forms is highly dependent on the SO_2 content. Sulphur dioxide has the ability to interact and combine with the anthocyanin molecule in position 4 of the central phenolic ring, causing the decolouration of the chromophore, leading to a colourless flavilium sulphonate [6]. The protective role of sulphur dioxide is due to its ability as antioxidant. In the case of the anthocyanins, SO_2 protects the non-coloured anthocyanin in solution until, due to the reversible nature of this reactions, the red anthocyanin chromophore is liberated.

Phenolic acids in grapes and wines include both hydroxycinnamic and hydoxybenzoic acids. Hydroxybenzoic acids, such as gallic acid, show a single intense absorption band at 280 nm, common to all phenolic substances (**Figure 4d**). On the other hand, hydroxycinnamic acids show an absorption band around 320 nm, characteristic of this group of compounds (**Figure 4e** (caftaric acid) and f (coutaric acid)). Finally, the flavonol group show also particular UV-visible absorption features with an additional absorption band around 360 nm (**Figure 4g** (rutin) and h (quercetin)). This absorption band together with the 280 nm absorption features define the UV-visible spectra of the flavonol group.

Grape phenolic compounds are released into the must after the crushing operation. Phenolic compounds are initially located in the solid parts of the berries. Seeds, skins and to a lesser extent, stems, are the main sources of phenolic compounds found in wines. During crushing the juice contained in the berries comes in contact with skins and seeds. Subsequently, during the maceration step this contact will lead to the diffusion of the phenolic substances into the must. While tannins are found in both skins and seed tissues, the anthocyanins are only located in the skins (also found in the flesh of a few tenturier cultivars). Hydroxycinnamic acids are, on the contrary, the only group of phenolic compounds that is found in high levels in the flesh, whereas hydroxybenzoic acids (seeds), stilbenes (skins) and flavonols (skins) are found mainly in the solid parts of the grape berries [4]. The winemaking strategy i.e. presence or absence of skin contact, length and conditions of the skin contact and grape characteristics will define the pool of phenolic compounds that will be present in the wine after the fermentation. Due to this phenolic extraction, important changes in the UV-visible spectral feature take place.

Figure 5 shows the average UV-visible spectral features of 13 different red wines during the first 15 days of the fermentation that included cultivars such as Cabernet Sauvignon, Shiraz, Grenache or Pinotage. Three main absorption bands are observed in the UV-visible spectral features. The first and more prominent band is observed around 280 nm. Following this, broad high intensity absorption properties are also observed around 320 nm. Finally, a third intense absorption band is identified in the visible region around 520 nm. As can be observed in **Figure 5**, right after crushing (Day 0) low absorption intensity bands are observed in the 280 and 320 regions,

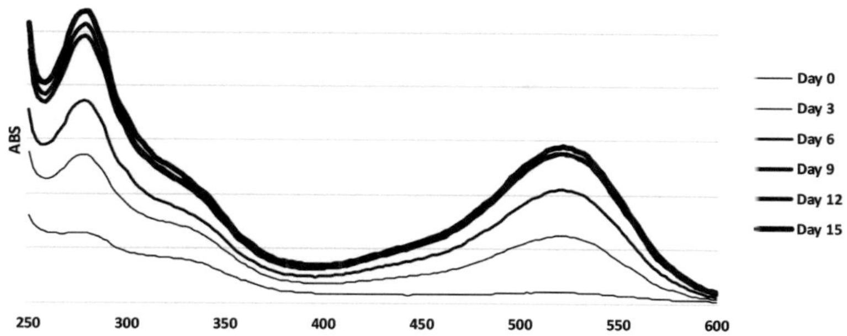

Figure 5.
UV-visible spectral features (250–600 nm) of red wines during fermentation.

whereas no absorption is observed at the visible anthocyanin absorbing 520 nm region. This can be explained by the instant release of some of the phenolic compounds located in the flesh such as the hydroxycinnamic acids. As fermentation progresses a hyperchromic effect is rapidly observed during the first days after crushing. The absorption band around 280 nm rapidly increases until Day 9 of fermentation. From then on, an increase is still identified but to a lesser extent than that initially observed. A different behaviour is observed for the absorption features around 320 and 520 nm. For these two regions, the intense hyperchromism is observed until Day 9 with no subsequent significant increase until the completion of fermentation.

Anthocyanins are water soluble compounds that are extracted during the early stages of fermentation. Alongside with the anthocyanins, the extraction of other skin-localised phenolics, such as flavonols and flavanols or tannins also takes place. However, as alcohol content increases, seed phenolics, mainly flavanols and tannins, are released into the must. The later extraction of seed flavanols and tannins requires the hydrolysis of the lipidic layer around the seed as well as the hydration of the seed tissue itself. Seed tannins have been defined as more astringent and bitter tannins while skin tannins have been described as softer or less reactive towards proteins [10]. The flavanol content in terms of individual composition (procyanidins or prodelphinidins), galloylated subunits and mean degree of polymerisation will provide the intensity and sub qualities of the bitterness and astringency perception of wines [9]. The intense absorption band at 230 nm is due to the extraction of flavonols, hydroxycinnamic acids, flavanols and the UV absorption part of the anthocyanins. The band observed around 320 nm is purely ascribed to the hydroxycinnamic acids. Finally, the band observed at 520 nm is due to the anthocyanin extraction during fermentation. The further increase in the absorption intensity at 280 nm after Day 9 may be due to further extraction of seed tannin content material.

Phenolic compounds are highly reactive and a large number of interactions and reactions can take place during wine ageing and storage. Some of these phenolic reactions benefit from the presence of oxygen during the barrel ageing period. This is the case for some of the direct tannin-anthocyanin complexes as well as the indirectly acetaldehyde mediated tannin-anthocyanin reactions. On the other hand, the absence or shortage of oxygen during the bottle ageing period will stimulate tannin polymerisation reactions and also some direct tannin-anthocyanin combinations. **Figure 6** shows the average UV-visible spectra of a number of commercial red wines after the fermentation process was completed as well as after a year of barrel ageing (12 months after fermentation is completed), followed by a year of bottle ageing (24 months of fermentation completion). In this case an average spectra of a large number of wines including Cabernet Sauvignon, Pinotage, Shiraz, Merlot,

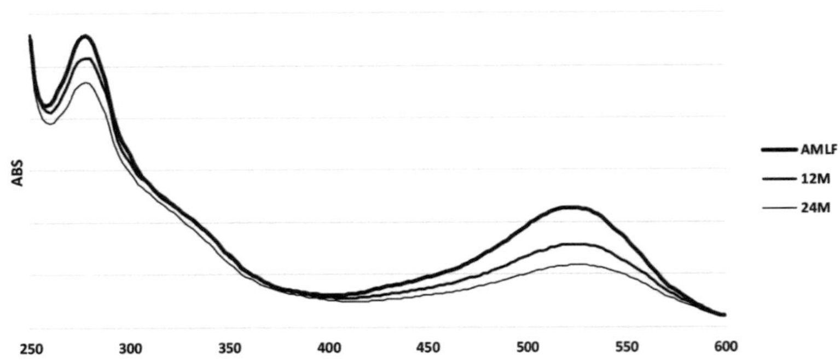

Figure 6.
UV-visible spectral features of wines after malolactic fermentation completion (AMLF) and at 12 months of barrel ageing (12M), followed by 12 months of bottle ageing (24M).

Ruby Cabernet, Petit Verdot, Cinsault, Malbec, Grenache, Pinot Noir and Cabernet Franc was evaluated. The most important features are observed at 280 and 520 nm, whereas the broad band at 320 nm remained constant over the ageing period. It is also important to mention that the bigger decrease in absorption intensity was observed at the 520 nm region which corresponds to the visible absorption part of the anthocyanins.

After reaching maximum levels during the fermentation process, anthocyanin content starts decreasing. Anthocyanins are involved in a large number of phenomena, such as degradation, oxidation, reabsorption into grape and yeast cell walls, precipitation with tartaric salts, interaction with SO_2 or reaction with tannins, among others [7]. Despite this, red wines still maintain an intense colour during ageing which is due to the transformation of anthocyanins into longer term stable polymeric pigments. Anthocyanins give rise to a number of pigments from acylation with diverse grape components, intra and intermolecular copigmentation reactions and interactions, occurring early during the process, to more complex reaction leading to pyranoanthocyanin or tannin-anthocyanin complexes formation [7]. The limited decrease observed around 280 nm is attributed to a larger extent to the decrease of the UV absorption ability of the anthocyanins and to a lesser extent to a decrease of tannin compounds through precipitation. Tannins are also highly reactive substances with high affinity for proteins and polysaccharides, which can lead to tannins precipitation. In addition, the polymerisation ability of these compounds may result in insoluble larger molecules that also precipitate from solution, thus reducing its content in wine. Finally, the absorption band around 320 nm remains stable during ageing, indicating stability of this region absorbing compounds during barrel and bottle ageing.

3. Spectrophotometric methods for phenolic analysis

3.1 Total phenolic content

Total phenolic index (TPI). The measurement of UV-visible absorption light to quantify phenolic compounds was first proposed in the late 1950's. The absorbance at 280 nm was selected as the best indicator of the phenolic content in wine due to the ability of phenolic substances, and more specifically the phenolic ring, to absorb UV light [20]. A simple wine or grape extract dilution is used to quantify the total phenolic content or total phenolic index (TPI). The TPI corresponds to the A280 nm times the dilution factor. The dilution factor might change depending on the sample under evaluation, as well as the path length of the cuvette. Dilution factors of 100 and 50 have been reported for red wines. Depending on the extraction methods dilution factors between 50 and 20 for grape extracts have been proposed. In the case of white and rose wines, with lower phenolic levels, the dilution factor needs to be adjusted. In this case dilution factors from 5 to 20 have been used. The TPI can also be expressed as gallic acid equivalents when used as a standard. This method has been reported to be simple, fast and reliable, although overestimation of the total phenolic content occurs due to the ability of other grape component that also absorb UV-light. A value of 4 units, that can be subtracted from the index, has been proposed to account for the interferences caused by these other UV absorbing material. Additionally, some other phenolic compounds such as cinnamic acids or chalcones do not show absorption features at 280 nm, however due to its low content in wines the expected differences are considered negligible [21].

Folin-Ciocalteu. The Folin-Ciocalteu assay for total phenolic content relies on the ability of the Folin-Ciocalteu reagent to strongly react with phenolic compounds. A mixture of two acids, namely phosphotungstic ($H_3PW_{12}O_{40}$) and phosphomolybdic ($H_3PMO_{12}O_{40}$) acids, react with mono and dihydroxylated phenolic substances due to their high ability to donate electrons. This reaction creates a blue coloured complex that is quantified at 750 nm [22]. After a simple wine dilution, the Folin-Ciocalteu reagent is added. A 20% $NaCO_3$ solution is then added to the mixture with some additional distilled water. The sample is then incubated for 30 min before absorbance measurement can be performed. Moreover, it is of crucial importance to maintain the order of the additions to ensure that the reaction takes place under alkaline conditions. In order to preserve accuracy, the A750 nm needs to be around 0.3 A.U. If this is not achieved, a different wine dilution needs to be performed. A blank with distilled water, to account for background interferences, is also included [23]. The results are commonly reported as gallic acid equivalents. Although the method is very often used, the ability of some other wine component to also donate electrons leads to potential overestimation of the phenolic content. This compromises the comparison of different samples containing varying phenolic and wine composition. In addition, the comparison of the Folin-Ciocalteu with the TPI is also possible by multiplying the A750 nm times the dilution factor times 20. A strong correlation between the two methods has been reported, thus making the total phenolic content between these two methods comparable [1].

3.2 Total anthocyanin content

Hydrochloric acid method. The estimation of the total concentration of anthocyanins in wine or grape extracts is possible due to the characteristic absorption band of this group of compounds around 520 nm. The coloration of anthocyanins are highly influenced by pH, with lower pH values leading to a higher proportion of anthocyanins in the red flavilium ion form. This property is thus exploited in this method to quantify the total anthocyanin content. Due to its ability to decrease pH, the method makes use of hydrochloric acid (HCl) i.e. the sample is diluted with a 1 M HCl solution. After a waiting period, to allow the free monomeric forms of the anthocyanin to be transformed into their red coloured forms, the A520 nm is measured [24]. The waiting period was initially reported to be longer than 3 hours but shorter than 24 hours, however later research confirmed that a waiting period of 1 hour is sufficient [25]. The values can be reported as A.U. or as malvidin-3-glucoside equivalents by making use of the molar extinction coefficient (commonly used 28,000 L/cm*mol) and the molecular weight (MW = 529 g/mol) of the major anthocyanin found in grapes and wines i.e. malvidin-3-glucoside.

Bisulphite bleaching method. Another property of the anthocyanins is in this case used to quantify this group of compounds. Sulphur dioxide is able to combine with the anthocyanin in the position 4 of the central phenolic ring, giving rise to a non-coloured flavene sulphonate. The decolouration ability of SO_2 is thus used to estimate the total content of free anthocyanins in the wine. The method also makes use of HCl with the aim of transforming the anthocyanins to their red coloured flavilium form. Two test samples are in this case compared. The control sample, with no SO_2 addition is compared against a treatment sample where the anthocyanins have been bleached by the SO_2 addition. After a waiting period, the A520 nm of both samples are compared and the total anthocyanin content calculated [26]. However, the ability of SO_2 to react and bleach some pigmented forms might lead to an overestimation of the total content [27].

pH differential method. Another method that exploits the effect of pH on the anthocyanin coloration was reported by Giusti and Worldstad [17]. This methodology compares a red flavilium form sample at pH 1 against a sample where the anthocyanins are transformed to its non-coloured hemiketal from at pH 4.5. Instead of measuring the anthocyanin content of both pH 1 and pH 4.5 samples at a fixed wavenumber (520 nm), the method measures the A_{max} observed around the 520 nm absorption band, which may not coincide with 520 nm. In addition, the method also includes the measurement of the A700 nm that is subtracted from the A_{max}, with the aim of accounting for possible light scattering caused by other sample components. By doing this the method ensures that the recorded absorption values only correspond to the anthocyanin content in the samples. The results are reported as malvidin-3-glucoside equivalents, by also using the molar extinction coefficient and the molecular weight of this anthocyanin. In addition, the method also allows for the calculation of additional indices by using the ability of sulphur dioxide to combine and bleach anthocyanins. A more complete picture of the anthocyanin content and composition is thus obtained after the inclusion of the pigment degradation, polymeric colour and browning indexes. In this case the method makes use of the absorbance at 420 nm to account for the polymeric anthocyanin material with colour properties closer to this region of the visible spectrum (orange colouration). The polymeric pigment colour is calculated as the proportion between the colour observed in the bleached samples at 420 nm and the A_{max} around 520 nm and that measured at the same wavelengths in the non-bleached samples. In order to ensure accuracy, measurements need to be taken between 15 min and 1 hour in line with what was reported earlier to avoid increased absorption properties at longer times [17].

Modified Somers assay. This methodology is based in the original method reported by Somers and Evans [21]. More recently a modified protocol, adapted to a high throughput format, using a microplate reader spectrophotometer was reported for both grape extract and wine samples [28]. The method presents a number of parameters and provides a broad overview of the status of the anthocyanin's equilibria in the sample. The method relies on the effect of hydrochloric acid, acetaldehyde and sulphur dioxide on the anthocyanins. Sulphur dioxide is added with the aim of calculating the levels of non-blanchable pigments, which includes more stable pigments such as tannin-anthocyanin complexes as well as pyranoanthocyanins. Moreover, acetaldehyde is used to negate the bleaching effect of SO_2 on anthocyanins and thus measure the total content of coloured anthocyanins. Finally, hydrochloric acid is added to account for those free anthocyanins that were not bleached or were derived from copigmentation complexes. The main advantage of the method relies on the fact that the pH adjustment, crucial to accurately estimate the state of the anthocyanins, is done by adjusting the pH of a buffer solution [28]. In the original protocol the pH of the samples was individually adjusted, with a considerable extension of the time of analysis. This method provides information on the wine "chemical age", which provides an estimation of the extent that the polymeric pigments has displaced the monomeric anthocyanins. Additional parameters report on the percentage of anthocyanins in its flavilium red form (% of ionisation), SO_2 resistant pigments (polymeric pigments), colour intensity, hue as well as total phenolic content.

Copigmentation assay. Anthocyanins interact with other wine components including other phenolic substances to form pigmented molecules through weak hydrophobic forces. The sandwich-like structure is composed of copigment molecules in between the anthocyanins [29]. The newly formed structure places the sugar moieties of the anthocyanin towards the external part of the complex, thus protecting the copigmented pigment from decolouration by water. These interactions account for a large part of the colour of young red wines with its contribution to wine colour decreasing over time, due to the weak nature of the copigmented structure [29]. Two main effects are characteristic of these complexes, which includes an increased absorption intensity in the visible absorption region of the anthocyanins (hyperchromic effect) accompanied by a shift into the absorption maxima towards higher wavelengths (blue colouration) through a bathochromic effect. The copigmentation assay was developed by Boulton and it is the only available method for the quantification of the colour due to copigmentation in red wines. The method relies on the ability of the anthocyanin complexes to avoid decolouration by water at constant pH i.e. measures the decolouration of the anthocyanins due to the dissociation of the copigmented forms [29].

3.3 Colour measurements

Colour density. Coloured anthocyanins and anthocyanin derived pigments are responsible for the colour properties of red wines. During the early stages of winemaking the colour properties of wines are mainly due to less complex monomeric forms of anthocyanins, however as the wine ages and anthocyanins start interacting with other wine components, more stable pigmented polymeric forms are responsible for the colour properties of red wines. The wine colour density was initially measured through the addition of the absorption values at 420 and 520 nm, which corresponds to the yellow and red colorations of wine [30]. Using this information, the hue of a wine samples was defined as the ratio between these two absorption values (A420 nm/A520 nm). More recently the absorption at 620 nm, which accounts for the blue wine colouration, was also added to the colour density parameter [31]. The method relies on a simple measurement (without dilution) and provides an estimation of the colour intensity of the wine. The results are often reported as %yellow, %red and %blue providing thus a more complete interpretation of wine colour properties. On the other hand, the A420 nm or A440 nm are commonly used to measure the colour properties of white wines including the brownish wine colour (browning index) [32].

CIElab colour space. Wine colour can also be measured through the information contained in the visible spectra of wines. Three colour components result from the integration of the visible absorption features. The Commission International de l'eclairage [33] proposed a method that uses three chromatic coordinates X, Y and Z to determine the chromatic characteristics of wines (also applicable to other beverages). The method aims to simulate the perception that real observers have for the colour properties of a sample. The calculation of the CIElab coordinates is based on measurement conditions given by a spectrophotometer with illuminant D65 and observed placed at 10°. The colour of a wine is thus described by the intensity of the wine colour (chromaticism), the luminosity of the wine and the colour itself based on the red, yellow, green and blue components (tonality). The colorimetric measurements are defined by the chromatic coordinates red/green component (a*) (a* > 0 red, a* < 0 green), blue/yellow component (b*) (b* > 0 yellow, b* < 0 blue), clarity (L*) (L* = 0 black and L* = 100 colourless) and its complementary magnitudes tone (H*) and chroma (C*). The ability to compare the colorimetric differences between two colours (ΔE*) makes it possible to directly compare the colour properties of wines. Moreover, it has been established that a colour difference higher than 2.7 indicates that the colour of two samples can be perceived different by the human eye [34].

3.4 Total tannin content

Acid hydrolysis. Due to the complex nature of proanthocyanidins or tannins the determination of these compounds is a difficult undertaking and has been challenging researchers for a long time. However, a number of methods, albeit with certain limitations, have been reported and will be discussed. The acid hydrolysis method is based on the transformation of proanthocyanidins in carbocations that are partially converted into anthocyanidins when exposed to heating under acidic conditions (Bate-Smith reaction). The total tannin content is thus estimated by using the red coloration of the resulting anthocyanin compounds at 550 nm and expressing it in cyaniding-3-glucoside equivalents. Although the method is widely used, a number of limitations have also been reported. First of all, the tannin concentration seems to be overestimated with higher values for tannins reported than those for total phenolic content. Moreover, it is also common to observe an increase in the total tannin content of wine during ageing and finally the method does not provide any information on the structure of the tannins [35].

Methylcellulose precipitable (MCP) tannins assay. This method falls under the precipitation based methods category as it uses the tannin precipitation ability of a methylcellulose polymer to estimate the total tannin content of grape extracts and wines. As mentioned the method relies on tannin-MCP interactions in the presence of ammonium sulphate, giving rise to an insoluble polymer-tannin complex that precipitates and is further separated by centrifugation [36]. This method has also been lately adapted and validated into a high throughput format leading to a considerable reduction of the analytical time [28]. A control sample without MCP addition (absence of tannin precipitation) is compared against a treated sample where the tannins have been removed after precipitation with MCP. The absorption difference measured at 280 nm is then used to quantify the total tannin content of a sample. The total tannin content is in this case estimated as epicatechin equivalents. In addition, one of the main benefits of precipitation based methods is that a theoretic positive correlation with astringency intensity is foreseen [37–39]. The hypothesis is based on the assumption that the method simulates the phenomena that naturally occurs in wine when it becomes in contact with the salivary proteins. An insoluble macromolecular complex is then formed that precipitates from solution causing the drying and puckering sensation known as astringency.

Bovine serum albumin (BSA) tannin assay. This precipitation based method exploits the ability of proteins to combine and precipitate tannins. The precipitation is achieved through the incorporation of bovine serum albumin protein. The precipitated protein-tannin complexes are then redissolved and quantified at 510 nm after the addition of ferric chloride [40, 41]. The accuracy of the method is based on obtaining the appropriate wine dilution as concentrated or very diluted samples tend to underestimate the tannin content. The BSA tannin assay, as part of the precipitation based methods for tannin analysis, has also been found to positively correlate with astringency intensities given by sensorial evaluation [37–39]. The total tannin content is in this assay calculated as catechin equivalents. In addition, the method also allows for the determination of additional parameters related to the anthocyanin and polymeric pigment fraction. Specifically, the method makes use of SO_2 to obtain information on the nature of the polymeric pigments by dividing them into small (SPP) (pigments that do not precipitate with BSA) and large polymeric pigments (LPP) that do precipitate with the protein. On the other hand, the comparison of both precipitations based methods has shown that MCP tannin values are on average three time higher than those found for BSA. However, a strong correlation (0.8) between the values obtained with the two methods has also been reported [42], whereas no correlation was observed between these two methods and the tannin content obtained with the acid hydrolysis method [37]. Finally, despite the differences in absolute values, attributable to the differences in both procedures, it has also been stated that both precipitants (BSA and MCP) precipitate the same amount of tannins when tested under the same conditions [39, 43].

4. UV-visible role in liquid chromatography

High liquid pressure chromatography (HPLC) is a suitable method to quantify individual phenolic compounds in grape extracts and wines. HPLC instruments make use of a diode array detector that allows for the quantification of phenolic substances at different wavelength within the UV-visible regions. The benefit of using diode array detectors in liquid chromatography is beyond using retention times for peak identification as it adds qualitative information by the incorporation of the UV-visible spectral features of a specific peak or compound [44]. It is thus nowadays possible to obtain a number of individual phenolic compounds by direct injection of wine samples without any sample pre-treatment. Based on its spectral features, phenolic compounds will be quantified at their absorption maxima, i.e. sub-families of phenolics are quantified at 280 nm for flavanol monomers and polymers and some phenolic acids, 320 nm for hydroxicinnamic acids, 360 nm for flavonols and finally 520 nm for anthocyanins. Although a considerable number of individual phenolics can be quantified using HPLC, the majority of the methods are not able to separate larger molecular structures such as polymeric phenols and pigments [13]. These two groups of compounds are commonly identified as broad absorption bands at later elution times at 280 nm for the polymeric phenols and at 520 nm for the polymeric pigments. Furthermore, in a previous study, the composition of the broad absorption band observed at 520 nm theoretically attributed to polymeric pigment material was investigated and confirmed [13]. Additionally, the polymeric pigments peak was also found to correlate with the spectrophotometric measurements of phenolic compounds and with wine age. In terms of polymeric phenols, it is believed that the phenolic compounds forming part of this broad absorption band correspond to a large extent to proanthocyanidins or tannins of high degree of polymerisation. The strong correlation (0.83) observed for a significant number of wines between the polymeric phenol peak area and the total tannin content, obtained with the MCP tannins assay, confirmed this [16]. HPLC methods for quantification of phenolic substances can also incorporate mass spectrometers. Mass spectrometry provides information about the molecular weight of the compounds and it is used to discern the identity of unknown compounds. The identification of phenolic compounds in chromatographic techniques using DAD is limited by co-elution (impure UV-visible spectra) or by similarities in the UV-visible properties of phenolic compounds belonging to the same phenolic family. These factors combined with similar elution times of some of the phenolic substances complicates the accurate quantification of chromatographic peaks. The use of mass-spectrometry provides thus a valid tool to confirm the identity of phenolic substances as well as the identification of novel compounds.

5. Fluorescence spectroscopy

An interesting and more recent technique to quantify phenolic compounds makes use of the ability of this group of substances to emit fluorescence light after the excitation/emission process. Fluorescence spectroscopy is able to measure the analyte concentration through its fluorescence properties, being thus suitable to measure compounds in solution, such as phenolics found in grape extracts or wines [14]. If phenolic compounds are excited at the appropriate light intensity and wavelength, generally through UV light exposure, the energy change occurring at electronic level will cause a light emission in the visible region of the electromagnetic spectrum [45]. Phenolic molecules are initially at ground levels at low energy state until light exposure elevate the vibrational levels to an elevated high energy state. After a period of time (in the order of milliseconds) the excited molecule while returning to its non-excited electronic state emits light (so-called fluorescence) at higher wavelengths than those absorbed during the excitation process. During the excitation/emission sequence both the absorbed and emitted light can be measured, with higher emission intensity corresponding to higher concentration of the analyte. Fluorescence spectroscopy has been commonly applied to the quantification of phenolic compounds in combination with liquid chromatography techniques. The main benefit of these applications rely on the increased sensitivity and selectivity of the method [45]. Additionally, fluorescence spectroscopy has been defined as a fast, non-destructive, easy to perform technique that can also be used for process monitoring purposes due to the versatility of the fluorescence spectrometers. Excitation emission spectral (EEM) properties might potentially be correlated with reference analytical data to establish regression calibrations for the quantification of phenolic compounds in a similar manner than what is reported for UV-visible or infrared spectroscopy calibrations.

6. UV-visible spectroscopy with chemometrics

The UV-visible spectra can alternatively be used in combination with powerful chemometric analysis to obtain spectroscopic calibrations for the prediction of phenolic content in grapes as well as in wines during the winemaking process [15]. In this case the totality or parts of the UV-visible spectra are correlated through multivariate regression approaches with reference phenolic data. After the spectral and phenolic content acquisition of a significant number of samples and in the case that strong correlations are found between the spectral data and the phenolic levels, a reliable prediction calibration can be obtained after the corresponding calibration and validation procedure. The advantage of these spectroscopy calibrations relies on the possibility of estimating the total content of phenolic substances through a simple spectral measurement, therefore avoiding the tedious reference method procedures. The main advantage of the spectroscopy calibrations is due to the rapidness, simplicity, reliability and cost-effectiveness ascribed to these techniques. Moreover, due to the multi-parametric nature of this approach a single spectral measurement is able to provide the levels of a number of phenolic compounds. Spectroscopic applications are also highly suitable to perform online measurement during the process of winemaking, allowing for improved process control strategies, through process monitoring, in line with a process analytical technologies (PAT) approach [46].

The first indication of the use of UV-visible spectroscopy calibrations to quantify some of the most important phenolic parameters was reported in 1995 [47]. In this first approach the total tannin and anthocyanin content was predicted using a limited number of samples. The UV-visible spectra was collected from 200 to 650 nm at 6 nm intervals. Errors in prediction (root mean standard error of prediction (RMSEP)) of 0.35 g/L (14% RMSEP%) and 29 mg/L (8%) where reported for tannins and anthocyanins respectively. Despite the relative small sample set and the limitations of the analytical reference method investigated (mainly due to non-specificity for phenolic compounds of the employed procedures) this publication reported for the first time the suitability of UV-visible spectroscopy to quantify phenolic content in wines through partial least squares (PLS) regression analysis.

In a further study the UV-visible spectral properties of a large dataset (400) were used to quantify phenolic content of samples collected at different stages of the winemaking process. The sample set included samples from a variety of different regions and cultivars. Spectral data was collected over the 230–900 nm at 0.17 nm intervals. The parameters derived from the BSA tannin assay including the anthocyanin and total phenolic related parameters were in this case evaluated. RMSEP of 87 mg/L (20% RMSEP%) for total anthocyanin content; 0.37 (26.4%), 0.46 (76.7%) and 0.48 (24%) A.U. for small, large and total polymeric pigments, respectively; 66 mg/L (30.1%) for tannin content; 99 (17.2%) mg/L for non-tannin phenols and 130 mg/L (16.4%) for total phenols were reported [48]. Later on, the same phenolic parameters were again investigated. A 100 samples of Cabernet Sauvignon and 100 samples of Shiraz were collected during the fermentation process over a single vintage to provide calibration that can be used for the prediction of phenolic content in must. In this case an adaptation of the BSA tannin assay was used for phenolic analysis. UV-visible spectral properties were collected in the 200–900 nm range. The results showed calibrations able to predict the phenolic content of Cabernet Sauvignon samples, but not for Shiraz, suggesting cultivar specificity of the predicted calibrations. Standard errors in cross validation (RMSECV) of 102.22 mg/L (23.8% RMSECV%) and 211.38 mg/L (25.6%) were reported for total tannin and iron reactive phenolic content, respectively for Cabernet Sauvignon samples. In terms of anthocyanin measurements, error in cross validation of 101 mg/L (43.3% RMSECV%), 0.46 A.U. (26.1%) and 0.48 A.U. (41.4%) for total anthocyanins, small and large polymeric pigments were observed [49].

Due to its characteristic absorption band at 280 nm the UV spectral properties of wines have also been used for the determination of phenolic content and more specifically for total tannin content. The MCP tannin levels of a significant number of samples from a variety of different locations, cultivars and during different steps of the winemaking process were successfully predicted with the use of multiple linear regression (MLR) and partial least square regression (PLS). In this case spectral properties were collected between the 230 and 350 nm range of the UV part of the electromagnetic spectrum. Errors in cross validation (RMSECV) of 0.2 g/L (9.3% RMSECV%) were reported for MLR models using the above-mentioned UV region. Moreover, the authors also reported calibrations but in this case using only a limited number of key wavelengths. Further calibrations were investigated using the UV absorption values at 250, 270, 280, 290 and 315 nm. The external validation calibrations showed errors in prediction (RMSEP) of 0.18 g/L (9.2%) which confirmed the suitability of the UV region spectral properties to quantify tannin content in wine samples [50].

In a more recent study the ability of UV-visible spectroscopy to predict tannin content in finished wines was reported. In this case two precipitation based methods, namely MCP and BSA tannin assays, were used to generate the spectral data. A large number of samples containing a varying number of cultivars from different regions as well as vintages were included in the model optimization procedure. UV-vis spectra was measured in the 260–610 nm region at 2 nm intervals. The best calibrations were found for both reference methods where the spectral properties in the UV region were used as spectral data (260–310 nm). A RMSEP of 0.16 g/L (9.9% RMSEP%) and 0.08 g/L (13.3%) were reported for MCP and BSA tannin content, respectively. In agreement with previous studies, accurate calibrations were also observed when a reduced number of wavelength were used as spectral data. Models optimised using the absorption values at 270, 280, 290, 300 and 314 nm lead to errors in prediction of 0.18 g/L (11.2% RMSEP%) and 0.11 g/L (18.3%) for MCP and BSA tannin content, respectively. Also in agreement with previous findings, cultivar and vintage specificity issues influenced to a certain extent the accuracy of the calibrations [42].

In a more recent study PLS calibrations based on UV-visible spectral data for the quantification of phenolic content in grapes, fermenting samples and wines have been reported. A large number of fermenting samples from 13 different vinifications over two consecutive vintages were included into the calibrations. Moreover, a number of finished wines from varying vintages and from a number of cultivars were also included. PLS validation calibrations showed prediction errors of 209 mg/L (14.3% RMSEP%), 14 mg/L (3.2%), 1.6 (3.2%) and 2.6 (14.7%) for total tannin content (MCP tannin assay), total anthocyanins, total phenolic content and colour density, respectively. In addition, individual phenolic compounds quantified using a HPLC method to generate the reference data were also reported, including flavanol monomers and the dimer B1, phenolic acids, flavonols as well as monomeric and acylated anthocyanins. Calibration for the estimation of polymeric phenol and pigment content were also reported. On the other hand, the same study reported PLS calibrations for determination of phenolic content in grapes extracts obtained through two extraction protocols. A phenolic extraction in high solvent content and after the entire berries being finely blended lead to successful calibrations for total tannin content, anthocyanins levels, total phenol index and colour density. The RMSEP reported was 0.22 mg/g (7% RMSEP%), 0.034 mg/g (3.1%), 0.17 (1.32%) and 0.72 (6.61%), for the above mentioned parameters, respectively. In addition, an alternative method with phenolic extraction performed under wine-like ethanol levels from hand crushed grapes was also reported. Validation errors of 0.12 mg/g (10.7% RMSEP%), 0.03 mg/g (8.33%), 0.42 (1%) and 6.2 (20%) for total tannins, total anthocyanins, total phenolic index and colour density, respectively were reported [16].

7. Conclusions

The role of UV-visible spectroscopy in wine science appears to be of high importance. A number of applications can be used to quantify the levels of phenolic compounds in grape extracts and wines. Apart from the conventional routine spectrophotometric methods for phenolic analysis, more advanced analytical techniques such as liquid chromatography can be also used to quantify individual phenolic substances using UV-visible spectroscopy. Moreover, fluorescence spectroscopy, making use of the ability of phenolic molecules to emit fluorescence light, appears to be a promising technique that can also be used to quantify phenolic content at different stages of the winemaking process and under different conditions. Finally, UV-visible spectroscopy calibrations are also a valid alternative as they allow for the efficient measurement of phenolics in grape extracts as well as wines during fermentation and ageing. These new developments in phenolic monitoring during the winemaking process opens exciting new possibilities for wine producers in their bid to obtain wines of a certain composition and style in a more controlled manner.

Author details

Jose Luis Aleixandre-Tudo* and Wessel du Toit
Department of Viticulture and Oenology, Stellenbosch University, Matieland, South Africa

*Address all correspondence to: joaltu@sun.ac.za

References

[1] Aleixandre-Tudo JL, Buica A, Nieuwoudt H, Aleixandre JL, du Toit W. Spectrophotometric analysis of phenolic compounds in grapes and wines. Journal of Agricultural and Food Chemistry. 2017;**65**:4009-4026

[2] Aleixandre R, Aleixandre-Tudó JL, Bolaños-Pizarro JL, Aleixandre-Benavent M. Mapping the scientific research on wine and health (2001–2011). Journal of Agricultural and Food Chemistry. 2013;**61**:11871-11880

[3] Cheynier V, Schneider R, Salmon J, Fulcrand H. Chemistry of wine. In: Comprehensive Natural Products II. The Netherlands: Elsevier Ltd.; 2010. pp. 1119-1172

[4] Teixeira A, Eiras-Dias J, Castellarin SD, Gerós H. Berry phenolics of grapevine under challenging environments. International Journal of Molecular Sciences. 2013;**14**:18711-18739

[5] Casassa LF, Harbertson JF. Extraction, evolution, and sensory impact of phenolic compounds during red wine maceration. Annual Review of Food Science and Technology. 2014

[6] He F, Liang NN, Mu L, Pan QH, Wang J, Reeves MJ, Duan CQ. Anthocyanins and their variation in red wines. I. Monomeric anthocyanins and their color expression. Molecules. 2012;**17**:1571-1601

[7] He F, Liang NN, Mu L, Pan QH, Wang J, Reeves MJ, Duan CQ. Anthocyanins and their variation in red wines. II. Anthocyanin derived pigments and their color evolution. Molecules. 2012;**17**:1483-1519

[8] Gomez-Plaza M, Cano-Lopez E. A review on micro-oxygenation of red wines: Claims, benefits and the underlying chemistry. Food Chemistry. 2011;**125**:1131-1140

[9] McRae JM, Kennedy JA. Wine and grape tannin interactions with salivary proteins and their impact on astringency: A review of current research. Molecules. 2011;**16**:2348-2364

[10] Smith PA, Mcrae JM, Bindon KA. Impact of winemaking practices on the concentration and composition of tannins in red wine. Australian Journal of Grape and Wine Research. 2015;**21**:601-614

[11] Boulet JC, Ducasse MA, Cheynier V. Ultraviolet spectroscopy study of phenolic substances and other major compounds in red wines: Relationship between astringency and the concentration of phenolic substances. Australian Journal of Grape and Wine Research. 2017;**23**:193-199

[12] Sanna R, Piras C, Marincola FC, Lecca V, Maurichi S, Scano P. Multivariate statistical analysis of the UV-vis profiles of wine polyphenolic extracts during vinification. The Journal of Agricultural Science. 2014;**6**:152-162

[13] Peng Z, Iland PG, Oberholster A, Sefton MA, Waters EJ. Analysis of pigmented polymers in red wine by reverse phase HPLC. Australian Journal of Grape and Wine Research. 2002;**8**:70-75

[14] Airado-Rodríguez D, Durán-Merás I, Galeano-Díaz T, Wold JP. Front-face fluorescence spectroscopy: A new tool for control in the wine industry. Journal of Food Composition and Analysis. 2011;**24**:257-264

[15] Cozzolino D. The role of visible and infrared spectroscopy combined with chemometrics to measure phenolic compounds in grape and wine samples. Molecules. 2015;**20**:726-737

[16] Aleixandre-Tudo JL, Nieuwoudt H, Olivieri A, Aleixandre JL, du Toit W. Phenolic profiling of grapes, fermenting samples and wines using UV-visible spectroscopy with chemometrics. Food Control. 2018;**85**:11-22

[17] Giusti M, Wrolstad R. Characterization and measurement of anthocyanins by UV-visible spectroscopy. Current Prvtocols in Food Analytical. 2001:1-13

[18] Hassane E, Gierschner J, Duroux J, Trouillas P. UV/visible spectra of natural polyphenols: A time-dependent density functional theory study. Food Chemistry. 2012;**131**:79-89

[19] Bueno JM, Ramos-Escudero F, Sáez-Plaza P, Muñoz AM, Navas MJ, Asuero AG. Analysis and antioxidant capacity of anthocyanin pigments. Part II: Chemical structure, color, and intake of anthocyanins. Critical Reviews in Analytical Chemistry. 2012;**42**:102-125

[20] Flanzy C, Poux M. Les possibilités de la microvinification, application à l'étude de la macération. Annales de Technologie Agricole. 1958:390-394

[21] Somers TC, Evans ME. Wine quality: Correlations with colour density and anthocyanin equilibria in a group of young red wines. Journal of the Science of Food and Agriculture. 1974;**25**:1369-1379

[22] Singleton VL, Rossi JA Jr. Colorimetry of total phenolics with phosphomolybdic-phosphotungstic acid reagents. American Journal of Enology and Viticulture. 1965;**16**:144-158

[23] Singleton VL, Orthofer R, Lamuela-Raventós RM. Analysis of total phenols and other oxidation substrates and antioxidants by means of folin-ciocalteu reagent. Methods in Enzymology. 1998;**299**:152-178

[24] Mazza G, Fukumoto L, Delaquis P, Girard B, Ewert B. Anthocyanins, phenolics, and color of cabernet franc, merlot, and pinot noir wines from British Columbia. Journal of Agricultural and Food Chemistry. 1999;**47**:4009-4017

[25] Bindon KA, Kassara S, Cynkar WU, Robinson EMC, Scrimgeour N, Smith PA. Comparison of extraction protocols to determine differences in wine-extractable tannin and anthocyanin in *Vitis vinifera* L. cv. Shiraz and cabernet sauvignon grapes. Journal of Agricultural and Food Chemistry. 2014;**62**:4558-4570

[26] Ribéreau-Gayon E, Stonestreet P. Le dosage des anthocyannes dans Je vin rouge. Bulletin de la Société Chimique de France. 1965;**9**:2649-2652

[27] De Beer D, Harbertson JF, Kilmartin PA, Roginsky V, Barsukova T, Adams DO, Waterhouse AL. Phenolics: A comparison of diverse analytical methods. American Journal of Enology and Viticulture. 2004;**55**:389-400

[28] Mercurio MD, Dambergs RG, Herderich MJ, Smith PA. High throughput analysis of red wine and grape phenolics—Adaptation and validation of methyl cellulose precipitable tannin assay and modified Somers color assay to a rapid 96 well plate format. Journal of Agricultural and Food Chemistry. 2007;**55**:4651-4657

[29] Boulton RB. The copigmentation of anthocynins and its role in the color of red wine: Comments on a critical review. American Journal of Enology and Viticulture. 2001;**52**:67-87

[30] Sudraud P. Interpretation des courbes de'absorption des vin rouges. Annals of Agricultural Sciences. n.d.;**7**:203-208

[31] Glories Y. La couleur des vins rouges, 2eme partie, Connaiss. La Vigne Du Vin. 1984;**18**:253-271

[32] Singleton VL, Kramling TE. Browning of white wines and an accelerated test for browning capacity. American Journal of Enology and Viticulture. 1976;**27**:4-7

[33] Commission Internationale de l'Eclairage. CIE Recommendations on Uniform Color Spaces, Color-Difference Equations, Psychometric Color Terms; CIE Public. Commission Internationale de l'Eclairage; 1978

[34] Martinez JA, Melgosa M, Perez MM, Hita E, Negueruela AII, Martínez JA, Pérez MM. Note. Visual and instrumental color evaluation in red wines. Food Science and Technology International. 2001;7:439-444

[35] Ribéreau-Gayón P, Stonestreet E. Dógase des tannins du vin rouges et détermination du leur structure. Chemia Analityczna. 1966

[36] Sarneckis CJ, Dambergs RG, Jones P, Mercurio M, Herderich MJ, Smith PA. Quantification of condensed tannins by precipitation with methyl cellulose: Development and validation of an optimised tool for grape and wine analysis. Australian Journal of Grape and Wine Research. 2006;**12**:39-49

[37] Cáceres-Mella A, Peña-Neira Á, Narváez-Bastias J, Jara-Campos C, López-Solís R, Canals JM. Comparison of analytical methods for measuring proanthocyanidins in wines and their relationship with perceived astringency. International Journal of Food Science and Technology. 2013;**48**:2588-2594

[38] Kennedy JA, Ferrier J, Harbertson JF, Peyrot Des C. Gachons, analysis of tannins in red wine using multiple methods: Correlation with perceived astringency. American Journal of Enology and Viticulture. 2006;**57**:481-485

[39] Mercurio MD, Smith PA. Tannin quantification in red grapes and wine: Comparison of polysaccharide- and protein-based tannin precipitation techniques and their ability to model wine astringency. Journal of Agricultural and Food Chemistry. 2008;**56**:5528-5537

[40] Harbertson JF, Yuan C, Mireles MS, Hanlin RL, Downey MO. Glucose, fructose and sucrose increase the solubility of protein-tannin complexes and at high concentration, glucose and sucrose interfere with bisulphite bleaching of wine pigments. Food Chemistry. 2013;**138**:556-563

[41] Harbertson JF, Mireles M, Yu Y. Improvement of BSA tannin precipitation assay by reformulation of resuspension buffer. American Journal of Enology and Viticulture. 2015;**66**:95-99

[42] Aleixandre-Tudo JL, Nieuwoudt H, Aleixandre JL, Du Toit WJ. Robust ultraviolet-visible (UV-vis) partial least-squares (PLS) models for tannin quantification in red wine. Journal of Agricultural and Food Chemistry. 2015;**63**:1088-1098

[43] Harbertson JF, Downey MO. Technical brief investigating differences in tannin levels determined by methylcellulose and protein precipitation. American Journal of Enology and Viticulture. 2009;**60**:246-249

[44] Lamuala-Raventós RM, Waterhouse A. A direct HPLC separation of wine phenolics. American Journal of Enology and Viticulture. 1994;**45**:1-5

[45] Cabrera-Bañegil M, Hurtado-Sánchez M d C, Galeano-Díaz T, Durán-Merás I. Front-face fluorescence spectroscopy combined with second-order multivariate algorithms for the quantification of polyphenols in red wine samples. Food Chemistry. 2017;**220**:168-176

[46] Aleixandre-Tudo JL, Nieuwoudt H, Aleixandre JL, du Toit W. Chemometric compositional analysis of phenolic compounds in fermenting samples and wines using different infrared spectroscopy techniques. Talanta. 2018;**176**:526-536

[47] Garcia-Jares C, Medina B, García-Jares C, Medina B. Prediction of some physico-chemical parameters in red wines from ultraviolet-visible spectra using a partial least-squares model in latent variables. The Analyst. 1995;**120**:1891-1896

[48] Skogerson K, Downey M, Mazza M, Boulton R. Rapid determination of phenolic components in red wines from UV-visible spectra and the method of partial least squares. American Journal of Enology and Viticulture. 2007;**58**:318-325

[49] Beaver CW, Harbertson JF. Comparison of multivariate regression methods for the analysis of phenolics in wine made from two vitis vinifera cultivars. American Journal of Enology and Viticulture. 2016;**67**:56-64

[50] Dambergs RG, Mercurio MD, Kassara S, Cozzolino D, Smith PA. Rapid measurement of methyl cellulose precipitable tannins using ultraviolet spectroscopy with chemometrics: Application to red wine and inter-laboratory calibration transfer. Applied Spectroscopy. 2012;**66**:656-664

Chapter 4

Probiotic, Prebiotic and Synbiotic Products in Human Health

Nicoleta-Maricica Maftei

Abstract

The health benefits imparted by probiotics and prebiotics as well as synbiotics have been the subject of extensive research in the past few decades. What is the real role of probiotics strains, prebiotics and synbiotics in influencing a health? To battle the increase in health care costs, in recent years has been developed a preventive approach to medicine with the development of new probiotics and prebiotics or symbiotic products. Many studies suggest that probiotics, prebiotics and synbiotics supplementation may be beneficial in prevention and management of nutritional and health. While these studies show promising beneficial effects, the long-term risks or health benefits of prebiotics, probiotics and synbiotics supplementation are not clear. In this chapter review the literature regarding available information and summarises the current knowledge on the effects of probiotics, prebiotics, and synbiotics on human health and explore recent trends and developments in this field.

Keywords: probiotics, prebiotics, synbiotics, health, functional food

1. Introduction

Probiotic, prebiotic and synbiotic are words of the modern era, bookmark "for life" and is in use to define bacterial association with beneficial effects on human health. In the world of highly processed food, both at the industrial and nutritional level clear consideration are paid to the composition and safety of the intake products. The nutrition quality is essential for human health because of the food poisoning, obesity, allergy, cardiovascular diseases, and cancer, that is consider the plague of the twenty-first century. Worldwide, many research reports underline the health advantages of using probiotics, prebiotics and also, synbiotics in human consumption [1]. In early 1990s, Metchnikoff [2] defined probiotics in a scientific context as the microorganisms that alter of floral/microbial diversity in human bodies and replaces the harmful microbes with useful ones. However, Tissier detected that the microbial population of a particular type of bacteria in stool samples of infected diarrheic children was significantly lower comparing to healthy children [3]. He suggested that patients with diarrhoea (infantile diarrhoea) should oral administration of live organisms (bifidobacteria) and in this way a healthy gut flora was restored. Havenaar and Huis in't Veld [4] have given the modern definition of probiotic: as a viable mono or mixed culture of bacteria which, when applied to animal or man, affects the host beneficially by improving the properties of the indigenous flora. In 2002, Food and Agriculture Organisation of the United Nations (FAO) and World Health Organisation (WHO) defined probiotics as being "live strains of strictly selected microorganisms which, when administered in adequate amounts, confer a health benefit on the host" [5]. The definition was preserved also, by the International Scientific Association for Probiotics and Prebiotics (ISAPP) in 2013 [6]. The vast majority of results of the clinical research underline the positive effect of the probiotics on the gastrointestinal diseases, such as: irritable bowel syndrome, gastrointestinal disorders, elimination of *Helicobacter*, inflammatory bowel disease, diarrhoeas, and allergic diseases, like as atopic dermatitis. Also, numerous clinical reports have demonstrated the efficiency of the probiotics for the treatment of diseases such as obesity, insulin resistance syndrome, type 2 diabetes, and non-alcoholic fatty liver disease. Increasing the body's immunity (immunomodulation) was the positive effect of probiotics on human health. Majority of scientific reports also show the benefits of the prophylactic use of probiotics in different types of cancer and side effects associated with cancer [1].

In 1995, Gibson and Roberfroid defined prebiotics were by as non-digested food components that, through the stimulation of growth and/or activity of a single type or a limited amount of microorganisms which residing in the gastrointestinal tract, improve the health condition of a host [7]. Instead, in 2004, prebiotics were described as selectively fermented compounds permitting precise changes in the composition and/or activity of the gastrointestinal tract microorganisms, these changes being useful for the host's health and wellbeing [8]. Recently, in 2007, FAO/WHO experts, designated prebiotics as a nonviable food constituent that confers a health advantage on the host linked to the microbiota modulation [9]. However, in the literature it is specified that prebiotics can be used as a probiotics substitute or as a supplementary support for them. Instead, numerous prebiotics can improve the growth of indigenous gut bacteria and have tremendous potential for changing the gut microbiota, but these variations occur just at the level of individual strains. Worldwide, numerous scientific studies underline the positively effects of the prebiotics for human health.

For the simultaneous use of probiotics and prebiotics high potential is attributed. In 1995, Gibson and Roberfroid introduced the term "synbiotic" to describe union between probiotics and prebiotics synergistically acting of health [7]. Synbiotic is a designated compound that introduced in the gastrointestinal tract can careful stimulates the growth and/or activates the metabolism of physiological intestinal microbiota, thus conferring beneficial result to the host's health [10]. As the word "synbiotic" is a synergy, the term can be attributed only to the products where a prebiotic compound selectively improves a probiotic microorganism [11]. The main aim of this type of combination is the improvement of probiotic microorganism's survival in the gastrointestinal tract. Therefore, synbiotic have both probiotic and prebiotic assets and were designed in order to solve the probiotics survival in the gastrointestinal tract [12]. An adequate combination of both components (prebiotic and probiotic) in a single product should guarantee a superior effect, compared to the action of the probiotic or prebiotic alone [13, 14].

Besides basic role of the nutrition consisting in the supply of necessary nutrients for growth and development of the organism, some additional aspects are becoming increasingly important, including the maintenance of health and counteracting diseases. The introduction of probiotics, prebiotics, or synbiotics into human diet is favourable for the intestinal microbiota and the human health. They may be consumed in the form of dairy products, raw vegetables and fruit or fermented pickles. Another source of probiotics, prebiotics, or synbiotics may be pharmaceutical formulas and functional food. Although probiotics, prebiotics and synbiotics have considerable potential in nutritional and clinical applications, considerable researches are required for the implementation of probiotics into human health, nutrition and regulation of different abnormalities. The screening of probiotics, prebiotics and synbiotics and their amounts is essential in gaining a therapeutic effect in health. However, further research focused on discovering new probiotic strains, the assortment of probiotics and prebiotics for synbiotics, dose setting, safety of use, and clinical trials is necessary. Also, the health benefits should be established in properly scheduled clinical trials conducted by independent research centres.

This chapter is an attempt to emphasise the possible benefaction of probiotics, prebiotics and synbiotics for improving human health and regulation of common metabolic disorders or abnormalities.

2. Probiotics

Gut bacterial colonisation starts since at birth when new-borns are exposed to a nonsterile climate. Henceforth, it changes and transforms over a lifetime, depends on a complex and dynamic interaction between the diet, genome, and lifestyle of the host, as well as antibiotic consumption. Remarkable bacterial colonisation of age-specific changes described in gut microbiota configuration include a decrease in the Bacteroidetes/Firmicutes ratio and a reduction in bifidobacteria in people aged over 60 years, when the immune system starts to decline [15]. Normally, the composition of the intestinal microflora is considered to be constantly throughout adulthood period.

Since the beginning of the twentieth century the interest in lactic acid fermentation was expressed by the Russian scientist and immunologist, Ilia Miecznikow, that worked at Pasteur Institute, Paris. In the book "Studies on Optimism" he affirmed that "with various foods undergoing lactic acid fermentation and consumed raw (sour milk, kefir, sauerkraut, pickles) humans introduced huge amounts of proliferating lactic acid bacteria to their alimentary tracts" [16].

2.1 Probiotic strains

The microorganisms that are used as probiotics can belong to different types, such as bacteria, yeast and mould. Selected probiotic bacteria strains can be as following:

a. *Lactobacillus: acidophilus, sporogenes, plantarum, rhamnosus, delbrueckii, reuteri, fermentum, brevis, casei, farciminis, paracasei, gasseri, crispatus*;

b. *Bifidobacterium*: *bifidum, infantis, adolescentis, longum, thermophilum, breve, lactis;*

c. *Streptococcus*: *lactis, cremoris, thermophilis, diacetylactis*;

d. *Leuconostoc mesenteroides*;

e. *Pediococcus* spp.;

f. *Propionibacterium* spp.;

g. *Enterococcus—Enterococcus faecium*;

The literature mentions as probiotics the following yeast and mould strains:

a. Yeast: *Saccharomyces cerevisiae, Saccharomyces bourlardii*, *Candida pintolopesii, and Sacaromyces boulardii*

b. Moulds: *Aspergillus niger, A. oryzae* [17].

The type of the microbes used as probiotics increased due to the increase in the research concerning the health but as well as by the increase of the newly discovered and identified microbes, which could be used as probiotics in different food and beverages with huge impact on human body.

With the development of better culturing methodologies, more affordable genome and metagenome sequencing, the probiotic research is in a fulminant era, one which permits designing adapted probiotics that address specific consumer needs and issues. Also, the data of the conformation and role of the human gut microbiome accelerated by massively parallel sequencing, has extended the range of microorganisms with possible human benefits, although many of these are still at the very early stage of research.

These organisms are sometimes referred to as next-generation probiotics (NGPs), but may also be termed live biotherapeutic products (LBPs). NPGs obviously follow to the standard classification of a probiotic, but mainly referring to those microorganisms that have not been used as agents to promote health till now, and which are more likely to be delivered under a drug regulatory framework. Next-generation probiotics fit well within the US Food and Drug Administration (FDA) definition of a live biotherapeutic products: "a biological product" that: comprises live microoorganisms, such as bacteria; it is not a vaccine; is applicable to the prevention, treatment, or cure of a disease or condition of human beings [18].

Examples of current NGP: *Faecalibacterium* spp., *Akkermansia* spp., *Bacteroides fragilis* strain ZY-312, *Bacteroides xylanisolvens* DSM 23964, *Clostridium butyricum* MIYAIRI 588, *Faecalibacterium prausnitzii* and other.

Probiotics are subject to regulations in the general food law worldwide, conforming to they should be safe for human and animal health. In the Unite State of America, microorganisms that are used for human consumption should have the Generally Regarded As Safe (GRAS) status, regulated by the Food and Drug Administration (FDA). Rather, in Europe, European Food Safety Authority (EFSA) introduced the term of Qualified Presumption of Safety (QPS). The term of QPS it is a concept which involves some additional criteria of the safety assessment of bacterial supplements, including the history of safe usage and absence of the risk of acquired resistance to antibiotics [19, 20]. Until this moment mechanism of action of probiotics has not been clearly understood, but research results are those obtained from animal models and in vitro experiments. From a medical point of view it is considered that action mode of probiotics may improve the barrier functions of the gut mucosa because several strains of *Lactobacillus* spp. and *Bifidobacterium* spp. as well as structural compounds, and microbial-produced metabolites are able to stimulate epithelial cell signalling pathways. Thomas and Versalovic [21] reported that the Nuclear FactorKappa-Light-Chain-Enhancer of activated B cells (NF-kB) pathway is controlled by probiotics at many different levels with effects seen on I Kappa B protein (IKB) degradation and ubiquitination, proteosome function [22] and nuclear-cytoplasmic movement of RelA through a PPAR-gamma dependent pathway. Also, it is known that probiotics can modulate the immune system functions for instance, *L. acidophilus* has been found to modulate toll-like receptors and the proteoglycan recognition proteins of enterocytes. This thing leads to activation of dendric cells and lymphocytes T-helper 1 responds. After stimulation of lymphocytes T-helper 1 cytokines can suppress lymphocyte T-helper 2 responses which provoke the atopic issues [23]. Another possible mechanism of action of probiotics may be their ability to suppress the growth of pathogenic bacteria by producing broad-spectrum bacteriocins [24]. After the latest research on probiotics we can conclude that molecular and genetic research allowed the determination of the beneficial effect of probiotics, involving four mechanisms:

1. Antagonism through the production of antimicrobial compounds [25];
2. Pathogens competition for adhesion to the epithelium and for nutrients [26];
3. Immunomodulation of the host [27];
4. Inhibition of bacterial toxin production [28].

The first two mechanisms are directly related with their effect on other microorganisms. Nevertheless, all four mechanisms, from medical point of view, play an important role in the infections prophylaxis and treatment and also, for maintenance a balanced host's intestinal microbiota [1]. The capability of probiotic strains to co-aggregate, as one of their mechanisms of action, can contribute to the development of a protective barrier preventing pathogenic bacteria from the colonisation of the gut epithelium [29]. Probiotics bacteria are able to adhere to epithelial cells, inhibiting the pathogens. This mechanism plays an important effect on the host's health condition. Also, the adhesion of probiotic microorganisms to epithelial cells can start a signalling cascade, leading to immunological modulation. Otherwise, the discharge of some soluble compounds may cause a direct or indirect (through epithelial cells) activation of immunological cells [30].

Probiotics may have an significant role in: chronic inflammation of the alimentary tract or of a part thereof, the prevention and treatment of contagious diseases, lactose intolerance and lactose digestion, cholesterol reduction, cardiovascular health, urogenital disease, allergic disease, oral health, gastrointestinal disease, obesity but and an possible role in the elimination of cancer cells.

2.2 Probiotics in human health

2.2.1 Probiotics in prevention and treatment of acute diarrhoea and diarrhoea associated with antibiotics

Diarrhoea induced by antibiotics is a very common complication in the hospital setting, representing a percentage by 13–60% and disease caused by Clostridium difficile is also a significant cause of nosocomial diarrhoea and colitis that prolongs the hospital stay by 3–7 days and increases the risk of new nosocomial infections with 20–65%, costs, and mortality (2- or 3-fold depending on reports) [31]. The roles of the probiotics used to treat these patients are:

1. restoration intestinal microflora;
2. increase immune response;
3. compete with pathogenic bacteria;
4. remove their toxins.

Saccharomyces boulardii, Lactobacillus acidophilus, Lactobacillus bulgaricus, Lactobacillus rhamnosus, Lactobacillus paracasei, Bifidobacterium longum, Bifidobacterium breve there were some of the most widely studied probiotics for treatment of acute diarrhoea. In a recent meta-analysis of 21 studies (4780 patients), the administration of *S. boulardii* decreased the risk of antibiotic-induced diarrhoea in both children and adults from 19 to 8.5%, with a relative risk of 0.47. In another meta-analysis of 82 randomised clinical trials using diverse species (usually

Lactobacillus spp., alone or combined with bifidobacteria, enterococci, or *S. boulardii*), a reduced risk of antibiotic-induced diarrhoea was also established, with a relative risk of 0.58 [31].

Floch et al. [32] reported that for the primary prevention of disease caused by *C. difficile* in patients treated with antibiotics, probiotics also decrease the incidence of such disease, especially when strains of *S. boulardii*, and possibly other *Lactobacillus*, such as GG, are administered. Instead, a recent meta-analysis settled that only four probiotic strains (not including *Lactobacillus* GG) have been shown to significantly decrease the incidence of diarrhoea induced by *C. difficile*, such as follows: *S. boulardii* (2×10^{10} CFU/day), *L. casei* DN114001 (probiotic drink twice daily), a mixture of *L. acidophilus* and *Bifidobacterium bifidum* (2×10^{10} CFU/day), and a mixture of *L. acidophilus*, *L. casei*, and *L. rhamnosus*) [33].

For patients that intake antibiotics to eradicate *Helicobacter pylori*, studies have been conducted based on probiotics adding in order to increase eradication rates and also to prevent side effects such as antibiotic-induced diarrhoea. Numerous meta-analyses showed that the addition of probiotics may increase the efficacy of eradication with an odds ratio (OR) ranging from 1.2 to 2 times compare to the control group. Although additional studies are needed, it appears that the most effective strains are *L. acidophilus* (1.25×10^9 CFU) (OR: 1.24), milk fermented with *L. casei* DN-114001 (2 packs daily) (OR: 1.47), yogurt with *Lactobacillus gasseri* (OR: 1.19) (2 packs daily), and *Bifidobacterium infantis* (2×10^9 CFU) (OR: 1.21) [31]. Also, in supplementary clinical researches where antibiotics are used, probiotics appear to decrease the incidence of diarrhoea (with an OR ranging from 0.16 to 0.47) [34].

Also, the efficiency of probiotic strains in the next therapy's: nosocomial, non-nosocomial, and viral diarrheas have been studied. The conclusion was as follows: it turns out that probiotics may increase the amount of IgA antibodies, which leads to the decrease number of a viral infection [35].

2.2.2 Probiotics in in diseases of the gastrointestinal apparatus

Inflammatory bowel disease (IBD) is a recurrent chronic condition in which an abnormal interaction exists between intestinal flora and the host. Patients with IBD have an increased risk of colorectal cancer [31]. Due to the growing area of disease spreading and ageing societies, the use of probiotic bacteria for human health is becoming increasingly important. The consumption of pre-processed food (fast food), often containing excessive amounts of fat and insufficient amounts of raw fruits and vegetables, is another factor of harmful modification of human intestinal microbiota. It seems that the system of intestinal microorganisms and its desirable modification with probiotic formulas and products may protect people against enteral problems, and improve health [1]. *L. plantarum* is a probiotic that has been used with good results in the management of some symptoms in patients with IBD. It has been reported that the DSM 9843 strain significantly reduced flatulence, and the LPO 1 and 299 V strains significantly reduced abdominal pain [36]. In many studies it has been reported that probiotics may be helpful in the treatment of inflammatory enteral conditions, Crohn's disease, ulcerative colitis, and non-specific ileitis. The aetiology of those diseases is not completely understood, but it is evident that they are associated with recurrent infections or chronic inflammations of the intestine. Using a complex probiotic, such as: VSL#3, which contains 4 lactobacilli strains—*L. acidophilus*, *L. casei*, *Lactobacillus delbrueckii* sp. *bulgaricus*, and *Lactobacillus plantarum;* 3 bifido bacterial strains: *B. longum*, *B. infantis*, and *Bifidobacterium breve;* and *Streptococcus salivarius* sp. *thermophilus*, revealed to decrease activity of pouchitis (a non-specific inflammation of the ileal pouch) in ulcerative colitis (UC) and after ileal anastomosis [37]. The frequent doses recommended in pouchitis are 2–4 sachets daily (each sachet contains 450,000 million live bacteria 4.5 × 10^{11} CFU; but there are also capsules containing 112,000 millions of bacteria) [31]. However, in additional research was described lower improvements in the reduction of disease in association with conventional treatment in patients with UC, and minor to moderate contribution, with the use of probiotic VSL#3, *Escherichia coli* Nissle, *Lactobacillus* GG, or milk fermented with bifidobacteria and/or lactobacilli (whether or not compared to placebo or other treatments, such as mesalazine) [38]. In trials with probiotics on remission induction or maintenance in Crohn's disease (using several strains such as *Lactobacillus* GG, VSL3, *L. johnsonii* LA1, *Escherichia coli* Nissle 1917, *S. boulardii*) have been reported less satisfactory results than in UC [32].

In a 2007 [39] demonstrated that administering probiotics may improve the rate of eradication and reduce the incidence of adverse events in case of infection with *Helicobacter pylori*. Zhang et al. [40] informed that the using the probiotics for standard eradication therapy in patients infected with *H. pylori* may increase the rate of eradication of the microorganism by approximately 13% and decrease the overall rate of adverse effects by approximately 41%, based on the patient's age, gender or probiotics dose. The probiotic used to improve the results of eradication therapies was *Lactobacillus reuteri*. In these therapies which demonstrated an ability to inhibit the colonisation of the human gastric mucosa with *H. pylori*, in addition to an ability to produce reuterin, a broad-spectrum antibiotic active against *H. pylori*, DSM 17648 strain of *L. reuteri* seemed especially effective for eradication therapies [36]. Also, *S. boulardii* seemed to significantly increase the rate of eradication, although under the desired success level (80% versus 71% in the control group) [36].

Few studies are, so far available, and, consequently much clinical evaluation is needed in the future of the most effective strains and of how host factors (such as the genetic characteristics of patients) influence therapeutic response.

2.2.3 Probiotics in liver disease

The researchers reported that probiotics can be useful in treating hepatic diseases due to their potential ability to modulate alterations in the gut microbiota, intestinal permeability, and immune and inflammatory responses. More studies based on murine and *in vitro* models show the role of probiotics in several liver diseases [41]. From medical point of view the pathogenic mechanism involved in liver damage secondary to alcohol abuse is endotoxemia. Researchers reported that through using *L. plantarum* encapsulated alginate beads induce a dose-dependent reduction of endotoxin level in rats exposed to alcohol [41].

Domingo [36] suggests that non-alcoholic fatty liver disease (NAFLD) comprises a varied range of pathological circumstances, from simple steatosis to cirrhosis, through steatohepatitis and fibrosis. It is known that probiotics (VSL#3) can modulate the intestinal flora, influencing the bowel-liver axis and improving NAFLD. Xu et al. [42] reported in a study that compared two types of probiotics (*L. acidophilus* and *B. longum*), neither improved intestinal permeability, but *B. longum* probiotic attenuated hepatic fat accumulation. However there are few human studies on the efficacy of probiotics in the prevention or treatment of NAFLD.

Hepatitis viruses, especially B and C, are known to cause long-term hepatocellular injury. As in other hepatic diseases, the plasma level of endotoxin increases in these patients because of changes in the gut microbiota [41]. Several studies evaluated the effects of probiotics in patients with hepatitis B virus (HBV) and hepatitis C virus (HCV). A research study achieved with *Bifidobacterium adolescentis* SPM0212 lead to increased expression of myxovirus (Mx) resistance A, an interferon (IFN)-inducible antiviral effector. Further, the extracellular surface antigen of HBV level decreased depend by the dose up to 50% and gene expression was inhibited by 40% in hepatoma *cell* line HepG2.2.15 [43].

Also, in the literature have been reported studies regarding treatment with probiotic of patients with cirrhosis. Zhang et al. [44] used a cirrhotic-rat model with modified gut microbiota. In this research it was observed that the effects on total bilirubin (BT) and the ratio between aerobic and anaerobic bacteria were similar in healthy and cirrhotic rats. After administration of norfloxacin and probiotics to modify the gut microbiota, BT, liver function and endotoxemia were estimated. Cirrhotic rats showed a higher population of *Enterobacteriaceae* compared to healthy rats. It was concluded that treatment with bifidobacteria decreased the amount of *Enterobacteriaceae* and endotoxin level and increased the amount of *Lactobacillus* compared with healthy rats [44]. There are limited studies suggesting the role of probiotics for hepatocellular carcinoma. Chávez-Tapia et al. [41] reported in his article that clinical data the next probiotics—*L. rhamnosus LC705* and *Propionibacterium freudenreichii subsp. Shermanii,* maybe reduce the biologically effective dose of aflatoxin exposure. Similar data from murine models with *L. rhamnosus GG* were reported. Particularly after aflatoxin exposure, lower expression of c-myc, cyclin D1, bcl-2 and rasp-21/g3pdh were found [41].

In recent years also, several studies have shown that probiotics have beneficial effects and after liver transplantation. In a research by [45] patients who suffered for liver transplant were allocated to groups that received one of three treatments: live *L. plantarum* 299 strain and prebiotics (fibre), heat-killed lactobacilli and fibre, or selective bowel decontamination. Also, all patients received early enteral feeding. Patients who intake live lactobacilli and fibre developed a lower amount of bacterial infections (e.g. 13%) when compared to patients that underwent selective bowel decontamination: 48% [45]. However, probiotic bacteria such as *Saccharomyces cerevisiae* and *Lactobacillus* have been associated in some studies to the development of sepsis but the use of probiotics in patients who underwent a liver transplant requires at this point, a much more careful analysis of their safety [41].

2.2.4 Probiotics in urogenital and vaginal disease

According to the Centers for Disease Control and Prevention (CDCP), more than 1 billion women around the world suffer from non-sexually transmitted urogenital infections, such as bacterial vaginitis (BV), urinary tract infection (UTI) and several other yeast infections [46]. The dominant microflora in a healthy human vagina is comprised from a variety of *Lactobacillus* species with crucial role in protecting women from genital infections. A slight change in lactobacilli concentration can result in microbial disproportion in the vagina, causing a quantitative and qualitative modification from normally occurring lactobacilli to a mixed microflora controlled by anaerobic bacteria such as *Gardnerella vaginalis*, *Bacteroides* spp., *Prevotella* spp., and *Mobiluncus* species [47]. Commane et al. [48] reported in a research study the importance of probiotics in a woman's urogenital wellbeing. It was confirmed that by supplementing with probiotics (*L. rhamnosus* GR-1 and *Lactobacillus reuteri)* it can stimulate the colonisation of beneficial microbiota and may improve the vaginal health. Daily oral consumption of probiotics such as *L. rhamnosus* and *L. fermentum* exhibited the modification of the vaginal flora [48]. It is well-known that there is an association between abnormal vaginal microbial flora and an increased incidence of urinary tract infection (UTI). When administered twice daily orally the only strains clinically shown to have an effect are *L. rhamnosus* GR-1 and *L. reuteri*, these strains reduce recurrences of UTI and restored a normal lactobacilli dominated vaginal flora in patients [49]. The smallest imbalance in the microbial composition greatly influences the health of the vaginal microenvironment, potentially leading to compromised state of BV and UTI. The primary solution for compromised state would be balancing the number of *Lactobacillus* spp. via the supplementation of probiotics [50].

2.2.5 Probiotics in cardiovascular diseases and lipid metabolism

Cholesterol is a precursor in many biochemical processes of the body and plays a vital role in many functions, like as production of steroidal hormones, while extreme cholesterol in the blood can lead to arterial clogging and increases the risk of heart disease and/or stroke. Patients with hypercholesterolemia showed the risk of heart attacks three times higher, compared to patients with normal blood lipid values [51]. The scientific literature reported some probiotic strains with hypocholerolemic effects, such as: *L. bulgaricus, L. reuteri, and B. coagulans*. Also, clinical research in humans with *L. acidophilus* L1 milk, revealed a significant reduction in serum cholesterol. Further, a clinical trial on 32 hypercholesterolemic patients that consumed low-fat yogurt with *B. longum* BL1 displayed a significant decline in triglycerides, total serum and LDL cholesterol. Also, HDL cholesterol was increased with 14.5% [52]. Thirty-two hyperc-holesterolemic men and women were intake *L. acidophilus* CHO-220 and inulin, during a randomised, double-blind, placebo-controlled, and parallel-designed trial. This research study demonstrated that plasma total cholesterol and low-density lipoprotein (LDL)-cholesterol reduced by 7.84 and 9.27%, respectively, after 12 weeks [53]. Worldwide, it is known that coronary heart disease (CHD) is one of the major causes of adult's death. The main coronary arteries supplying the heart are no longer able to provide sufficient blood and oxygen to the myocardium, mainly because of the accumulation of plaques in the intimae of arteries [54]. Ranjbar et al. [54] concluded that in recent years, several foods enriched with probiotics were produced industrially. These foods have recently been subject to more research for their beneficial effects on the gut microflora and links to their systemic effects on the lowering of lipids known to be risk factors for CHD.

2.2.6 Probiotics in oral health

The human mouth harbours diverse microbiomes in the human body such as viruses, fungi, protozoa, archaea and bacteria and they cause different diseases. From a dental point of view the bacteria cause two common diseases: dental caries and the periodontal (gum) diseases. The most used probiotics for oral health are species of *Lactobacillus* and *Bifidobacterium*. In a double-blind, placebo-controlled trial the consumption of *Streptococcus salivarius* K12 decreased the occurrence of plaque and also, reduced the concentration of *Streptococcus mutans* [55]. It is known that *Streptococcus uberis* and *S. oralis* also can inhibit the periodontal pathogens [56]. Additionally, the halitosis and the volatile sulphur compounds synthesis could be prevented by probiotics consumption.

Bowen [57] declared that the evidence for periodontitis is less than dental caries, but the use of probiotics to manage the oral microflora appears tobe an effective method to control oral conditions [57]. Many more studies are needed to understand the mechanism by which these probiotics colonise and affect the oral cavity. Is needed to better understand how they improve oral health.

2.2.7 Probiotics in lactose intolerance

Daliria and Lee [58] supposed that lactose is an important nutrient in all mammalian neonates, almost all of them have the capability to metabolise lactose to glucose and galactose. It is known that in humans, lactase activity decreases during mid-childhood [58]. Medical research reports that lactose intolerance is determined by blood glucose concentrations, and breath hydrogen test following ingestion of a lactose load [58] and symptoms include: abdominal distress like diarrhoea, bloating, abdominal pain and flatulence. The researchers noticed that treatment with probiotics (such as *Lactobacillus bulgaricus* and *Streptococcus thermophiles*) relieves symptoms of lactose intolerance. It is also observed that consumption of milk containing *Bifidobacterium longum* and *L. acidophilus* cause significantly less hydrogen production and flatulence. In researches where was used a combination of *Lactobacillus casei shirota* and *Bifidobacterium breve* Yakult has shown better effect on patients and improved the symptoms of lactose intolerance significantly [59].

2.2.8 Probiotics in cancer

Kerry et al. [50] declared that as per World Health Organisation (WHO) cancer fact sheet this is a dreadful disease affecting peoples all over the globe. Approximately 14 million new cases and 8.2 million cancer-related deaths added till 2012. The global cancer deaths are from Asian, African, and American continents (more than 70%) [60]. *In vitro* studies, probiotic strains, *Lactobacillus fermentum* NCIMB-5221 and -8829, revealed the highly potential in destroying the colorectal cancer cells and promoting normal epithelial colon cell growth by producing the SCFAs (ferulic acids). This probiotics were compared to other probiotics (*L. acidophilus* ATCC 314 and *L. rhamnosus* ATCC 51303) known with tumorigenic properties [61]. Also, *L. acidophilus* is known to prolong the induction of colon tumours. It was demonstrated that feeding milk and colostrum fermented with *L. acidophilus* resulted in 16–41% reduction in tumour proliferation [62]. Also, the other probiotic *L. bulgaricus* has also been reported to induce antitumor activity against sarcoma-180 and solid Ehrlich ascites tumours [63]. Probiotics could play a significant role in neutralising cancer but research is limited only to *in vitro* tests.

3. Prebiotics

Like probiotics, prebiotics is also being widely explored for their utility in the various field of applied science, more specifically as nutrients and supplements [50]. Food and Agriculture Organisation (FAO)/WHO defines prebiotics as a nonviable food component that confer health benefit(s) on the host associated with modulation of the microbiota [62].

Sources of prebiotics are as follows: breast milk, soybeans, inulin from diverse sources (Jerusalem artichoke, chicory roots), raw oat, wheat bran, barley bran, yacon roots, non-digestible carbohydrates (non-digestible oligosaccharides). From prebiotics, only bifidogenic, non-digestible oligosaccharides, especially inulin, and its hydrolysis products, such as oligofructose, and (trans) galactooligosaccharides (GOS), achieve all the criteria for prebiotics term [64]. Prebiotics can be obtained naturally from sources like vegetables, fruits, and grains consumed in our daily life but are also artificially prebiotic products such as: lactulose, galactooligosaccharides, fructooligosaccharides.

Kuo [65] reported that an ideal prebiotic should be:

- resistant to the actions of acids in the stomach, bile salts and other hydrolysing enzymes in the intestine;
- not be absorbed in the upper gastrointestinal tract;
- be easily fermentable by the beneficial intestinal microflora.

Prebiotics not only serve as an energy source because their presence of prebiotics in the diet may lead to numerous health benefits. Several health benefits are reported in scientific literature, such as inhibition of the development of pathogens, reducing the prevalence and duration of diarrhoea, increases the absorption of minerals, mostly of magnesium and calcium, exerting protective effects to prevent colon cancer and providing relief from inflammation and other symptoms associated with intestinal bowel disorders.

Several studies demonstrated that the colorectal carcinoma was less present at people who consume a lot of vegetables and fruits. The inulin and oligofructose from fruits and vegetables could suppress the disease [66]. When it comes to the advantages of prebiotics, it can be mention the reduction of the blood LDL (low-density lipoprotein) level, stimulation of the immunological system, increased the calcium absorbability, preservation of adequate intestinal pH value, low caloric value, and alleviation of symptoms of peptic ulcers and vaginal mycosis [67]. Other benefits of inulin and oligofructose on human health could be the prevention of carcinogenesis, as well as the support of lactose intolerance or dental caries treatment [68]. Also, prebiotics are useful in combating pathogenic microorganisms, such as *Salmonella enteritidis* and *Escherichia coli*, and reduce odour compounds and [69] confirmed a positive effect of fructooligosaccharides (FOS) on protection against *Salmonella typhimurium* and *Listeria monocytogenes* infections. Pokusaeva et al. [70] said that prebiotics are also implicated in enhancing the bioavailability and uptake of minerals, lowering of some risk factors for cardiovascular disease, and promoting satiety and weight loss.

Prebiotics have been reported to play a beneficial role in controlling the IBD. A major reduction in the number of bacteriodetes in faeces was reported in patients with chronic pouchitis treated with 24 g per day of inulin [71]. In another study, 10 Crohn's Disease patients receiving 15 g of FOS demonstrated a reduced disease activity index [72]. In another randomised study involving 103 Crohn's Disease patients who received FOS 15 g/day these showed no clinical improvement however, though no change in IL-12 was observed it was able to reduce IL-6 of lamina propria dendritic cells [1].

Kerry et al. [50] suggests that even with their enormous nutritional and medicinal benefits, research concerning screening new versatile prebiotics is quite deficient. Therefore, the research should be focused on identifying new healthy supplements, while screening novel prebiotic strains should be a major concern.

4. Synbiotics

Due to the expansion of microbial research were discovered synbiotics as a combination of probiotics and prebiotics products which provide the survival and the implantation of the live microorganism dietary supplements in the gut [73]. The synergistic welfares are more proficiently promoted when both the probiotic and prebiotic act together in the living system. It is known that the symbiotic association between prebiotics and probiotics significantly improve the human health [50]. From the medical point of view the term of synbiotic product positively influence the host through improving the survival and implantation of live microbial dietary supplements in to the gastrointestinal tract and stimulating the growth and/or activating the metabolism of health promoting bacteria [62]. Since the word synbiotics suggests synergism, this term should be reserved for products in which the prebiotic compound(s) positively influence the probiotic organism(s) [74]. Markowiak and Śliżewska [1] suggests that when develop a synbiotic product, the most important aspect that have taken into account, is the selection of an appropriate probiotic and prebiotic, that can act separately on the host's health. The prebiotic compounds should selectively stimulate the growth of probiotics, with beneficial effect on human health and not to be able to stimulate the other microorganisms.

Lactobacillus spp., *Bifidobacteria* spp., *S. boulardii*, *B. coagulans* are one of the probiotic strains that are used in synbiotic formulations, whereas the prebiotics used are as follows: oligosaccharides (fructooligosaccharide (FOS), GOS and xyloseoligosaccharide (XOS)), and inulin (from natural sources like chicory and yacon roots) [62]. Synbiotics consumption by humans includes the following beneficial effects:

- Increased levels of lactobacilli and bifidobacteria and balanced gut microbiota.
- Prevention of bacterial translocation and reduced incidences of nosocomial infections in surgical patients.
- Improvement of liver function in cirrhotic patients.
- Improvement of immunomodulating ability [75].

In adult subjects with non-alcoholic steatohepatisis (NASH) in a randomised study what used of a synbiotic product which contained five probiotics namely: *Lactobacillus plantarum*, *L. delbrueckii* spp. *bulgaricus*, *L. acidophilus*, *L. rhamnosus*, *Bifidobacterium bifidum* and inulin as a prebiotic has been demonstrated a significant reduction of intrahepatic triacylglycerol (IHTG) within 6 months [1]. Fifty-two adults participated for 28 weeks in a research trial based on the effects of the synbiotic product. The synbiotic comprised a mix of probiotic strains: *Lactobacillus casei, L. rhamnosus, Streptococcus thermophilus, Bifidobacterium breve, L. acidophilus, B. longum, L. bulgaricus* and fructooligosccharides, as prebiotic. The authors stated that consumption of the synbiotic product resulted in the inhibition of nuclear factor-kB (NF-kB) and a condensed production of tumour necrosis factor α (TNF-α) [76].

Moreover, synbiotics seems to be quite attractive for improving the immune system. A significant decrease in the levels of C-reactive protein and also increase the glutathione levels was obtained through combination of *B. coagulans* with inulin, in diet for 6 weeks [77].

Recently, commercial interest in functional foods based on synbiotics has improved due to the awareness of the welfares for gut health, disease prevention and therapy. Investigates in this scientific zone is presently concentrated on designing new functional foods, as well as on screening new strains with capability to inhabit the human gut, along with their aptitude to metabolise new prebiotics [50]. Trials and investigation *in vitro* and *in vivo* demonstrated that the beneficial effects of using probiotics, prebiotics, and synbiotics in health are much more active than their unitary use known till present. Nevertheless, more investigates concerning the designing new mixtures of probiotics, prebiotics and synbiotics are imperative necessary for achieve further opportunities of improving nutritional and clinical health.

5. Conclusion

The use of probiotics, prebiotics, and synbiotics in health is emerging as a promising therapy which is generally safe in different disease. Probiotics, probiotics and synbiotics have systemic effects on the urogenital disease, liver disease, oral health and immune system. There are many published reports on the use of probiotics in humans but information on prebiotics and synbiotics is quite a few. It seems that we will see and in the coming years further studies on combinations of probiotics and prebiotics, and further development of synbiotics. It is possible that future studies may explain the mechanisms of actions of those components, which may confer a beneficial effect on human health. However, the health claims made needs to be substantiated and firmly established by properly designed large scale clinical trials on human body. Therefore, current focus is on evaluating new strains of probiotics, a new prebiotics and new synbiotics products and their applicability in biomedical/clinical research, paving a new direction for exploration and exploitation of probiotics, prebiotics and synbiotics aimed at improving human health. There is a need for more randomised, placebo-controlled clinical trials with adequate statistical power. I encourage researchers to submit possible publications in peer-reviewed journals of all clinical trials, whether the outcome is positive, negative or adverse, because the scientific and medical world needs it relevant information on the dose–response effects, efficacy, and safety of probiotic, prebiotic and synbiotic products. At present, the available information on current probiotics, prebiotics and synbiotics provides convincing safety records. I believe it is highly likely that in the near future, the vast amount of research on the beneficial impact of the probiotics, prebiotics and synbiotics on human wellbeing will suppose discovery and development of innovative products derived from our microbiota. Further, these may belong to uncommon and formerly uncharacterized microorganisms with rare assets, or perhaps could be microorganisms formerly known as pathogens or pathobionts. These progresses will represent new trends but also significant challenges for scientific and medical research, for industrial exploitation and for human health and clinical nutrition.

Conflict of interest

Author declares no conflict of interest.

Author details

Nicoleta-Maricica Maftei
Faculty of Medicine and Pharmacy, “Dunărea de Jos” University of Galati, Galați, România

*Address all correspondence to: nicoleta.aron@ugal.ro

References

[1] Markowiak P, Śliżewska K. Effects of probiotics, prebiotics, and synbiotics on human health. Nutrients. 2017;**9**(1021):1-30. DOI: 10.3390/nu9091021

[2] Metchnikoff E, Mitchell PC, editors. Essais Optimistes. London: Heinemann; 1907

[3] Tissier H. Tritement des infections intestinales par la methode de translormation de la flore bacterienne de lintestin. Comptes Rendus Social Biology. 1906;**60**:359-361 (in French)

[4] Havenaar R, Huis in't Veld JHJ. Probiotics: A general view. In: Wood BJB, editor. The Lactic Acid Bacteria in Health and Disease. London: Elsevier Applied Science; 1992. pp. 151-170

[5] Food and Agriculture Organization (FAO). Guidelines for the Evaluation of Probiotics in Food; Report of a Joint FAO/WHO Working Group on Drafting Guidelines for the Evaluation of Probiotics in Food. London, ON, Canada: FAO; 2002

[6] Hill C, Guarner F, Rei G, Gibson GR, Merenstein DJ, Pot B, et al. Expert consensus document: The International Scientific Association for Probiotics and Prebiotics consensus statement on the scope and appropriate use of the term probiotic. Nature Reviews Gastroenterology & Hepatology. 2014;**11**:506-514. DOI: 10.1038/nrgastro.2014.66

[7] Gibson RG, Roberfroid MB. Dietary modulation of the human colonic microbiota: Introducing the concept of prebiotics. The Journal of Nutrition. 1995;**125**:1401-1412. DOI: 10.1093/jn/125.6.1401

[8] Gibson GR, Probert HM, van Loo J, Rastall RA, Roberfroid M. Dietary modulation of the human colonic microbiota: Updating the concept of the prebiotics. Nutrition Research Reviews. 2004;**17**:259-275. DOI: 10.1079/NRR200479

[9] Food and Agriculture Organization. FAO Technical Meeting on Prebiotics: Food Quality and Standards Service (AGNS), Food and Agriculture Organization of the United Nations (FAO). Rome, Italy: FAO Technical Meeting Report; FAO; 2007. pp. 15-16

[10] Skalkam ML, Wiese M, Nielsen DS, van Zanten G. In Vitro Screening and Evaluation of Synbiotics. Copenhagen, Denmark: University of Copenhagen; 2016 (Chapter 33). pp. 477-486

[11] Cencic A, Chingwaru W. The role of functional foods, nutraceuticals, and food supplements in intestinal health. Nutrients. 2010;**2**:611-625. DOI: 10.3390/nu2060611

[12] Rioux KP, Madsen KL, Fedorak RN. The role of enteric microflora in inflammatory bowel disease: Human and animal studies with probiotics and prebiotics. Gastroenterology Clinics of North America. 2005;**34**:465-482. DOI: 10.3390/nu2060611

[13] Bengmark S. Bioecological control of the gastrointestinal tract: The role of flora and supplemented probiotics and synbiotics. Gastroenterology Clinics of North America. 2005;**34**:413-436. DOI: 10.1016/j.gtc.2005.05.002

[14] Panesar PS, Kaur G, Panesar R, Bera MB. Synbiotics: Potential Dietary Supplements in Functional Foods. Berkshire, UK: IFIS; 2009. DOI: 10.1136/gut.2005.074971

[15] Lloyd-Price J, Abu-Ali G, Huttenhower C. The healthy human microbiome. Genome

Medicine. 2016;**8**:1-11. DOI: 10.1186/s13073-016-0307-y

[16] Miecznikow E. O naturze ludzkiej—Zarys Filozofii Optymistycznej (Translation F. Wermiński). Warszawa, Poland: Wydawnictwo Biblioteka Naukowa; 1907

[17] Amara AA, Shibl A. Role of probiotics in health improvement, infection control and disease treatment and management. Saudi Pharmaceutical Journal. 2015;**23**:107-114. DOI: 10.1016/j.jsps.2013.07.001

[18] O'Toole PW, Marchesi JR, Hill C. Next-generation probiotics: The spectrum from probiotics to live biotherapeutics. Nature Microbiology. 2017;**2**:1-6 (article number: 17057). DOI: 10.1038/nmicrobiol.2017.57 Available from: www.nature.com/naturemicrobiology

[19] Anadón A, Martínez-Larrañaga MR, Martínez MA. Probiotics for animal nutrition in the European Union. Regulation and safety assessment. Regulatory Toxicology and Pharmacology. 2006;**45**:91-95. DOI: 10.1016/j.yrtph.2006.02.004

[20] Gaggia F, Mattarelli P, Biavati B. Probiotics and prebiotics in animal feeding for safe food production. International Journal of Food Microbiology. 2010;**141**:S15-S28. DOI: 10.1016/j.ijfoodmicro.2010.02.031

[21] Thomas CM, Versalovic J. Probiotics-host communication: Modulationof signaling pathways in the intestine. Gut Microbes. 2010;**1**(3): 148-163. DOI: 10.4161/gmic.1.3.11712

[22] Shiou R, Yu Y, Guo Y, He SM, Andrew CHM, Hoenig J, et al. Synergistic protection of combined probiotic con-ditioned media against neonatal necrotizing enterocolitis-like intestinalinjury. PLoS One. 2013;**8**(5): e65108. DOI: 10.1371/journal.pone.0065108

[23] Cosmi L, Maggi L, Santarlasci V, Liotta F, Annunziato F. T helper cells plasticity in inflammation. Cytometry. Part A. 2014;**85**(1):36-42. DOI: 10.1002/cyto.a.22348

[24] Hardy H, Harris J, Lyon E, Beal J, Foey A. Probiotics, prebiotics and immunomodulation of gut mucosal defences: Homeostasis andimmunopathology. Nutrients. 2013;**5**:1869-1912. DOI: 10.3390/nu5061869

[25] Vandenbergh PA. Lactic acid bacteria, their metabolic products and interference with microbial growth. FEMS Microbiology Reviews. 1993;**12**:221-238. DOI: 10.1111/j.1574-6976.1993.tb00020.x

[26] Guillot JF. Probiotic feed additives. Journal of Veterinary Pharmacology and Therapeutics. 2003;**26**:52-55. DOI: 10.1046/J.1365-2885.26

[27] Isolauri E, Sutas Y, Kankaanpaa P, Arvilommi H, Salminen S. Probiotics: Effects on immunity. American Journal of Clinical Nutrition. 2001;**73**:444-450. DOI: 10.1093/ajcn/73.2.444s

[28] Brandao RL, Castro IM, Bambirra EA, Amaral SC, Fietto LG, Tropia MJM. Intracellular signal triggered by cholera toxin in *Saccharomyces boulardii* and *Saccharomyces cerevisiae*. Applied and Environmental Microbiology. 1998;**64**:564-568

[29] Schachtsiek M, Hammes WP, Hertel C. Characterization of *Lactobacillus coryniformis* DSM 20001T surface protein CPF mediating coaggregation with and aggregation among pathogens. Applied and Environmental Microbiology. 2004;**70**:7078-7085. DOI: 10.1128/AEM.70.12.7078-7085.2004

[30] Oelschlaeger A. Mechanisms of probiotic actions—A review. International Journal of Medical Microbiology. 2010;**300**:57-62. DOI: 10.1016/j.ijmm.2009.08.005

[31] Olveira G, González-Moleroa I. An update on probiotics, prebiotics and symbiotics in clinical nutrition. Endocrinología y Nutrición. 2016;**63**(9):482-494. DOI: 10.1016/j.endoen.2016.10.011

[32] Floch MH, Walker WA, Sanders ME, Nieuwdorp M, Kim AS, Brenner DA, et al. Recommendations for probiotic use-2015update: Proceedings and consensus opinion. Journal of Clinical Gastroenterology. 2015;**49**(Suppl. 1):S69-S73. DOI: 10.1016/j.iccn.2010.07.001

[33] McFarland LV. Probiotics for the primary and secondary preven-tion of *C. difficile* infections: A meta-analysis and systematic review. Antibiotics. 2015;**4**:160-178. DOI: 10.3390/antibiotics4020160

[34] Dang Y, Reinhardt JD, Zhou X, Zhang G. The effect of probioticssupplementation on *Helicobacter pylori* eradication rates andside effects during eradication therapy: A meta-analysis. PLoS One. 2014;**9**:e111030. DOI: 10.1371/journal.pone.0111030

[35] Parvez S, Malik KA, Ah Kang S, Kim HY. Probiotics and their fermented food products are beneficial for health. Journal of Applied Microbiology. 2006;**100**:1171-1185. DOI: 10.1111/j.1365-2672.2006.02963.x

[36] Domingo JJS. Review of the role of probiotics in gastrointestinal diseases in adults. Gastroenterología y Hepatología. 2017;**40**(6):417-429. DOI: 10.1016/j.gastre.2016.12.001

[37] Guslandi M. Role of probiotics in Crohn's disease and in pouch-itis. Journal of Clinical Gastroenterology. 2015;**49**(1):S46-S59. DOI: 10.1097/MCG.0000000000000351

[38] Chibbar R, Dieleman LA. Probiotics in the management of ulcerative colitis. Journal of Clinical Gastroenterology. 2015;**49**(1):S50-S55. DOI: 10.1097/MCG.0000000000000368

[39] Tong JL, Ran ZH, Shen J, Zhang CX, Xiao SD. Meta-analysis: The effect of supplementation with probiotics on eradication rates and adverse events during *Helicobacter pylori* eradication therapy. Alimentary Pharmacology & Therapeutics. 2007;**25**:155-168. DOI: 10.1111/j.1365-2036.2006.03179.x

[40] Zhang MM, Qian W, Qin YY, He J, Zhou YH. Probiotics in *Helicobacter pylori* eradication therapy: A systematic review and meta-analysis. World Journal of Gastroenterology. 2015;**21**:4345-4357. DOI: 10.3748/wjg.v21.i14.4345

[41] Chávez-Tapia NC, González-Rodríguez L, Jeong MS, López-Ramírez Y, Barbero-Becerra V, Juárez-Hernández E, et al. Current evidence on the use of probiotics in liver diseases. Journal of Functional Foods. 2015;**17**:137-151. DOI: 10.1016/j.jff.2015.05.009

[42] Xu RY, Wan YP, Fang QY, Lu W, Cai W. Supplementation with probiotics modifies gut flora and attenuates liver fat accumulation in rat nonalcoholic fatty liver disease model. Journal of Clinical Biochemistry and Nutrition. 2012;**50**(1):72-77. DOI: 10.3164/jcbn.11-38

[43] Lee DK, Kang JY, Shin HS, Park IH, Ha NJ. Antiviral activity of Bifidobacterium adolescentis SPM0212 against hepatitis B virus. Archives of Pharmacal Research. 2013;**36**(12):1525-1532. DOI: 10.1007/s12272-013-0141-3

[44] Zhang W, Gu Y, Chen Y, Deng H, Chen L, Che S, et al. Intestinal flora

imbalance results in altered bacterial translocation and liver function in rats with experimental cirrhosis. European Journal of Gastroenterology & Hepatology. 2010;**22**(12):1481-1486. DOI: 10.1097/MEG.0b013e32833eb8b0

[45] Rayes N, Seehofer D, Hansen S, Boucsein K, Müller AR, Serk S, et al. Early enteral supply of lactobacillus and fiber versus selective bowel decontamination: A controlled trial in liver transplant recipients. Transplantation. 2002;**74**(1):123-128 12134110

[46] Waigankar SS, Patel V. Role of probiotics in urogenital healthcare. Journal of Midlife Health. 2011;**2**:5-10. DOI: 10.4103/0976-7800.83253

[47] Petricevic L, Domig K, Nierscher F, Sandhofer M, Fidesser M, Krondorfer I, et al. Characterisation of the vaginal *Lactobacillus* microbiota associated with preterm delivery. Scientific Reports. 2014;**4**:1-6 (article number: 5136). DOI: 10.1038/srep05136

[48] Commane D, Hughes R, Shortt C, Rowland I. The potential mechanisms involved in the anti-carcinogenic action of probiotics. Mutation Research. 2005;**591**:276-289. DOI: 10.1016/j.mrfmmm.2005.02.027

[49] Reid G, Bruce A. Probiotics to prevent urinary tract infections: The rationale and evidence. World Journal of Urology. 2006;**24**:28-32. DOI: 10.1007/s00345-005-0043-1

[50] Kerry GR, Patra JK, Gouda S, Park Y, Shin HS, Das G. Benefaction of probiotics for human health: A review. Journal of Food and Drug Analysis. 2018;**26**(3):927-939. DOI: 10.1016/j.jfda.2018.01.002

[51] Ghosh AR. Appraisal of probiotics and prebiotics in gastrointestinal infections. Webmed Central Gastroenterology. 2012;**3**(10):WMC003796. DOI: 10.9754/journal.wmc.2012.003795

[52] Homayouni A, Payahoo L, Azizi A. Effects of probiotics on lipid profile: A review. American Journal of Food Technology. 2012;**7**(5):251-265. DOI: 10.3923/ajft.2012.251.265

[53] Ooi LG, Liong MT. Cholesterol-lowering effects of probiotics andprebiotics: A review of *in vivo* and *in vitro* findings. International Journal of Molecular Sciences. 2010;**11**:2499-2522. DOI: 10.3390/ijms11062499

[54] Ranjbar F, Akbarzadeh F, Homayouni A. Probiotics usage in heart disease and psychiatry, chapter 61, in book: Probiotics, Prebiotics, and Synbiotics Bioactive Foods in Health Promotion: Probiotics and Prebiotics, Edited by R. Ross Watson and V. R. Preedy. Elsevier Inc., Academic Press, London, UK, 2016, pp.807-811

[55] Burton J, Drummond B, Chilcott C, Tagg J, Thomson W, Hale J, et al. Influence of the probiotic *Streptococcus salivarius* strain M18 on indices of dental health in children: A randomized double-blind,placebo-controlled trial. Journal of Medical Microbiology. 2013;**62**:875-884. DOI: 10.1099/jmm.0.056663-0

[56] Hillma J, McDonell E, Hillman C, Zahradnik R, Soni M. Safety assessment of ProBiora3, a probiotic mouthwash: Subchronic toxicity study in rats. International Journal of Toxicology. 2009;**28**:357-367. DOI: 10.1177/1091581809340705

[57] Bowen DM. Probiotics and oral health. Journal of Dental Hygiene. 2013;**87**:5-9

[58] Daliria EBM, Lee BH. New perspectives on probiotics in health and disease. Food Science and Human Wellness. 2015;**4**(2):56-65. DOI: 10.1016/j.fshw.2015.06.002

[59] Vonk RJ, Reckman GA, Harmsen HJ, Priebe MG. Probiotics and lactose intolerance. In: Rigobelo EC, editor. Probiotics. Rijeka, Crotatia: InTech; 2012. DOI: 10.5772/51424

[60] Vidya S, Thiruneelakandan G. Probiotic potentials of lactobacillus and its anti-cancer activity. International Journal of Current Research. 2015;7:20680-20684

[61] Kahouli I, Malhotra M, Alaoui-Jamali MA, Prakash S. *In-vitro* characterization of the anti-cancer activity of the probiotic bacterium *Lactobacillus fermentum* NCIMB 5221 and potential against colorectal cancer cells. Journal of Cancer Science and Therapy. 2015;7:224-235. DOI: 10.4172/1948-5956.1000354

[62] Pandey KR, Naik SR, Vakil BV. Probiotics, prebiotics and synbiotics—A review. Journal of Food Science and Technology. 2015;**52**(12):7577-7587. DOI: 10.1007/s13197-015-1921-1

[63] Lee JH, Nam SH, Seo WT, Yun HD, Hong SY, Kim MK, et al. The production of surfactin during the fermentation of *cheonggukjang* by potential probiotic B*acillus subtilis* CSY191 and the resultant growth suppression of MCF-7 human breast cancer cells. Food Chemistry. 2012;**131**(4):1347-1354. DOI: 10.1016/j.foodchem.2011.09.133

[64] Pokusaeva K, Fitzgerald GF, van Sinderen D. Carbohydrate metabolism in Bifidobacteria. Genesis Nutrition. 2011;**6**(3):285-306. DOI: 10.1007/s12263-010-0206-6

[65] Kuo SM. The interplay between fiber and the intestinal microbiome in the inflammatory response. Advances in Nutrition: Journal of Internal Medicine. 2013;**4**(1):16-28. DOI: 10.3945/an.112.003046

[66] Mojka K. Probiotyki, prebiotyki i synbiotyki—Charakterystyka i funkcje. Problemy Higieny i Epidemiologii. 2014;**95**:541-549

[67] Socha P, Stolarczyk M, Socha J. Wpływ probiotyków i prebiotyków na gospodarke̜ lipidowa̜. Pediatria Współczesna Gastroenterologia Hepatologia I Żywienie Dziecka. 2002;**4**:85-88

[68] Jakubczyk E, Kosikowska M. Nowa generacja mlecznych produktów fermentowanych z udziałem probiotyków i prebiotyków, produkty synbiotyczne. Przegląd Mleczarski. 2000;**12**:397-400

[69] Buddington KK, Danohoo JB, Buddington RK. Dietary oligofructose and inulin protect mice from enteric and systemic pathogens and tumour inducers. The Journal of Nutrition. 2002;**132**:472-477. DOI: 10.1093/jn/132.3.472

[70] Pokusaeva K, Fitzgerald GF, Sinderen D. Carbohydrate metabolism in bifidobacteria. Genes & Nutrition. 2011;**6**:285-306. DOI: 10.1007/s12263-010-0206-6

[71] Langen LV, Mirjam AC, Dieleman LA. Prebiotics in chronic intestinal inflammation. Inflammatory Bowel Diseases. 2009;**15**(3):454-462. DOI: 10.1002/ibd.20737

[72] Lindsay JO, Whelan K, Stagg AJ, Gobin P, HO A-H, Rayment N, et al. Clinical, microbiological, and immunological effects of fructo-oligosaccharide in patients with Crohn's disease. Gut. 2006;**55**(3):348-355. DOI: 10.1136/gut.2005.074971

[73] Tufarelli V, Laudadio V. An overview on the functional food concept: Prospectives and applied researches in probiotics, prebiotics and synbiotics. Journal of Experimental Biology and Agricultural Sciences. 2016;**4**:274-278. DOI: 10.18006/2016.4(3S).273.278

[74] Cencic A, Chingwaru W. The role of functional foods, nutraceuticals, and food supplements in intestinal health. Nutrients. 2010;**2**(6):611-625. DOI: 10.3390/nu2060611

[75] Zhang MM, Cheng JQ, Lu YR, Yi ZH, Yang P, Wu XT. Use of pre-, pro-and synbiotics in patients with acute pancreatitis: A metaanalysis. World Journal of Gastroenterology. 2010;**16**(31):3970. DOI: 10.3748/wjg.v16.i31.3970

[76] Eslamparast T, Poustchi H, Zamani F, Sharafkhah M, Malekzadeh R, Hetmatdoost A. Synbiotic supplementation in nonalcoholic fatty liver disease: A randomized, double-blind, placebo-controlled pilot study. The American Journal of Clinical Nutrition. 2014;**99**:535-542. DOI: 10.3945/ajcn.113.068890

[77] Panda AK, Rao SVR, Raju MV, Sharma SR. Dietary supplementation of Lactobacillus sporogenes on performance and serum biochemico-lipid profile of broiler chickens. The Journal of Poultry Science. 2006;**43**(3):235-240

Chapter 5

African Fermented Food Condiments: Microbiology Impacts on Their Nutritional Values

Nurudeen Ayoade Olasupo and Princewill Chimezie Okorie

Abstract

Fermented food flavoring condiments are products usually derived from the fermentative activities of microorganisms on vegetable proteins of legumes or oil seeds. Africa is a continent that is endowed with many fermented food condiments. These condiments, apart from their flavoring properties, serve as a cheap source of plant protein to the populace, especially the rural dweller whose staple foods are mainly carbohydrate based. The production dynamics of these condiments vary from country to country. However, the microbial interplay during their production and their nutritional qualities appear to be same. This chapter seeks to evaluate the range of substrates employed in the production of fermented condiments of African origin, the microbial interplay in their production and their nutritional values.

Keywords: microbiology, nutrition, fermentation, African fermented condiments

1. Introduction

Fermented foods constitute a significant component of African diets. There are many fermented foods known in Africa. These foods are classified into five major categories based on the substrate from which they are derived [1] and they include fermented food condiments among others.

Condiment is defined as a spice, sauce or other food preparation that is added to food to impart a particular flavor or enhance its taste (example salt). Fermented food flavoring condiments are products usually derived from the fermentative activities of microorganisms on vegetable proteins of legumes or oil seeds origin [2, 3]. They include *iru* from Africa locust bean, *ugba* from African oil bean seed and *ogiri* from melon seeds among others. These fermented food condiments are known to be good sources of proteins and vitamins [1, 4].

The use of fermented vegetable proteins as seasonings is wide spread in Africa, especially among the rural dwellers. In West Africa, some of the common fermented vegetable condiments include *iru or dawadawa* from locust bean (*Parkia biglobosa*) (**Figure 1**), *ogiri* from melon seeds (*Citrullus vulgaris*) (**Figure 2**), *daddawa* from soybean (*Glycine max*), *soumbala* from soybean (*Glycine max*) (**Figure 3**), *ugba* from African oil bean seed (*Pentaclethra macrophylla*) (**Figure 4**) and *owoh* from

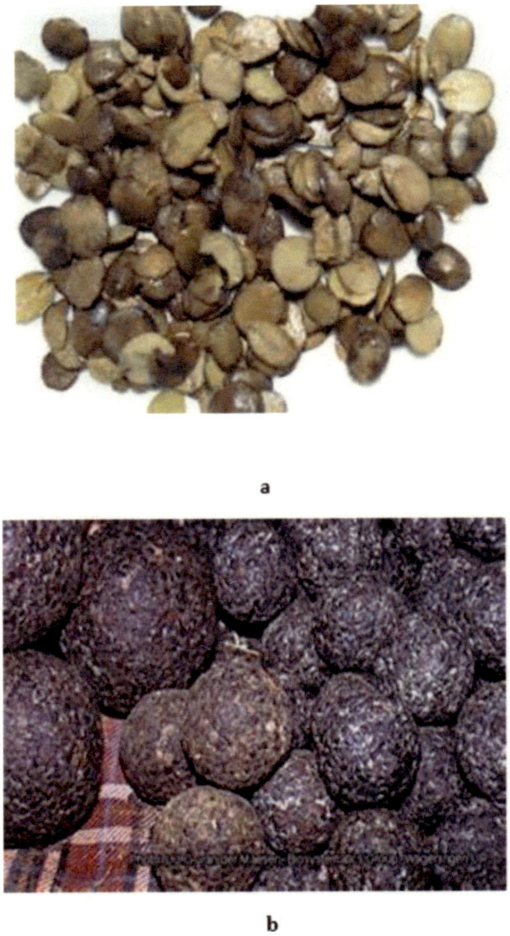

Figure 1.
Unfermented seeds of African locust bean (a) and fermented seeds of African locust bean (b) (iru/ dawadawa/ Afitin/Sonru/soumbala). Source: [31].

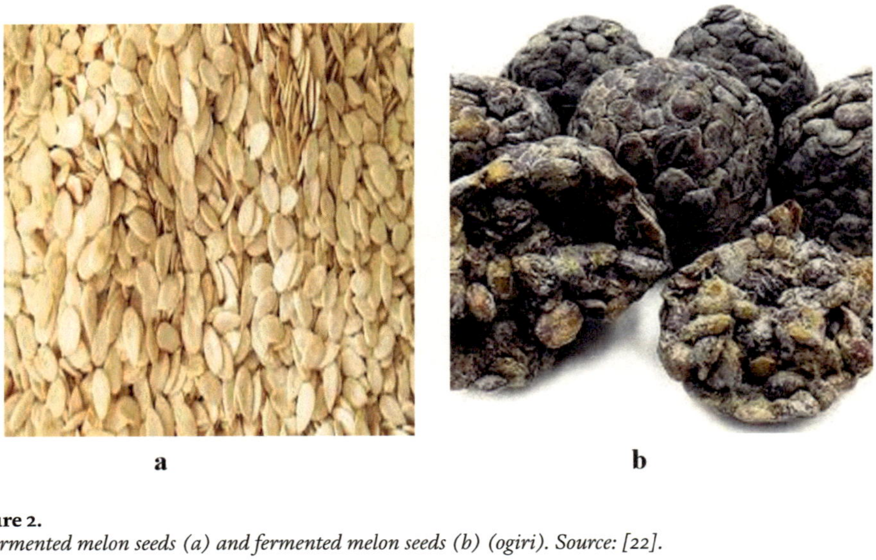

Figure 2.
Unfermented melon seeds (a) and fermented melon seeds (b) (ogiri). Source: [22].

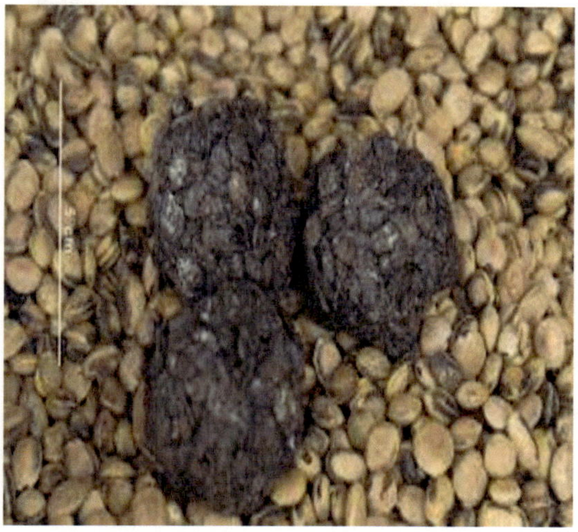

Figure 3.
Soumbala (in balls) and the seeds used for their preparation. Source: [11].

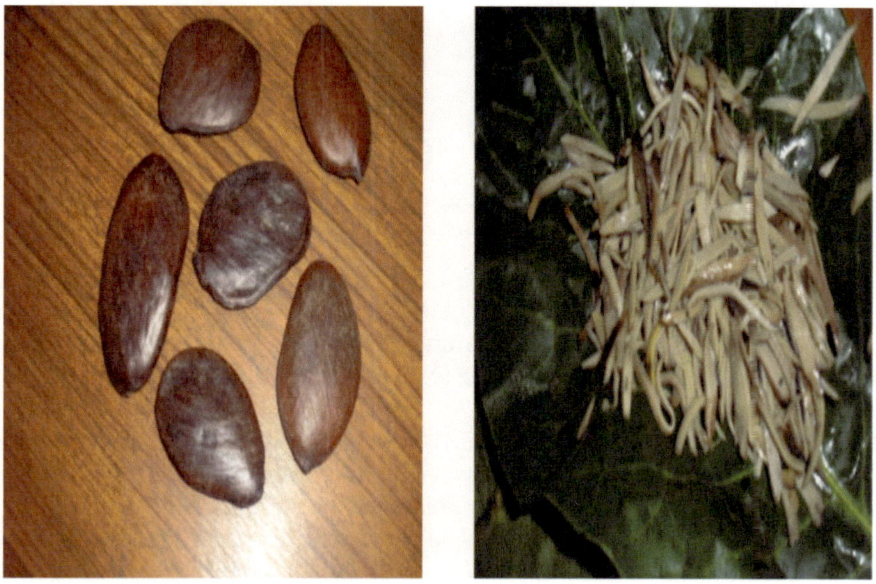

a b

Figure 4.
African oil bean seeds (a) and fermented slices of the oil bean cotyledon (b) ugba. Source: [57].

cotton seeds (*Gossypium hirsutum*). **Table 1** presents a comprehensive list of fermented food condiments of African origin.

These fermented condiments bear different names according to the country or region of the continent from which they are produced. African locust bean tree (*Parkia biglobosa*), for instance, is one of the most common plants whose seeds are used as protein source condiment after fermentation. It is consumed by various socioethnic groups in the West African subregion, and it bears different names across the region. It is popularly known as *afitin/sonru/iru* in Benin [5–7], *iru/dawadawa* in Nigeria [8, 9], *soumbala* in Burkina Faso [10, 11] and *netetu* in Senegal [12].

Raw material	Product	Country	Reference
Soy bean	*Dawadawa*	Nigeria	[19]
	Soumbala	Burkina Faso	[11]
	Tempeh	Ghana	[19]
Melon seed	*Ogiri*	Nigeria	[23]
Castor oil seed	*Ogiri igbo*	Nigeria	[26]
Fluted pumpkin seed	*Ogiri ugu*	Nigeria	[27]
African locust bean	*Dawadawa/iru*	Nigeria	[17]
	Afitin/Sonru	Benin	[5]
	Soumbala	Burkina Faso	[10]
	Netetu	Senegal	[12]
African oil bean seed	*Ugba*	Nigeria	[38]
African yam bean	*Ogiri*	Nigeria	[38]
Cotton seed	*Owoh*	Nigeria	[95]
Bambara groundnut	*Ogiri okpei*	Nigeria	[31]
Prosopis africana seed	*Okpehe*	Nigeria	[28]
Roselle plant	*Bikalga*	Burkina Faso	[14]
	Dawadawa botso	Niger	[14]
	Furundu	Sudan	[14]
	Mbuja	Cameroon	[14]
Fish	*Lanhouin*	Benin	[15]

Table 1.
Common fermented food condiments of African origin.

The Roselle plant (*Hibiscus sabdariffa* L.) is another herbal shrub whose seeds are rich in protein, oil and dietary fiber [13]. The seeds of this plant are widely used in alkaline fermentation for the production of food condiment popularly known as *bikalga* (Burkina Faso), *dawadawa botso* (Niger), *datou* (Mali), *furundu* (Sudan) and *mbuja* (Cameroon) [14].

Even within a country, the names of these condiments vary from one part to another. The origin of such names, however, could be attributed to a number of factors which include (a) the region or area of manufacture of the condiment, (b) the type of legume or oil seed used and (c) the spelling according to the region or area. In Nigeria, for instance, the Yorubas of the Southwestern Nigeria locally call fermented condiments *iru*, the Hausas of the Northern part call it *dawadawa* and the Ibos of the Eastern part call it *ogiri* [1]. *Owoh*, on the other hand, is a popular name for fermented condiments among the Urhobos and Itsekiris in the Niger Delta region, while the Igala and Idoma people of the Middle Belt region call it *okpiye* [3].

The conventional substrates for these condiments production are diverse but are mainly legumes and oil seeds. *Lanhouin* is, however, a fish-based condiment, which is common in Benin [15]. *Lanhouin* is used as a taste- and flavor-enhancing condiment in some main dishes such as vegetable, slimy vegetable and tomato sauces. One condiment can be produced from more than one raw material. For instance, in Nigeria, *dawadawa* and *iru* are locally produced from three materials: African locust bean (*Parkia biglobosa*), soybean (*Glycine max*) or Bambara groundnut (*Vigna subterranea*) [16–21]. *Ogiri* is traditionally prepared by fermenting melon seeds (*Citrullus vulgaris*) and fluted pumpkin (*Telfairia occidentalis*) or castor oil seed (*Ricinus communis*) [22–27]. *Owoh* is produced from fermented seeds of the cotton plant (*Gossypium hirsutum*) or African yam bean (*Sphenostylis stenocarpa*)

DOI: http://dx.doi.org/10.5772/intechopen.83466

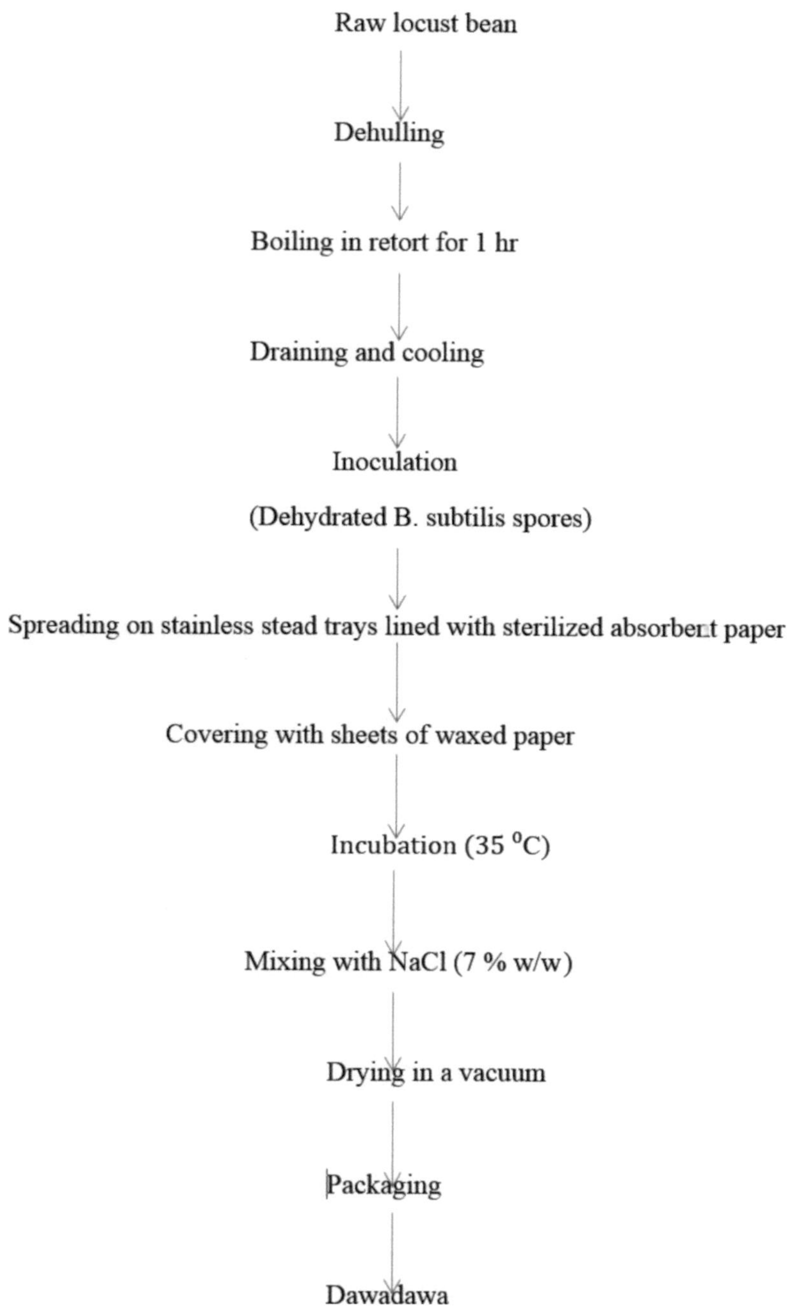

Figure 5.
Flowchart for the preparation of dawadawa. Source: [31].

[28–30]. On the other hand, *okpiye* is prepared from the seeds of *Proscpis africana* [31–33]. Almost any edible plant material can be subjected to fermentation to produce condiment.

Fermented food condiments play very important role in the diet of many Africans. They are used to enhance the flavor of many dishes including soups and sauces [6, 34]. These fermented food condiments are also known to be good sources of protein and vitamins [1, 4]. Apart from the flavoring attributes, they contribute to the protein intake of the consumers. The significance of this fact is better appreciated when you realize that most of the meals in many parts of West, Central, and

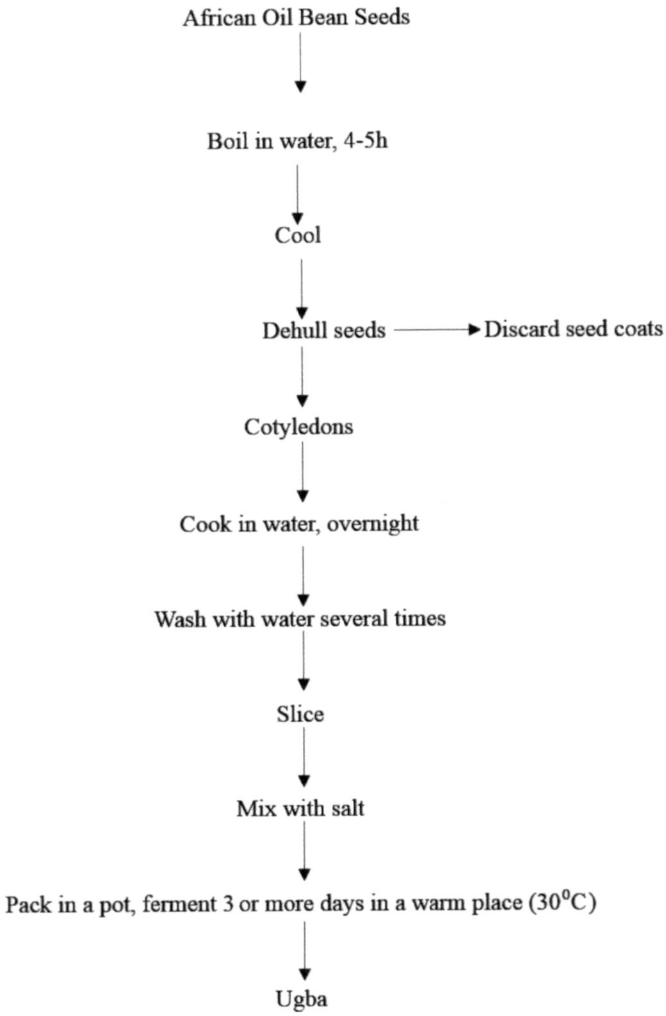

Figure 6.
Flowchart for the preparation of ugba. Source: [97].

Southern Africa are made of starchy roots and grains and have to be taken with soups to which these condiments are an essential input [3].

The traditional methods of preparation of these condiments are generally very laborious, time and energy consuming and are usually carried out with rudimentary utensils. The essential steps in the preparation of these condiments are similar with minor differences occurring from one condiment to another and among different localities [30]. In Benin Republic, for instance, *ikpiru* and *yanyanku* are two additives used for traditional alkaline fermentation of African locust bean (*Parkia biglobosa*) to obtain the popular *afitin/sonru/iru* condiment [35]. These additives are, however, not involved in the production of the same condiment in the other neighboring countries. The basic steps in the production of these condiments involve shelling/decorticating and dehulling of the seeds, the seeds are washed and wrapped in several layers of leaves and left to ferment. In some other methods, the seeds are spread in calabashes that are stacked together and wrapped in several jute bags and left to ferment. These conditions create low oxygen tension and help to maintain the optimum conditions of temperature and humidity necessary for the fermentation process. The fermentation time varies from one product to another

Castor oil seed.

↓

Boil for two to three hours.

↓

De-hull

↓

Rinse in clean water.

↓

Boil for one hour.

↓

Allow to cool.

↓

Wrap with enough banana leaves.

↓

Pack in clean containers, ferment for four days.

↓

Ogiri

Figure 7.
Flowchart for the preparation of ogiri. Source: [98].

Prosopia africana seeds

↓

Boiled for 1-2 days

↓

De-hulled by processing with finger tips or pounding on the mortar

↓

Washed and seed coat removed

↓

Cotyledons boiled again for 1-2 h

↓

Cotyledons wrapped with paw-paw/traditional leaves

↓

Wrapped cotyledons packed in nylon

↓

Fermentation for 5-6 days

↓

Okpehe/Afiyo

Figure 8.
Flowchart for the preparation of okpehe. Source: [43].

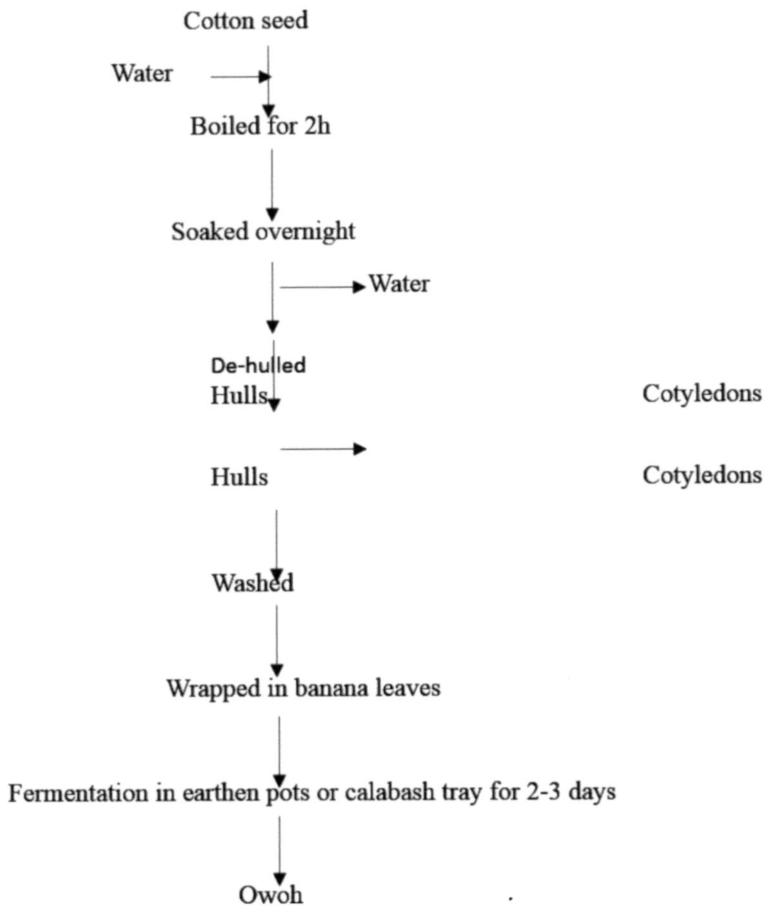

Figure 9.
Flowchart for the preparation of owoh. Source: [28].

and from one processor to another. Generally, it ranges from 48 to 120 h (2–5 days). **Figures 5–9** show the flowcharts for the fermentation of African locust bean seeds, African oil bean seeds, castor oil seeds, *Prosopis africana* seeds and cotton seeds, respectively, into various food condiments.

2. Microbiology of African fermented condiments

The microbiota in any fermenting food matrix is a function of the hygienic status of the production environment, the utensil and the raw material used and the handlers. The traditional fermentation method employed in the processing of most fermented African condiments is by chance inoculation [2, 30, 36]. The microbial interaction during their production is, therefore, determined by the microbiological status of the raw material, utensils, handlers and production environment. These factors vary from one community to the other and from one processor to another. The microbial interplay in the fermenting mash, therefore, may also vary from one processing community to the other and from one processor to another and even from one batch of production to another (**Table 2**). During fermentation of these condiments, the microorganisms use the nutritional components of the substrates, converting them into products that contribute to the chemical composition and taste of the final product [30, 37].

Food	Area of production/ consumption	Raw material	Microorganisms
Dawadawa or *iru*	Most of West Africa especially northern African parts	African locust bean (*Parkia biglobosa*) Soybean (*Glycine max.*)	*Bacillus subtilis* *B. licheniformis*
Ogiri	Southwestern Nigeria	Melon (*Citrullus vulgaris*)	*Bacillus* sp.(predominant), *Proteus*, *Pediococcus*
Ogiri-nwan	Southwestern Nigeria	Fluted pumpkin bean (*Telfairia occidentalis*)	*Bacillus* sp. (proteolytic)
Ogiri-igbo (ogiri-agbor)	Southeastern Nigeria	Castor oil seed (*Ricinus communis*)	Various *Bacillus* species: *B. subtilis, B. megaterium, B. firmus*
Ogiri-saro (sigda)	Sierra Leone, Sudan	Sesame seed (*Sesamum indicum*)	*Bacillus* sp.
Ogiri-okpei/Okpehe	Middle belt Nigeria	Mesquite (*Prosopis africana*)	*Bacillus* sp.
Ugba (apara)	Eastern Nigeria	African oil bean (*Pentaclethra macrophylla*)	*Bacillus subtilis* *Micrococcus* sp.
Owoh	Midwestern Nigeria	Cotton seeds (*Gossypium hirsutum*)	*Bacillus* sp.
Bakalga	Niger, Mali, Sudan, Burkina Faso	Kartade red sorrel (*Hibiscus sabdariffa*)	*Bacillus subtilis*

Source: [3].

Table 2.
Some important fermented vegetable foods of Africa and their fermenting organisms.

The major fermenting microorganisms involved in the fermentation process of most vegetable protein (fermented condiments) have been identified as proteolytic *Bacillus* species, e.g., *B. subtilis, B. megaterium, B. circulans* [2, 30, 33, 38]. *Bacillus subtilis*, however, appears to be the most predominant of all the *Bacillus* species. The endospores of these bacilli are believed to be associated with the cotyledons of these seeds from the onset of the fermentation process.

Proteolysis is the major biochemical activity taking place during the fermentation of most fermented food condiments that are of plant origin [39, 40]. Proteolytic activity has been found to steadily increase with increase in the fermentation period during the production of these food condiments [39, 41]. Due to the high level of hydrolytic enzyme production by *Bacillus* species, all the species have been reported to have one or more enzymatic hydrolytic properties during legume fermentation [42, 43]. However, it appears that *Bacillus subtilis* is the most adapted and dominant species. *Bacillus subtilis* produces high levels of protease, amylase and polyglutamic acid (responsible for mucilage production that is common in fermented vegetable protein) [43].

Protein has been identified as one of the major components of the legumes and oil bean seeds used for the fermentation of these condiments [38]. Metabolic and enzymatic hydrolytic activities of the *Bacillus* species serve to break down the protein into amino acids [39, 40, 43–46]. An increase in the population of *Bacillus* species from the beginning of the fermentation process till the end had been reported [41]. Microorganisms belonging to other groups of bacteria are also associated with the fermentation of these condiments. They include species of *Escherichia, Proteus, Pediococcus, Micrococcus, Staphylococcus, Streptococcus, Alcaligenes, Pseudomonas, Corynebacterium and Enterococcus* [17, 18, 20, 37, 41, 47–49]. *Staphylococcus* and

Micrococcus species are very active at the early stage of the fermentation process. They multiply rapidly within 24 h of fermentation and then decrease as fermentation progresses [41]. Their role in the fermentation process is, however, lower compared to that played by the *Bacillus* species. Species of *Escherichia*, *Proteus* and *Pediococcus* generally play a minor role in the fermentation process [38, 50, 51].

Besides proteolysis, other biochemical changes mediated by microorganisms during the production of these condiments include production of flavor-enhancing compounds, production of vitamins and essential fatty acids and degradation of indigestible oligosaccharides responsible for flatus factors [45]. A significant increase in vitamins, such as thiamine and riboflavin, has been observed in these condiments, which is possibly due to riboflavin synthase associated with the *Bacillus subtilis* [45]. A reduction in the content of flatus factors [stachyose, raffinose and melibiose] in fermented condiments of African origin has been reported [52]. The reduction is as a result of sucrase activities of the *Bacillus* group and possibly by the α-galactosidase activities of other microorganisms in the fermenting mash [39, 53].

Members of the *Enterobacteriaceae* have also been associated with the ecology of fermenting plant protein especially at the early stages of production [31, 54]. These species do not survive until the end of the fermentation, presumably because of the modified environment [41]. It is evident that production of these fermented condiments is initially mediated by a diverse microbial flora, which eventually becomes Gram-positive flora (a reflection of many African fermented foods) [26].

The identification of these organisms have been based on phenotypic approach with its inherent shortcomings, especially its inability to isolate and identify viable, but unculturable, microorganisms. Unculturable, yet viable, microorganisms are known to be in most food matrix [55, 56]. In a recent study [57] on the processing methods and safety of a fermented food condiment in Nigeria (*ugba*), the author deployed both phenotypic and molecular tools in his study. New bacterial species of *Arthrobacter, Empedobacter, Providencia, Brevibacterium, Elizabethkingia, Acinetobacter, Burkholderiales, Proteobacterium, Wautersiella, Dysgomonas, Zymomonas* and *Flavobacterium* were uniquely identified by the clone library technique employed. The study, therefore, underscores the need to deploy molecular techniques in the evaluation of the microbiology of these African fermented food condiments. It is possible that the microbial structure reported for these products could be wider than is currently recorded.

3. Nutritional properties

Fermentation has generally been observed to improve the nutritional qualities and safety of fermented food products [58–63]. Proximate analyses of most fermented vegetable protein of African origin have shown that these condiments are rich sources of protein, essential amino acids, vitamins and minerals. These components have been found to increase during the fermentation of these condiments [4, 63–65].

The substrates for the fermentation of these condiments harbor diverse microorganisms from the environment [66–68]. These microorganisms transform the chemical constituents of the raw materials during fermentation. The transformation has the following advantages: [i] enhance nutritive value of the products; [ii] enrich bland diets with improved flavor and texture; [iii] preserve perishable foods; [iv] fortify products with essential amino acids, health promoting bioactive compounds, vitamins and minerals; [v] degrade undesirable compounds and antinutritional factors; [vi] impart antioxidant and antimicrobial properties; [vii] improve digestibility and [viii] stimulate probiotic functions. Fermentation of these products also results in a lower proportion of dry matter in the food products, and the concentration of the vitamins, minerals and protein appears to increase when measured on dry weight basis [4, 63–65, 69, 70].

A large percentage of Africa's population live below poverty line with diets that are poor in protein and other essential nutrients [3, 71]. Fermented food condiments have been found to be rich in proteins and other essential nutrients and, therefore, serve as supplements for these nutrients outside their usage as flavoring agents [72–75] (**Table 3**). *Bikalga*, for instance, is a popular fermented food condiment in Benin Republic, which is considered as an excellent source of protein with essential amino acids. It also contains lipids, carbohydrates, essential fatty acids and vitamins [11, 76]. Many families often use *Bikalga* as a meat substitute. Most African fermented food condiments are used to improve nutritional values of foods as well as their sensory properties and as taste enhancer [70].

Generally, a significant increase in the soluble fraction of amino nitrogen of a food is observed during fermentation [77]. Investigation by Niba [78] showed that protein quality in grain cereals is improved during fermentation due to depletion of trypsin inhibitors, which increases the digestibility of various amino acids.

Fermentation markedly improves the digestibility, nutritive value and flavor of raw seeds [79–81]. Studies on the effect of fermentation on the nutrient content of some unfermented leguminous seeds (locust beans and oil bean seeds) showed that protein and fat increased when fermented, whereas the quantity of carbohydrates decreased [82]. Increased levels of the amino acids were also reported except for arginine, leucine and phenylalanine. Similar results have been reported for other seed legumes [26, 52]. The organisms involved in the fermentation processes, especially *Bacillus* sp., produce proteolytic enzymes, which hydrolyze proteins to amino acids and peptides [18, 23, 26, 50, 83–85]. *Bacillus* strains obtained from fermenting African oil bean seed and locust beans have been found to produce glutamic acid and extracellular proteinases, which play active role in the fermentation process of these seeds [42, 86].

The proximate composition of some fermented vegetable protein (FVP) and their raw materials indicate that the major components are protein and fat (**Table 3**). The most significant reaction/change in the fermentation of proteins is their hydrolysis to free amino acids and other soluble nitrogen compounds. The amino acids produced vary, depending on the type of seed [fermenting substrate]. The peptides and amino acids are important in the evolution of the flavor of the condiments. Glutamic acid, an important flavoring component, has been observed in the fermentation of *ugba, iru* and *dawadawa* [87].

The major component of the carbohydrate content of legumes is starch, raffinose, melibiose and stachyose [26, 50]. During fermentation, these oligosaccharides

Proximate composition (%)						
Condiments	**Moisture**	**Ash**	**Crude fiber**	**Crude protein**	**Carbohydrate**	**Fat**
Iru/Dawadawa	52.0 ± 5.0	3.6 ± 0.1	4.0 ± 0.1	32.9 ± 0.1	16.3 ± 0.8	24.2 ± 0.1
Ogiri	44.1 ± 0.8	3.0 ± 0.0	15.6 ± 0.4	19.9 ± 0.8	25.2 ± 1.2	—
Owoh	46.6	2.21	6.01	16.37	14.06	20.76
Ugba	34.4	1.11	2.93	7.13	17.48	19.72
Okpehe	9.46	4.84	2.99	36.88	47.18	11.35

Source: Adapted from [4, 64, 99].

Table 3.
Proximate composition of some African fermented condiments.

Mineral composition (mg/100 g)								
Condiments	**P**	**K**	**Na**	**Ca**	**Mg**	**Zn**	**Fe**	**Mn**
Iru	80.00	205.00	—	9.01	35.00	—	3.31	—
Ogiri	91.17	1075.00	369.36	78.60	58.72	1.17	14.50	1.15
Owoh	—	464.50	416.50	246.0	150.0	119.7	16.0	—
Ugba	291.02	110.39	172.06	208.92	334.98	9.23	42.46	26.87
Okpehe	—	183.1	—	45.3	—	14.2	10.2	4.2

Source: Adapted from [4, 64, 99].

Table 4.
Mineral composition of some African fermented condiments.

are hydrolyzed to simple digestible sugars [88]. Assay of the fermenting mash of African oil bean seed and African locust bean showed activities of α- and β-galactosidases and sucrase [89], with α- and β-galactosidases being the highest. Other enzymes present are galactanase, glucosidases and fructofuranosidases and polygalacturonases. These enzymes are produced by *Bacillus* species, *Staphylococcus* species and lactic acid bacteria, the latter group producing α-galactosidase, and they play very active role in the hydrolysis of these oligosaccharides. The nutritional significance of hydrolysis of oligosaccharides is evident in the drastic reduction of the level of indigestible carbohydrates, which cause flatulence [89].

Oil constitutes a major component of the legumes and oil seeds, but lipolytic activities are minimal during the production of most African fermented food condiments. Low lipolytic activities were detected during *ugba* and *dawadawa* production. The lipolytic activities are attributed to *Staphylococcus* species in the fermentation medium [39, 90]. During fermentation, the free fatty acid fractions [FFA] are reduced from 0.6 to 0.1% w/w in the fermented seeds. No significant differences were observed between the fatty acid content of the raw seeds and the fermented seeds; the major components are palmitic acid, stearic acid, oleic acid and linoleic acid [91].

Many reports confirm that vitamin levels are higher in fermented vegetable protein foods than in the raw materials, especially for riboflavin, thiamine, niacin, vitamin C and folic acid [1, 89]. Food condiments made from vegetable proteins may be a good source of certain B vitamins, but they are found to be deficient in ascorbate and some fat-soluble vitamins, which are lost during fermentation. Fermentation significantly increases the content of thiamine, riboflavin and niacin in the African oil bean [92]. Similar changes were observed during the fermentation of melon seed and fluted pumpkin seed [93, 94].

Calcium, phosphorus and potassium have been observed to increase when African oil bean seed and African yam bean were fermented for condiment production [95, 96]. Similar observation has been made on other fermented condiments (**Table 4**). It is evident that most fermented food condiments of African origin are good sources of essential nutrients and could be used to produce complementary food supplements and macronutrients in fermented legumes and therefore enhance food quality. However, issues of quality inconsistency, poor keeping quality and safety observed with these products must be addressed.

4. Conclusion

Fermented condiments constitute an important part of diet of most Africans. These condiments, apart from their flavoring properties, serve as cheap source of protein and other essential micronutrients to the consumers. The production process of most of these condiments is still based on spontaneous fermentation process with its inherent shortcomings. There is need, therefore, for more microbiological studies of their production process with the aim of establishing standardized protocols for their production.

Author details

Nurudeen Ayoade Olasupo[1]* and Princewill Chimezie Okorie[2]

1 Department of Microbiology, Faculty of Science, Lagos State University, Lagos, Nigeria

2 Department of Biotechnology, Federal Institute of Industrial Research Oshodi, Lagos, Nigeria

*Address all correspondence to: naolasupo@yahoo.com

References

[1] Olasupo NA. Fermentation biotechnology of traditional foods of Africa. In: Shetty K, Pometto A, Paliyath G, Levi RE, editors. Food Biotechnology. 2nd ed., revised and expanded ed. Boca Raton, New York: CRC Press, Taylor and Francis Group; 2006. pp. 1705-1739

[2] Isu NR, Ofuya CO. Improvement of the traditional processing and fermentation of African oil bean (*Pentaclethra macrophylla* Bentham) seeds into a food snack ugba. International Journal of Food Microbiology. 2000;**59**:235-239. DOI: 10.1016/S0168-1605(00)00318-4

[3] Olasupo NA, Obayori OS, Odunfa SA. Ethnic African fermented foods. In: Tamang JP, editor. Fermented Foods and Beverages of the World. Boca Raton, London, New York: CRC Press, Taylor and Francis Group; 2010. pp. 323-352

[4] Okechukwu RI, Ewelike N, Ukaoma AA, Emejulu AA, Azuwike CO. Changes in the nutrient composition of the African oil bean meal "ugba" (*Pentaclethra macrophylla* Benth) subjected to solid state natural fermentation. Journal of Applied Bioscience. 2012;**51**:3591-3595

[5] Azokpota P, Hounhouigan DJ, Annan N, Nago MC, Jakobsen M. Diversity of volatile compounds of Afitin, iru and sonru, three fermented food condiments from Benin. Western Journal of Microbiology and Biotechnology. 2008;**24**:879-885

[6] Azokpota P, Hounhouigan DJ, Nago MC, Jakobsen M. Esterase and protease activities of *Bacillus* spp. from afitin, iru and sonru: Three African locust bean (*Parkia biglobosa*) condiments from Benin. African Journal of Biotechnology. 2006;**5**(3):265-272

[7] Hongbété F. Valorisation de la technologie du Afitin: Amélioration de la fermentation et mis au point d'exhausteur de goût. Thèse d'ingénieur agronome. Bénin: Faculté des Sciences Agronomiques, Université d'Abomey-Calavi; 2001. 75p

[8] Ajayi OA, Akinrinde IM, Akinwunmi OO. Towards the development of shelf stable 'iru' (*Parkia biglobosa*) condiment bouillon cubes using corn, cassava and potato starch extracts as binders. Nigerian Food Journal. 2015;**33**:67-72. DOI: 10.1016/j.nifoj.2015.04.006

[9] Daramola B, Fasominu OA, Oje OJ, Makanju OO. Influence of dietary supplementation on biotransformation of locust beans (*Parkia biglobosa*) to condiment. African Journal of Biotechnology. 2009;**8**:1116-1120

[10] Diawara B, Sawadogo L, Amoa-Awua WKA, Jakobsen M. Quality system for the production of soumbala. The HACCP System for Traditional African Fermented Foods: Soumbala. Taastrup; 1998. ISBN 87= 90737=00=8 WAITRO Danish Technological Institute

[11] Ouoba LII, Rechinger KB, Diawara B, Traore AS, Jakobsen M. Degradation of proteins during the fermentation of African locust bean (*Parkia biglobosa*) by strains of Bacillus subtilis and *Bacillus pumilus* for production of *soumbala*. Journal of Applied Microbiology. 2003;**94**:396-402. DOI: 10.1046/j.1365-2672.2003.01845.x

[12] Ndir B, Lognay G, Wathelet B, Cornelius C, Marlier M, Thonart P. Composition chimique du nététu, condiment alimentaire produit par fermentation des graines du caroubier africain *Parkia biglobosa* (Jacq.) Benth. Biotechnology, Agronomy and Social Environment. 2000;**4**(2):101-105

[13] Ismail A, Ikram MKE, Nazri MSH. Roselle (*Hibiscus sabdariffa L.*) seeds—Nutritional composition,

protein quality and health benefits. Food Science. 2008;**2**(1):1-16

[14] Parkouda C, Nielsen DS, Azokpota P, Ouob LII, Amoa-Awua WK, Thorsen L, et al. The microbiology of alkaline fermentation of indigenous seeds used as food condiments in Africa and Asia. Critical Review in Microbiology. 2009;**35**(1):139-156

[15] Kindossi JM, Anihouvi VB, Vieira-Dalodé G, Akissoé NH, Jacobs A, Dlamini N, et al. Production, consumption, and quality attributes of Lanhouin, a fish-based condiment from West Africa. Food Chain. 2012;**2**(1):117-130

[16] Campbell-platt G. African locust bean (*Parkia* species) and its West African fermented food products, Dawadawa. Ecology and Food Nutrition. 1980;**9**:123-132

[17] Odunfa SA. Microorganisms associated with fermentation of African locust bean (*Parkia filicoidea*) during iru preparation. Journal of Plant Foods. 1981a;**91**:219-223

[18] Antai SP, Ibrahim MH. Microorganisms associated with African locust bean (*Parkia filicoidea*) fermentation for dawadawa production. Journal of Applied Biotechnology. 1986;**61**:145-148

[19] Popoola TOS, Akueshi CO. Microorganisms associated with the fermentation of soybean for the production of soybean daddawa (as condiment). Nigerian Food Journal. 1984;**283**:194-196

[20] Ogbadu CO, Okagbue RN. Bacterial fermentation of soybean for dawadawa production. Journal of Applied Bacteriology. 1988;**65**:353-356. DOI: 10.1111/j.1365-2672.1988.tb01902

[21] Barimalaa IS, Achinewhu SC, Yibatima I, Amadi EN. Studies on the solid substrate fermentation of bambara groundnut (*Vigna subterranea* (L) Verdc). Journal of Science, Food and Agriculture. 1989;**66**:443-446

[22] Ogundana SK. The production of ogiri a Nigerian fermented food condiment. Lebensmittel Wissenschaft und Technologie. 1981;**13**:334-336

[23] Odunfa SA. Microbiology and amino acid composition of ogiri—A food from fermented melon seeds. Die Nahrung. 1981;**25**:811-816

[24] Odibo FJC, Umeh AI. Microbiology of the fermentation of *Telfferia rosopis* seeds for ogiri production. MIRCEN Journal of Applied Microbiology and Biotechnology. 1989;**5**:217-222

[25] Anosike EO, Egwuatu CK. Biochemical changes during the fermentation of castor oil (*Ricinus communis*) seeds for use as a seasoning agent. Plant Foods for Human Nutrition. 1981;**30**:181-184

[26] Odunfa SA. African fermented foods. In: Wood BJB, editor. Microbiology of Fermented Foods. Vol. 2. London/New York, NY: Elsevier Applied Science; 1985. pp. 155-191

[27] Barber L, Achinewhu SC, Ibiama EM. The microbiology of ogiri production from castor seed (*Ricinus communs*). Food Microbiology. 1988;**5**:177-182

[28] Sanni AI, Ogbonna DN. The production of owoh—A Nigerian fermented seasoning agent from cotton seed (*Gossypium hirsitium*). Food Microbiology. 1991;**8**:223-229

[29] Sanni AI, Ogbonna DN. Biochemical studies on owoh—A Nigerian fermented soup condiment from cotton seed. Food Microbiology. 1992;**9**:177-183

[30] Sanni AI, Onilude AA, Fadahunsi IF, Ogubanwo ST, Afolabi RO. Selection of starter cultures for the production

of ugba, a fermented soup condiment. European Food Research Technology. 2002;**215**:176-180. DOI: 10.1007/s00217-002-0520-3

[31] Achi OK. Microorganisms associated with natural fermentation of Prosopis Africana seed for the production of okpehe. Plant Foods for Human Nutrition. 1992;**42**:304-309

[32] Odibo FJC, Ugwu DA, Ekeoha DC. Microorganisms associated with the fermentation of Prosopis seeds for ogiri-okpei production. Journal of Food Science Technology. 1992;**29**:306-307

[33] Sanni AI. Biochemical changes during production of okpehe—A Nigerian fermented food condiment. Chemical Microbiological Technology Lebensmittel. 1993;**15**:97-100

[34] Gutierrez ML, Maizi P, Nago CM, Hounhouigan J. Production et commercialisation de l'Afitin dans la région d'Abomey-Bohicon au Bénin. CERNA, CNEARC, CIRAD Librairie du CIRAD; 2000. 124 p

[35] Agbobatinkpo PB, Dabade SD, Laleye F, Akissoe N, Azokpota P, Hounhouigan JD. Softening effect of Ikpiru and Yanyanku, two traditional additives used for the fermentation of African Locust Bean (*Parkia biglobosa*) seeds in Benin. International Journal of Biology and Chemical Science. 2012;**6**(3):1281-1292

[36] Ogueke CC, Anosike F, Owuamanam CI. Prediction of amino nitrogen during *ugba* (*Pentaclethra macrophylla*) production under different fermentation variables: A response surface approach. Nigerian Food Journal. 2015;**33**(1):61-66

[37] Njoku HO, Okemadu CP. Biochemical changes during the natural fermentation of the African oil bean for the production of ugba. Journal of Food Science and Agriculture. 1989;**49**:457-465. DOI: 10.1002/jsfa.2740490408

[38] Obeta JAN. A note on the microorganisms associated with the fermentation of seeds of African oil bean (*Pentaclethra macrophylla*). Journal of Applied Biotechnology. 1983;**54**:433-435

[39] Odunfa SA, Oyewole OB. Identification of *Bacillus* species from iru. a fermented African locust bean product. Journal of Basic Microbiology. 1986;**26**:101-108. DOI: 10.1002/jobm.3620260212

[40] Ghosh D, Chattora DK, Chattopadhyay P. Studies on changes in microstructure and proteolysis in cow and soy milk curd during fermentation using lactic cultures for improving protein bioavailability. Journal of Food Science Technology. 2013;**50**:979-985

[41] Ogueke CC, Aririatu LE. Microbial and organoleptic changes associated with ugba stored at ambient temperature. Nigerian Food Journal. 2004;**22**:133-140

[42] Aderibigbe EY, Schink B, Odunfa SA. Extracellular proteinases of *Bacillus* sp isolated from African locust bean, iru. Food Microbiology. 1990;**7**:281-293. DOI: 10.1016/0740-0020(90)90033-E

[43] Oguntoyinbo FA, Sanni AI, Franz CMAP, Holzapfel WH. *In-vitro* fermentation studies for selection and evaluation of *Bacillus* strains as starter cultures for production of *okpehe*, a traditional African fermented condiment. International Journal of Food Microbiology. 2007;**113**:208-218

[44] Isu NR, Njoku HO. An evaluation of the microflora associated with fermented African oil bean (*Pentaclethra macrophylla* Bentham) seeds during *ugba* production. Plant Foods for Human Nutrition. 1997;**51**:145-157

[45] Odunfa SA. Dawadawa. In: Raddy NR, Pierson MD, Salunkhe DK, editors. Legume Based Fermented Foods. Boca Raton, FL: CRC Press; 1986. pp. 173-189

[46] Wang J, Fung DYC. Alkaline fermented foods. A review with emphasis on pidan fermentation. Critical Review in Microbiology. 1996;**22**:101-138

[47] Eze VC, Onwuakor CE, Ukeka E. Proximate composition, biochemical and microbiological changes associated with fermenting African oil bean (*Pentaclethra macrophylla* Benth) seeds. American Journal of Microbiology. 2014;**2**:674-681

[48] Ogbulie TE, Nsofor CA, Nze FC. Bacteria species associated with ugba (*Pentaclethra macrophylla* Bentham) produced traditionally and in the laboratory and the effect of fermentation on product of oligosaccharide hydrolysis. Nigerian Food Journal. 2014;**32**(2):73-80

[49] Anyanwu NCJ, Okonkwo OL, Iheanacho CN, Ajide B. Microbiological and nutritional qualities of fermented ugba (*Pentaclethra macrophylla* Bentham) sold in Mbaise, Imo state, Nigeria. Annual Research Review in Biology. 2016;**9**(4):1-8. DOI: 10.9734/ARRB/2016/23610

[50] Odunfa SA. Biochemical changes in fermenting African locust bean (*Parkia biglobosa*) during iru fermentation. Journal of Food Technology. 1985;**20**:295-303. DOI: 10.1111/j.1365-2621.1985.tb00379.

[51] Odunfa SA, Komolafe OB. Nutritional characteristics of Staphylococcus species from fermenting African locust bean (*Parkia biglobosa*). Die Nahrung. 1989;**33**:607-615

[52] Sarkar PK, Morrison E, Tinggi U, Somerset SM, Craven GS. B-group vitamin and mineral contents of soybeans during kinema production. Journal of Science Food and Agriculture. 1998;**78**:498-502

[53] Aderibigbe EY, Odunfa SA. Growth and extracellular enzyme production by strains of *Bacillus* species isolated from fermenting African locust bean, iru. Journal of Applied Bacteriology. 1990;**69**:662-671. DOI: 10.1111/j.1365 2672.1990.tb01560

[54] Mulyowidarso RK, Fleet GH, Buckle KA. The microbial ecology of soybean soaking for tempe production. International Journal of Food Microbiology. 1989;**8**:35-46. DOI: 10.1016/0168-1605(89)90078-0

[55] Davey HM, Kell DB. Flow cytometry and cell sorting of heterogeneous microbial populations: The importance of single cell analyses. Microbiological Review. 1996;**60**:641-696

[56] Gunasekera TS, Dorasch MR, Slado MB, Veal DA. Specific detection of *Pseudomonas* spp in milk by fluorescent in situ hybridization using ribosomal RNA directed probes. Journal of Applied Microbiology. 2003;**94**:936-945

[57] Okorie PC. Studies on the processing methods and safety of ugba: An indigenous Nigerian fermented condiment [PhD thesis]. Ojo, Lagos, Nigeria: Lagos State University; 2018

[58] Anukam KC, Reid G. African traditional fermented foods and probiotics. Journal of Medicine and Food. 2009;**12**:1177-1184

[59] Chelule PK, Mbongwa HP, Carries S, Gqaleni N. Lactic acid fermentation improves the quality of mahewu, a traditional South African maize-based porridge. Food Chemistry. 2010;**122**(3):656-661

[60] Charles MAP, Franz M, Huch JMM, Hikmate A, Nabil B, Gregor R, et al. African fermented foods and

probiotics. International Journal of Food Microbiology. 2014;**6**:248-256

[61] Chen P, Li C, Li X, Li J, Chu R, Wang H. Higher dietary folate intake reduces the breast cancer risk: A systematic review and meta-analysis. British Journal of Cancer. 2014;**110**:2327-2338

[62] Reid G, Nduti N, Sybesma W, Kort R, Kollmann TR, Adam R, et al. Harnessing microbiome and probiotic research in sub-Saharan Africa: Recommendations from an African Workshop. Microbiome. 2014;**2**:12

[63] Chung SK, Mee SL, Se IO, Sang CP. Discovery of novel sources of vitamin B12 in traditional Korean foods from nutritional surveys of centenarians. Current Gerontology Geriatrics Research. 2010;**2010**(3):374897. DOI: 10.1155/2010/374897

[64] Makanjuola OM, Ajayi A. Effect of natural fermentation on the nutritive value and mineral composition of African locust beans. Pakistian Journal of Nutrition. 2012;**11**(1):11-13

[65] Tofalo R, Schirone M, Perpetuini G, Angelozzi G, Suzzi G, Corsetti A. Microbiological and chemical profiles of naturally fermented table olives and brines from different Italian cultivars. International Journal of Biotechnology. 2012;**102**:121-131. DOI: 10.1007/s10482-012-9719-x

[66] Daeschel MA, Anderson RE, Fleming HP. Microbial ecology of fermenting plant materials. FEMS Microbiological Review. 1987;**46**:357-367. DOI: 10.1111/j.1574-6968.1987.tb02472

[67] Ouba LII, Diawara B, Moa-Awua WK, Traore AS, Moller PL. Genotyping of starter cultures of *Bacillus subtilis* and *Bacillus pumilus* for fermentation of African locust bean (*Parkia biglobosa*) to produce Soumbala. International Journal of Food Microbiology. 2004;**90**:197-205

[68] Ling J, Wu Q, Xu Y, Fan W. Interactions between *Bacillus licheniformis* and *Saccharomyces cerevisiae* in the fermentation of soy-sauce flavor liquor. Microbiology China. 2013;**40**:2014-2021

[69] Adams MR. Topical aspect of fermented foods. Trends in Food Science & Technology. 1990;**1**:141-144. DOI: 10.1016/0924-2244(90)90111-B

[70] Savadogo A, Tapi A, Chollet M, Wathelet B, Traoré AS, Jacques PH. Identification of surfactin producing strains in Soumbala and Bikalga fermented condiments using polymerase chain reaction and matrix assisted laser desorption/ionization-mass spectrometry methods. International Journal of Food Microbiology. 2011;**151**:299-306. DOI: 10.1016/j.ijfoodmicro.2011.09.022

[71] Oguntoyinbo FA. Safety challenges associated with traditional foods of West Africa. Food Review International. 2014;**30**:338-358. DOI: 10.1080/87559129.2014.940086

[72] Mbadiwe EI. Nutritional evaluation of seeds of *Pentaclethra macrophylla*. Plant Foods for Human Nutrition. 1978;**28**:261-269

[73] Mba AV, Njike MC, Oyenuga VA. Proximate chemical composition and amino acid content of Nigerian oil seeds. Journal of Food Science and Agriculture. 1974;**25**:1547-1553. DOI: 10.1002/jsfa.2740251216

[74] Odoemelam SA. Proximate composition and selected physicochemical properties of the seeds of African oil bean (*Pentaclethra marcrophylla*). Pakistian Journal of Nutrition. 2005;**4**:382-383. DOI: 10.3923/pjn.2005.382.383

[75] Ogueke CC, Nwosu JN, Owuamanam CI, Iwouno JN. Ugba, the fermented African oil bean seeds; its production, chemical composition, preservation, safety and health benefits. Pakistian Journal of Biological Science. 2010;**13**:489-496

[76] Yagoub AG, Mohamed BE, Ahmed AH, El Tinay AH. Study on Furundu, a traditional Sudanese fermented roselle (*Hibiscus sabdariffa*) seed: Effect on in vitro protein digestibility, chemical composition and functional properties of the total proteins. Journal of Agriculture and Food Chemistry. 2004;**52**(20):6143-6150

[77] Sahlin P. Fermentation as a method of food processing, production of organic acid, pH development and microbial growth in fermenting cereals [licenciate thesis]. Lund, Scania, Sweden: Lund Institute of Technology, Lund University; 1999

[78] Niba LL. The relevance of biotechnology in the development of functional foods for improved nutritional and health quality in developing countries. African Journal of Biotechnology. 2003;**2**:631-635

[79] Kiers JL, Van Laeken AEA, Rombouts FM, Nout MJR. In vitro digestibility of Bacillus fermented soybean. International Journal of Food Microbiology. 2000;**60**:163-169

[80] Oboh G. Nutrient and anti-nutritional composition of condiments produced from some fermented underutilized legumes. Journal of Food Biochemistry. 2006;**30**:579-588

[81] Ng'ong'ola-Manani TA, Østlie HM, Mwangwela AM, Wicklund T. Metabolite changes during natural and lactic acid bacteria fermentations in pastes of soybeans and soybean–maize blends. Food Science and Nutrition. 2014;**2**(6):768-785

[82] Eka OU. Effect of fermentation on the nutrient status of locust beans. Food Chemistry. 1980;**5**:305-308

[83] Steinkraus KH. African alkaline fermented foods and their relation to similar foods in other parts of the world. In: Wesby A, Reilly PJA, editors. Proceedings of a Regional Workshop on Traditional African Foods – Quality and Nutrition. Stockholm, Sweden: International Foundation for Science; 1991. pp. 87-92

[84] Addy EOH, Salami LI, Igboeli LC, Remawa HS. Effect of processing on nutrient composition and anti-nutritive substances of African locust bean (*Parkia filicoidea*) and Baobab seed (*Adansonia digitata*). Plant Foods for Human Nutrition. 1995;**48**:113-117

[85] Leejeerajumnean AA, Duckham SC, Owens JD, Ames JM. Volatile compounds of *Bacillus* fermented soybeans. Journal of Science, Food and Agriculture. 2001;**81**:525-529

[86] Ogbadu CO, Okagbue RN, Ahmed AA. Glutamic acid production by *Bacillus* isolates from Nigerian fermented vegetable proteins. World Journal of Microbiology and Biotechnology. 1990;**6**:377-382

[87] Beaumont M. Flavouring composition prepared by fermentation with *Bacillus* species. International Journal of Food Microbiology. 2002;**75**:189-196

[88] Adebayo-Tayo B, Elelu T, Akinola G, Oyinloye I. Screening and production of mannanase by *Bacillus* strains isolated from fermented food condiments. Food Biotechnology. 2013;**13**:53-62, in Roman

[89] Odunfa SA. Carbohydrate changes in fermenting African locust bean (*Parki filicoidea*) during iru preparation. Plant Foods for Human Nutrition. 1983;**32**:3-10

[90] Ikenebomeh MJ. The solid substrate fermentation of African locust bean (*Parkia filicodea*) [PhD thesis]. Montreal, Quebec, Canada: McGill University; 1982

[91] Odunfa SA, Adesomoju AA. Effects of fermentation on the free fatty acids of African locust bean during iru production. Journal of Plant Foods. 1985;**6**:111-115

[92] Achjnewhu SC, Ryley J. Effects of fermentation on thiamin, riboflavin and niacin content of melon seed (*Citrullus vulgaris*) and the African oil bean seed (*Pentaclethra macrophylla*). Food Chemistry. 1987;**20**:243-252

[93] Achinewhu SC. The effect of fermentation on carbohydrate and fatty acid composition of the African oil bean (*Pentaclethra macrophylla*) seed. Food Chemistry. 1986;**19**:105-116. DOI: 10.1016/0308-8146(86)90104-4

[94] Achinewhu SC. Some biochemical and nutritional changes during the fermentation of fluted pumpkin (*Telferia occidentale*). Plant Foods for Human Nutrition. 1986;**36**:97-106

[95] Ogbonna DN, Sokari TG, Achinewhu SC. Development of owoh-type product from African yam bean (*Sphenostylis stenocarpa*) seeds by solid state fermentation. Plant Foods for Human Nutrition. 2001;**56**:183-194. DOI: 10.1023/A:1011185513717

[96] Nwokeleme CO, Ugwuanyi JO. Evolution of volatile flavour compounds during fermentation of African oil bean (*Pentaclethra macrophylla* Benth) seed for "ugba" production. International Journal of Food Science. 2015;**2015**:706328. DOI: 10.1155/2015/706328

[97] Odunfa SA, Oyeyiola GF. Microbiological study of the fermentation of ugba: A Nigerian indigenous fermented food flavor. Journal of Plant Foods. 1985;**6**:155-163

[98] Omafuvbe BO, Olumuyiwa SF, Osuntogun B, Adewusi SRA. Chemical and biochemical changes in African locust bean (*Parkia biglobosa*) and melon (*Citrullus vulgaris*) seeds during fermentation to condiments. Pakistan Journal of Nutrition. 2004;**3**(3):140-145. DOI: 10.3923/pjn.2004.140.145

[99] Omafuvbe BO, Abiose SH, Shonukan OO. Fermentation of soybean (*Glycine max*) for soy-daddawa production by starter cultures of Bacillus. Food Microbiology. 2003;**19**:561-566

Chapter 6

Pursuing the Perfect Performer of Fermented Beverages: GMMs vs. Microbial Consortium

Jesús Alejandro Aldrete-Tapia,
Dalia Elizabeth Miranda-Castilleja,
Sofia Maria Arvizu-Medrano,
Ramón Álvar Martínez-Peniche, Lourdes Soto-Muñoz
and Montserrat Hernández-Iturriaga

Abstract

Fermented beverages are widely diverse around the world and their quality is largely based on the organoleptic characteristics developed by the metabolism of the microorganisms present during fermentation. In order to achieve controllable processes in fermented beverages along with organoleptic complexity, two divergent approaches have been followed in terms of inoculum development: (1) the inoculation of multiple microorganisms, intending to promote synergism and favor organoleptic complexity derived from the metabolic diversity, and (2) the genetic modification of a single strain with the intention that it performs multiple functions. In this chapter, we discuss these divergent approaches, their achievements and perspectives.

Keywords: microbial consortium, genetic modified microorganism, biochemical changes, fermented beverages, organoleptic characteristics

1. Introduction

The induction of fermentation on raw materials provides new products with added nutrients and organoleptic complexity vastly appreciated by consumers. The changes in the components of the raw materials are mainly caused by the main and secondary metabolism of the microorganisms present during the fermentation processes. The microorganisms need carbon and nitrogen sources to obtain energy and structural blocks to maintain cell integrity and functions and to proliferate. However, some of the carbon and nitrogen are transformed and released to the medium as by-products of the metabolism which generate the characteristics of the fermented food. Spontaneous fermentation harbors complex evolving and diverse microbiota that provides organoleptic complexity, mainly in aromas and flavors. However, it is hard to control and usually derives in inconsistent and even defective products. This is why commercial starter cultures emerged, allowing a better control of fermentation. Nevertheless, some argue that commercial inoculation leads to a loss of unique regional style. In these cases, flavors often considered superior are achieved, at the cost of consistency and occasional production losses. The microorganism core that causes the expected characteristics of several beverages has been studied widely, indicating the participation of multiple microorganisms through different stages of the fermentation. Two divergent approaches have been proposed to improve fermentation by the controlled inoculation of multiple microorganisms each causing different expected changes in the fermentation, or by the manipulation of the genome of single strains to perform multiple tasks by themselves. Both approaches have their strengths and weaknesses, and it seems that the next step is the combination of both strategies to provide a holistic solution.

2. Metabolism in fermented beverage processes

Fermentation is the metabolic process carried out by microorganisms to obtain energy by oxidizing carbohydrates in which the final electron acceptors are organic molecules rather than O_2 [1]. The catabolism of sugars results in the production of reduced pyridine nucleotides (nicotinamide adenine dinucleotide NADH); and to regenerate it in anaerobic conditions, pyruvate acts as the electron acceptor to reoxidate NADH [2]. The different fates of pyruvate are ethanol, lactic acid, or acetate, depending on the microorganism and environmental conditions [3].

2.1 Alcoholic fermentation

Alcoholic fermentation is the transformation of the sugars, mainly glucose and fructose, into ethanol and CO_2. This process is carried out by yeast such as *Saccharomyces cerevisiae* and *S. bayanus* [4], as well as by some bacteria, including *Zymomonas mobilis*, used in Central America in the fermentation of *Agave* to produce *pulque* [5] or palm wine (Toddy) [6]. The pyruvate is decarboxylated before a final reduction by NADH, to yield ethanol. The recovery of NAD maintains the flux of glycolysis reactions [7].

In addition, other by-products of fermentation are generated, such as glycerol, acetate, succinate, higher alcohols, and esters. The production of glycerol can be considered beneficial in some cases, that is, wine production, but is undesirable in the production of distilled beverage since it represents a waste of substrate [8]. Likewise, succinate production by yeast can have an important beneficial effect on the quality of *sake*, while it produces a negative effect on wine favoring a salty and bitter taste [9]. Esters represent an important group of flavor-active compounds with beneficial fruity/floral flavors and aromas in fermented beverages [7].

It should be noted that alcoholic fermentation could occur in aerobic environments. For example, even in the presence of abundant oxygen, yeast cells greatly prefer fermentation to oxidative phosphorylation, as long as sugars are readily available for consumption, a phenomenon known as the Crabtree effect [10].

2.2 Lactic and malolactic fermentation

Lactic acid fermentation is mainly a bacterial process that plays important roles in fermented beverages, enhancing its nutritional value and organoleptic quality. A group of morphologically and physiologically diverse bacteria has been designated the term lactic acid bacteria (LAB), due to the main production of lactic acid generated from the catabolism of carbohydrates [11]. They can be divided into two physiological groups, homo- and heterofermentative, depending on the hexose metabolic pathways used. Homofermentative LAB (*Lactobacillus delbrueckii* and

Streptococcus thermophilus) ferment hexoses via glycolysis (the Embden-Meyerhof pathway), producing lactic acid as the major end product, whereas the heterofermentative LAB (*Oenococcus oeni, Lactobacillus brevis, Lactobacillus hilgardii*, and *Lactobacillus buchneri*) and facultative homofermentative bacteria (*Lactobacillus plantarum*), in contrast, ferment hexoses and pentoses via the pentose phosphate or phosphoketolase pathway to produce acid lactic, CO_2, and ethanol and/or acetic acid [12].

Malolactic fermentation, the second important stage in winemaking, normally takes place after alcoholic fermentation. The malolactic fermentation is also conducted by LAB, preferably *Oenococcus oeni*, which reduce acidity of the wine or cider by transforming malic acid (dicarboxylic acid) to lactic acid (monocarboxylic acid) resulting in a softer taste [7]. In addition, the malolactic fermentation also affects the final aroma and taste balance by modifying and producing aroma-active compounds [12].

2.3 Acetic fermentation

Acetic fermentation, also called oxidative fermentation, is a process in which alcohol is oxidized to acetic acid by the action of a group conveniently called acetic acid bacteria (AAB). These are strict aerobic bacteria found in high-sugar, alcoholic and acidic environments, characteristics found in fermented beverage processes [13]. The AAB partially oxidate carbohydrates to generate aldehydes, ketones, and organic acids in the fermentative media [14]. AAB are evidently involved in the production of vinegar and participate in fermentation of other beverages, such as palm wine, pulque, and kombucha [15]. However, the main concern with this type of microorganisms is that they are involved in the spoilage of wine, cider, and beer, where the production of acid acetic is undesired [16].

2.4 Secondary metabolism

The metabolism of microorganisms is not a straightforward pathway, and other compounds are produced in lower concentrations during the metabolization of substrates, the so-called secondary metabolites.

Higher alcohols, polyols, esters, organic acids, vicinal ketones, and aldehydes are the main secondary metabolites produced in lower concentrations, as low as ng/L, althougth human senses are able to detect them due to the low perception threshold of these compounds, providing flavor and aroma to the fermented beverages [7].

Superior alcohols, also called fusel oils, are generated as by-products of the catabolism of amino acids, specifically by transamination reaction, which yields α-keto acid that enters the Ehrlich pathway, resulting in decarboxylation forming an aldehyde, and it is then oxidized to generate an alcohol [17]. Also, the aldehyde could be released or reduced to generate an acid.

Glycerol, the most important polyol, is formed during fermentation, as one molecule of glucose at some point is divided in two molecules of three carbons, one yielding glycerol and the other pyruvate [18].

Esters are formed by the reaction of an alcohol group and an acid group. The most important are the acetate esters, in which the acid group is originated from acetic acid and ethyl esters, where the alcohol group is from ethanol. Yeast produce esters to achieve the transport from cytosol to the fermenting medium as they are able to passively diffuse the cellular membrane [19].

Vicinal diketones are formed as intermediates of the biosynthesis of branched amino acids valine, leucine, and isoleucine [20].

2.5 Microbial stress and adaptation process during fermentation

During the fermentation process, yeast and LAB must respond to several adverse conditions, mainly low pH, increasing ethanol concentration, nutrient limitations, fluctuations of oxygen concentration, and the presence of diverse compounds with antimicrobial effects [21, 22]. One of the major stress response pathways is the global stress response, including the expression of heat shock factors [23]; this is activated by several environmental conditions, as a general non-specific cell response to adverse conditions. Likewise, specific adaptation strategies are triggered under certain circumstances. Adaptation of *S. cerevisiae* environmental conditions involves the activation and repression of different sets of genes during fermentation. For example, macromolecules transport and glucose signaling are repressed at initial stages of fermentation in synthetic must, while vacuolar activity is important as far as the beginning of stationary phase [24].

Yeast viability in stationary phase is fundamental to an efficient fermentation, some reactive oxygen species (ROS) could be produced and cause oxidative damage on lipids, proteins, and nucleic acids, including mitochondrial DNA. Cells respond with the production of proteins like superoxide dismutase and rhodanases [25]. Cellular accumulation of trehalose has been associated with increased resistance to oxidative stress and survival to low temperatures [22].

Assimilable nitrogen in must have a great influence over fermentation rate in wine—low nitrogen concentration leads to a low biomass yield and slow fermentation rate [26]. During nitrogen depletion different pathways are activated such as ammonium permease, nitrogen catabolic genes, post diauxic shift elements, and autophagy; all depending of target of rapamycin signaling [27].

LAB are recognized by their high acid tolerance, and indeed, malolactic fermentation is an adaptation response to reduce wine acidity, improving its survival [28]. Other strategies to respond to high acidity are citrate fermentation, amino acid degradation to produce alkaline substances, active proton pump, accumulation of trehalose and glutathione, and degradation of phenolic acids [12].

3. Strategies to improve desirable characteristics

In the past, the main objective for the selection of microorganisms was that they achieve fermentation in a relatively short time, with high conversions from substrates to the metabolites of interest and without the generation of compounds detrimental to the quality of the fermented food [29]. Nowadays, the characteristics sought for in fermentation processes have increased to satisfy the needs of more customers and producers which aim to increase flavor and aroma rather than ethanol concentration [30]. The focus on the use of a single strain to perform such deeds is considered impossible. This is why two main strategies have been proposed and evaluated, the use of multiple microorganisms each carrying out a specific function and as a whole produce the desired change, or the use of single microorganisms genetically modified to perform several tasks by themselves.

4. Microbial consortium

During beverage fermentations, two or more microbial groups living symbiotically define a consortium [31]. In food fermentation consortia, many aspects that are summarized as follows need to be considered: (1) different strains fulfill different and complex tasks, dividing work; (2) an adequate dynamic of the interactions between microorganisms leads to stronger adaptability and stability of the consortium; (3) the participation of different microorganisms increases complexity in microbial dynamism, metabolism, transcriptomics, and interactions, that ultimately affect organoleptic characteristics of the product. Thus, along with the evolution of the medium, these microorganisms will establish relationships that will modify their individual behavior, determining temporal dominances, proportion of the participants, and thus major metabolites, which according to the substrate, will give organoleptically complex, microbiologically stable, and healthy products that consumers desire.

4.1 Main microorganisms present in some fermented beverages and their roles

It is still unclear how much mankind has intervened in the evolution of certain groups of microorganisms in fermented foods; however, it is clear that each substrate itself exerts a different selection pressure on them. In order to determine the diversity and evolution of a microbial consortium in any type of substrates, two approaches are available nowadays. First, the traditional microbiological methods, defined as culture-dependent, which may be biased by selectivity of culture media, low populations, and the presence of viable but non-culturable cells; however, it allows to further study individual behavior of isolates. The second approach is the culture-independent or molecular methods, which nevertheless may be affected by the specificity of primers, conditions of the reaction, detection of death cells, and database availability. Culture-independent methods have allowed to obtain a more complete scene, and combining with selective flow cytometry, metabolomics, and transcriptomic studies, a further comprehensive vision of microbial biodiversity of fermented foods can be reached [32]. Some of the most important fermented beverages are presented in **Table 1**, according to the type of dominant microorganisms and the raw materials used for their preparation.

Main microorganism	Raw material (substrate)	Examples	References
Saccharomyces yeasts	Fruit	Fermented teas, wine, cider, perry, fruit-fermented beverages.	[33–35]
	Dairy	Kumis, kefir	[36]
	Grains	Beer and distillates	[37]
Non-*Saccharomyces* yeasts	Fruits	Pulque and mezcal	[5]
	Dairies	Kumis, kefir	[36]
	Grains	African fura, Mexican pozol, South American champú, Asian rice wine, among others.	[38–41]
Lactic acid bacteria	Fruits	Pulque, Taberna, tomato juice, pomegranate juice	[5, 42–44]
	Dairies	Yogurt, kefir	[45, 46]
	Grains	Sourdough, Cocoa beans, Lambic beer	[47]
Acetic acid bacteria	Fruits	Kombucha, Water kefir	[33, 48]
Molds	Grains	Sake and soy sauce	[49]

Table 1.
Classification of some of the most common fermented foods produced worldwide according to the main groups of microorganisms and the starting substrate.

4.2 Interaction between microorganisms in mixed cultures

In order to survive in an environment, a group of different type of microorganisms need to adapt and specialize through the time they spend in it. Microbial relationships are needed to establish and maintain the microbial consortium; the type of interaction that can emerge may be positive as mutualism or synergism, in which both parts benefit from being together. However, the relationships can also be negative or antagonistic, when one microorganism inhibits another, for instance by nutrients or space competition; or by producing a metabolite that harms the other; or by presenting parasitism, in which one microorganism benefits at the expense of other, damaging and even killing it [50, 51]. Any type of interaction starts by recognizing the environment, then transferring the information to others. The phenomenon is regulated by mechanisms such as quorum sensing, which consists in a stimuli-response system that regulates gene expression in response to population density [51].

In the particular environment of beverage fermentations, as exhaustively reviewed by [50], microorganisms manifest a variety of interactions. During fermentation, the environment generated maintains most of human pathogenic or food spoilage microorganisms. This role is achieved through competition and antagonism, through the fast consumption of nutrients and production of inhibitory compounds, mainly ethanol and organic acids, usually acting together with medium, short-chain fatty acids and proteinaceous toxins such as yeast's killer toxin in wine. On the other hand, throughout the evolution of the original substrate, the limiting factors change and the dominant microorganisms also change along with them. This succession of species has been reported in almost every fermented food studied. Positive interactions determine largely the succession of microbes in a particular substrate, for instance in *sake* production, where the saccharification of starch by *Aspergillus flavus* var. *oryzae* is first required in order to let *S. cerevisiae* conduct the alcoholic fermentation [52].

Besides the simply descriptive craving to know the diversity and roles that each microorganism plays, by understanding the types of interactions and how they emerge, a more controllable process can be achieved and the quality of the products can be improved. Finding the combination of microorganisms (species and strains) that will give desired characteristics is a strategy vastly explored in wine [53, 54], and also in *cachaça* [55], prickly pear wine [56] where mixed populations of *Saccharomyces*, non-*Saccharomyces* yeast, and even LAB have been explored.

One important aspect to consider when a proper combination of microorganisms is sought is to investigate their compatibility, that is, not negative type of interaction, as well as to determine if the intended promoting role actually occurs during the fermentation process. For instance, regarding compatibility, a study was conducted to observe synergism, antagonism, or no apparent interaction between selected native yeasts and LAB strains for the production of wine in the region of Queretaro, Mexico [57]. For this, yeast strains were grown in a medium resembling must, after 12 h yeast biomass was removed and the resulting broth was used to incubate the different strains of LAB and to observe their growth by means of optical density (OD) (**Figure 1**).

Positive values indicate a growth promotion from yeast to LAB observed in different extent, showing synergism superior in the combinations of native yeast strains compared with the growth promotion given by the commercial yeast (K1-V1116). It is also observable that the behaviors were strain-combination dependent, an aspect cited by other authors [58]. This test allowed to foresee and select compatible strains in order to further analyze their performance in a traditional winemaking process, where LAB strain is inoculated after the alcoholic fermentation performed by the yeast strain.

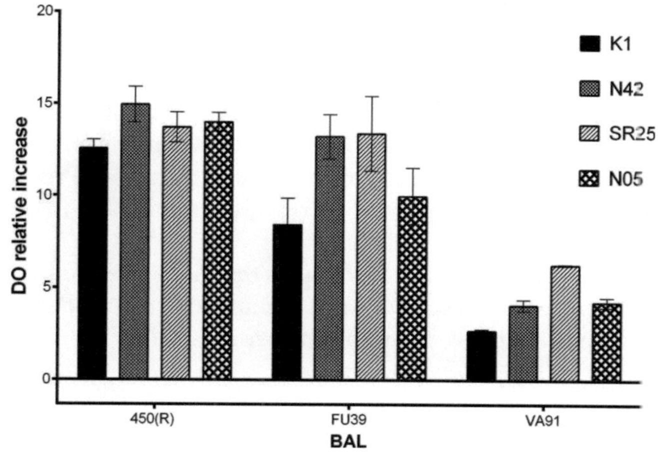

Figure 1.
Compatibility of four native LAB grown into the medium produced by five native S. cerevisiae *strains (N42, SR25, N05), measured as relative optical density increase* $\left[ODi = \frac{ODi_{afteryeast} - ODi_{withoutyeast}}{DOi_{withoutyeast}}\right]$. *Strain 450®* (O. oeni) *and K1-V1116® (K1) were used as commercial references.*

In a different context, regarding a particular metabolic interest or synergism, a study carried out in tequila fermentation is briefly presented. An important safety issue in the consumption of tequila (and in general, distillates) to take into account is the elevated concentration of ethyl carbamate generated by the reaction between urea and ethanol driven by the elevated temperatures occurring during the distillation stage. While ethanol is the desired metabolite in this process, urea is the by-product of nitrogen metabolism of *S. cerevisiae* and thus its production cannot be totally eliminated. On the other side, bacteria are capable of consuming urea as nitrogen source [59]. Taking advantage of the usual symbiosis across yeast, LAB, and AAB, an alternative approach that has been explored to reduce ethyl carbamate production is the use of mixed cultures, combining a selected *S. cerevisiae* strain and bacteria strains isolated from spontaneously fermenting agave juice (**Figure 2**).

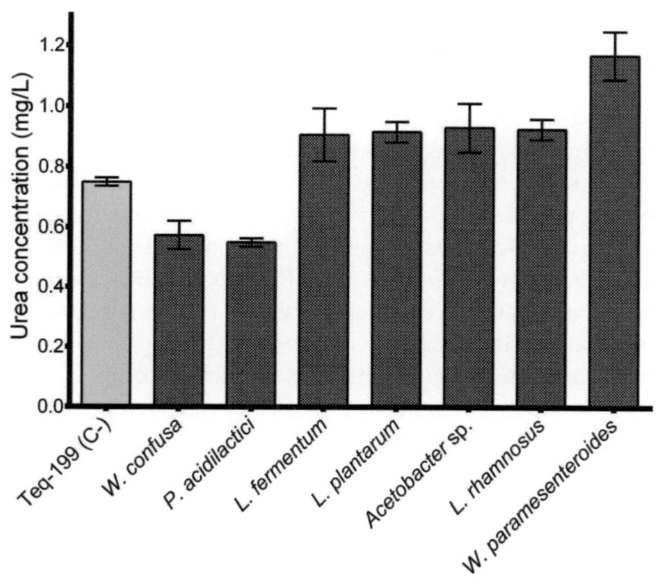

Figure 2.
Urea concentration produced by S. cerevisiae *strain Teq-199 individually (C-) or in combination with seven native bacteria species (data not published).*

Compared with fermentation individually carried out by *S. cerevisiae* strain, a clear tendency to decrease urea concentration of approximately 0.2 mg/L was observed when *Weissella confusa* and *Pediococcus acidilactici* were co-inoculated with the *S. cerevisiae* strain. Conversely, a moderate increase was obtained with the rest of the bacterial strain, especially with *Weissella paramesenteriodes*, with an increase of about 0.4 mg/L compared with the control. These changes are respectively associated with a consumption and production of the metabolite in question, depending on the species used.

These cases exemplify some of the strategies that have been followed in order to choose or validate the use of mixed cultures, seeking to achieve particular objectives and trying to ensure the success of combining certain strains.

5. Genetically modified microorganisms

Natural genetic differences are shown in strains of the same species. This variability can be replicated under laboratory conditions intended to improve characteristics of microorganisms [60]. These traits could be modified by directed or by “natural” methodologies. Even though both approaches result in genetically modified microorganisms (GMMs), the laws that dictate the feasibility on food production depend on the strategy used [61].

It is necessary to consider that the strains to be modified for food fermentation must be labeled as generally recognized as safe (GRAS) or qualified presumption of safety (QPS), not related with pathogens; so, they should be taxonomically identified, as well as being genetically stable under industrial processes [62]. Under these considerations the most investigated eukaryotic microorganism is *S. cerevisiae*, used for several centuries for food and alcoholic production; thus, their metabolic pathways and gene-related regulation are well known. Furthermore, the genome of this species has been completely sequenced, providing the basis for applications of genetic engineering [63]. Meanwhile, technological improvement investigation has been carried out mainly on LAB (**Table 2**).

5.1 Directed genetic modifications

The directed modification is carried out by genetic engineering causing a punctual manipulation in a known region in the genome that in turn will improve a characteristic of interest or the repression of a negative trait. The changes usually involve the promoter region to induce or repress gene translation, or the deletion or insertion of new genes from other microorganisms. This approach presents several drawbacks in food industry. First, it requires the global knowledge of metabolic pathways, genes involved, and their regulation [79]. Second, a single gene modification cannot produce the expected result, since some pathways are regulated by several genes, making a complex process to obtain the desirable trait [61]. And third, the use of microorganisms modified this way is prohibited in foods by law in the European Union, USA, and other countries [80].

The only permitted directed genetically engineered strain used in USA is a *S. cerevisiae* strain able to fully carry out a malo-alcoholic fermentation. This strain was generated by the integration of a malate permease gene from *Schizosaccharomyces pombe* and malic enzyme from *O. oeni* to the constitutive promoter of the 3-phosphoglycerate kinase of *S. cerevisiae* [81].

Modification technique	Species	Modified trait	Reference
Adaptive evolution	*S. cerevisiae*	Flocculation in the surface	[64]
	S. cerevisiae	Ethanol reduction and flavor increase	[65]
	S. cerevisiae	Ethanol reduction	[66]
Random mutagenesis	*L. lactis*	Domestication from plant to milk fermentation	[67]
	Yeast (species not identified)	Reduction of acetic acid	[68]
	O. oeni	Malolactic efficiency and sensory properties	[69]
Natural conjugation	*S. cerevisiae* *S. bayanus*	Fermentation at low temperature	[70]
	S. cerevisiae *S. bayanus*	Stress resistance and fermentation performance	[71]
	S. cerevisiae *S. paradoxus* *S. pastorianus*	Aroma production	[60]
	S. cerevisiae	Determine gene implicated in nitrogen requirements	[72]
	S. cerevisiae	Acid- and thermo-tolerance	[73]
Genome shuffling	*S. cerevisiae*	Improve fermentation performance, affected negatively the flocculation capacity	[74]
	S. cerevisiae	Improve fermentation performance	[75]
	S. cerevisiae	Improve fermentation performance	[76]
	Candida krusei	Improve acetic acid tolerance	[77]
	Acetic acid bacterium	Improve tolerance of ethanol	[78]

Table 2.
Examples of genetic modifications applied to microorganisms for fermented beverages improvement.

5.2 Natural genetic modifications

To obtain microorganisms with desired genetic characteristics using natural techniques, growth conditions are guided in the laboratory to improve the probability of inducing the desired genome modifications. All these natural techniques target the whole genome of the strain, generating several different genotypic changes and, thus, generating the need to further select the strains with the phenotypic variation desired. These methodologies are "allowed," or at least not prohibited by the law as they do not enter in the legal definition of GMM [30]. Among other strategies, some of the most important are described below.

5.2.1 Adaptive evolution

In this methodology, strains are grown in a medium exerting an increasing selective pressure to allow the most adapted generations to become dominant. During the replication of DNA, mutations could accumulate in the offspring without causing an evident modification. However, in a selective condition, only strains with the genetic pool needed to maintain the homeostasis of the cell under the stress pressure will be able to grow [82].

Adaptive evolution has been applied to divert ethanol to glycerol production, then reducing ethanol graduation in wine. It was achieved by increasing osmotic stress with salts in growth media. Glycerol is produced and accumulated in the interior of the yeast cell to counteract the osmotic pressure in the environment [66].

5.2.2 Random mutagenesis

The exposure of microorganisms to physical factors such as UV light, or chemical mutagens as alkylating agent, allows increasing the rate of mistakes in the replication. The offspring then are screened to select colonies with improved characteristics. The randomness of the mutations causes a big drawback, and the modification of regions other than the target of interest could impact negatively on the performance [83]. Also, as the genes occur in more than one copy in the genome, the mutation should be present in all the copies to obtain a strain with changed phenotype [84].

5.2.3 Natural conjugation

This methodology mainly has been applied to yeast, in which two strains, both having an interesting characteristic are crossed using their sexual cycle, thus also receiving the name of direct mating [60]. The resulting hybrid strain contains half genes from each parental strain, meaning that it will obtain some characteristics and lose others [85]. To discriminate the new hybrids from the parental strains, the latter must be differentiated, usually using respiratory-deficient and auxotrophic strains, which in turn only hybrids with prototrophy and respiratory proficiency would be able to grow in a selective media [60].

The most famous yeast strain generated by natural hybridization is the lager beer *S. pastorius*, having characteristics of *S. cerevisiae* and cryotolerance of *S. eubayanus*, which gave the desired fermentative proficiency at low temperatures [37]. Laboratory hybridization of *S. cerevisiae* x *S. mikatae* has also generated strains with improved and diverse volatile compounds that provide complexity to wines [86]. In addition, a hybrid of *S. cerevisiae* and *S. kudriavzevii* accumulated more glycerol, providing more cryotolerance, osmotolerance, and ethanol tolerance [87].

The major drawback of the sexual reproduction in yeast is that industrial strains poorly sporulate [61]. Rare mating is applied in these cases, switching the mating type of diploid or polyploid cells, and then being able to hybridize with the contrary mating type, to generate a new hybrid [88].

5.2.4 Cell fusion

In this methodology, the cell wall is disrupted generating spheroplasts that will spontaneously fuse to other cells, integrating their DNA into a single cell and, then, recombination occurs. The insertion of genetic material could be done even from microorganisms of other kingdoms [89].

Genome shuffling is based on protoplast fusion and nowadays several methodologies are integrated to provide complex phenotypes. It involves the induction of mutagenesis in a population of a specific strain, and then this new genetically diverse population could be screened by the evaluation of individual isolates or by applying a selective pressure to the media containing the mutants. The resulting exceptional mutants are hybridized by protoplast fusion or by mating. The resulting combinations could be further hybridized repeatedly to improve characteristics of interest [75]. As this methodology is relatively new, their evaluation at industrial level to provide certainty of the results is still needed.

5.2.5 Horizontal gene transfer

In nature, horizontal gene transfer occurs in fungi and bacteria kingdoms, it involves the insertion of sequence elements, conjugation, transformation, and transduction from one microorganism to another [90]. These transferences could happen in non-taxonomically related microorganisms. In yeast, this mechanism is not well known; however, it has provided important features such as the identified in a *S. cerevisiae* strain by whole genome sequencing, in which a total of 34 genes were found to be transferred from non-*Saccharomyces* and *Zygosaccharomyces bailii*, providing important fructose fermentation capability [30].

Regarding bacteria, mating process involves close physical contact between a strain that donates its genetic material, mainly a plasmid, to a recipient. The vast majority of the plasmids transferred do not contain any technological use [91]. In LAB, important plasmids naturally present provide the ability to ferment lactose, gain resistance to bacteriophages, and produce bacteriocins [92]. Plasmids could also encode for antibiotic resistance and further transferring could occur to other species of importance to pathogenic bacteria [93].

6. Trends and perspectives

During the last years, there has been an increase in the demand of natural, artisanal, and organic-labeled products, leading to a rise in the request for autochthonous starters, which reflect the biodiversity of a particular area, supported by the idea of microbial "terroir."

An alternative to the use of single-strain starter cultures, which leads to very standardized products, is the use of autochthonous mixed starters (consortia), able to mimic the natural biodiversity, increasing organoleptic properties, but still maintaining controllable processes [52, 53].

On the other hand, considering the fact that mixed populations can perform functions that are difficult or even impossible for individual strains or species to do, nowadays the theoretical support to successfully obtain synthetic microbial consortium exists and presents a wider application potential than single synthetic cells. Taking into consideration the knowledge acquired on naturally occurring microbial interactions, the application of such technology seems feasible and attractive for many industries. This approach would make it possible to efficiently complete many tasks and to acquire a specific product profile compartmentalizing molecular components of each pathway, transcriptional regulators, and chemical intermediates in each different microbial individual. Nevertheless, the use of this technology would face many drawbacks until it is approved to be used in fermented foods, in spite of being the focus of several studies in other similar fields [94-96].

7. Conclusions

The genetic modification of strains and the development of mixed starter cultures aim for similar objectives, to improve the characteristics of fermented beverages maintaining control of the process and quality of the products. Both approaches possess strengths and weaknesses. While some advocate that changes in the genome open a vast opportunity to achieve all the desired characteristics in fermented beverages, the other groups remark that only natural diversity and traditional methods could generate best products with typicity. Furthermore, the application of genetic modifications is badly perceived by consumers and legally prohibited in some cases. It seems that the next step in the improvement agenda is the combination of both approaches, the incorporation of mixtures of natural, genetically modified microorganisms and native strains to provide a holistic solution to the existing difficulties in fermentation.

Acknowledgements

The authors thank the Universidad Autónoma de Querétaro for their financial support, and CONACYT for the scholarships given to Dalia Miranda-Castilleja and Alejandro Aldrete-Tapia.

Conflict of interest

The authors state that there is not conflict of interest.

Author details

Jesús Alejandro Aldrete-Tapia, Dalia Elizabeth Miranda-Castilleja, Sofia Maria Arvizu-Medrano, Ramón Álvar Martínez-Peniche, Lourdes Soto-Muñoz and Montserrat Hernández-Iturriaga*
Universidad Autónoma de Querétaro, Queretaro, Mexico

*Address all correspondence to: montshi@uaq.mx

References

[1] El-Mansi E, Bryce C, Hartley B, Demain A. Fermentation microbiology and biotechnology: An historical perspective. In: El-Mansi E, Bryce C, Dahhou B, Sanchez S, Demain A, Allman A, editors. Fermentation Microbiology and Biotechnology. Boca Raton: CRC Press; 2012. pp. 2-4

[2] Stanbury P, Whitaker A, Hall S. Principles of Fermentation Technology. Butterworth-Heinemann; 2016. pp. 1-20

[3] Kamal-Eldin A, Mehta B, Iwanski R. Fermentation: Effects on food properties. Boca Raton: CRC Press; 2012. pp. 8-44

[4] Hui Y. Fermented plant products and their manufacturing. In: Hui Y, Evranuz E, editors. Handbook of Plant-based Fermented Food and Beverage Technology. Burlington: CRC Press; 2012. pp. 1-3

[5] Escalante A, Giles-Gómez M, Hernández G, Córdova-Aguilar M, López-Munguía A, Gosset G, et al. Analysis of bacterial community during the fermentation of pulque, a traditional Mexican alcoholic beverage, using a polyphasic approach. International Journal of Food Microbiology. 2008;**124**: 126-134. DOI: 10.1016/j.ijfoodmicro.2008.03.003

[6] Weir P. The ecology of *Zymomonas*: A review. Folia Microbiologica. 2016;**61**: 385-392. DOI: 10.1007/s12223-016-0447-x

[7] Walker G, Stewart G. *Saccharomyces cerevisiae* in the production of fermented beverages. Beverages. 2016;**2**:30. DOI: 10.3390/beverages2040030

[8] Nicol D. Rum. In: Lea A, Piggott J, editors. Fermented Beverage Production. Boston: Springer; 2003. p. 265. DOI: 10.1007/978-1-4615-0187-9

[9] Swiegers J, Saerens S, Pretorius I. The development of yeast strains as tools for adjusting the flavor of fermented beverages to market specifications. In: Havkin-Frenkel D, Dudai N, editors. Biotechnology in Flavor Production. Chichester: John Wiley & Sons; 2008. pp. 6-7. DOI: 10.1002/9781444302493.ch1

[10] Hagman A, Säll T, Compagno C, Piskur J. Yeast "make-accumulate-consume" life strategy evolved as a multi-step process that predates the whole genome duplication. PLoS One. 2013;**8**:e68734. DOI: 10.1371/journal.pone.0068734

[11] Muñoz R, Moreno-Arribas M, de las Rivas B. Lactic acid bacteria. In: Carrascosa AV, Muñoz R, González R, editors. Molecular Wine Microbiology. 1st ed. 2011. pp. 191-226

[12] Liu S. Malolactic fermentation in wine—Beyond deacidification. Journal of Applied Microbiology. 2002;**92**: 589-601. DOI: 10.1046/j.1365-2672.2002.01589.x

[13] Gullo M, Giudici P. Acetic acid bacteria in traditional balsamic vinegar: Phenotypic traits relevant for starter cultures selection. International Journal of Food Microbiology. 2008;**125**:46-53. DOI: 10.1016/j.ijfoodmicro.2007.11.076

[14] Sengun I, Karabiyikli S. Importance of acetic acid bacteria in food industry. Food Control. 2011;**22**:647-656. DOI: 10.1016/j.foocont.2010.11.008

[15] Kersters K, Lisdiyanti P, Komagata K, Swings J. The family *Acetobacteraceae*: The genera *Acetobacter*, *Acidomonas*, *Asaia*, *Gluconacetobacter*, *Gluconobacter* and *Kozakia*. In: Dworkin M, Falkow S, Rosenberg E, Schleifer K, Stackebrandt E, editors. The Prokaryotes. 3. New York: Springer; 2006. pp. 163-200. DOI: 10.1007/0-387-30745-1_9

[16] Bartowsky E, Henschke P. Acetic acid bacteria spoilage of bottled red wine—A review. International Journal of Food Microbiology. 2008; **125**:60-70. DOI: 10.1016/j.ijfoodmicro.2007.10.016

[17] Hazelwood W, Daran J, van Maris A, Pronk J, Dickinson R. The Erhlich pathway for fusel alcohol production: A century of research on *Saccharomyces cerevisiae* metabolism. Applied and Environmental Microbiology. 2008;**74**: 2259-2266. DOI: 10.1128/AEM.02625-07

[18] Wang Z, Zhuge J, Fang H, Prior B. Glycerol production by microbial fermentation: A review. Biotechnology Advances. 2001;**19**:201-223. DOI: 10.1016/S0734-9750(01)00060-X

[19] Saerens S, Delvaux F, Verstrepen K, Van Dijck P, Thevelein J, Delvaux F. Parameters affecting ethyl ester production by *Saccharomyces cerevisiae* during fermentation. 2008;**74**:454-461. DOI: 10.1128/AEM.01616-07

[20] Krogerus K, Gibson B. Influence of valine and other amino acids on total diacetyl and 2,3-pentanedione levels during fermentation of brewer's wort. Applied Microbiology and Biotechnology. 2013;**97**:6919-6930. DOI: 10.1007/s00253-013-4955-1

[21] Alegría E, López I, Ruiz JI, Sáenz J, Fernández E, Zarazaga M, et al. High tolerance of wild *Lactobacillus plantarum* and *Oenococcus oeni* strains to lyophilisation and stress environmental conditions of acid pH and ethanol. FEMS Microbiology Letters. 2004;**230**: 53-61. DOI: 10.1016/S0378-1097(03)00854-1

[22] Gibson BR, Lawrence SJ, Leclaire JPR, Powell CD, Smart KA. Yeast responses to stresses associated with industrial brewery handling. FEMS Microbiology Reviews. 2007;**31**: 535-569. DOI: 10.1111/j.1574-6976.2007.00076.x

[23] Nussbaum I, Weindling E, Jubran R, Cohen A, Bar-Nun S. Deteriorated stress response in stationary-phase yeast: Sir2 and Yap1 are essential for Hsf1 activation by heat shock and oxidative stress, respectively. PLoS One. 2014;**9**:e111505

[24] Novo M, Mangado A, Quirós M, Morales P, Salvadó Z, Gonzalez R. Genome-wide study of the adaptation of *Saccharomyces cerevisiae* to the early stages of wine fermentation. PLoS One. 2013;**8**:e74086. DOI: 10.1371/journal.pone.0074086

[25] Tesnière C, Delobel P, Pradal M, Blondin B. Impact of nutrient imbalance on wine alcoholic fermentations: Nitrogen excess enhances yeast cell death in lipid-limited must. PLoS One. **8**:e61645. DOI: 10.1371/journal.pone.0061645

[26] Tesnière C, Brice C, Blondin B. Responses of *Saccharomyces cerevisiae* to nitrogen starvation in wine alcoholic fermentation. Applied Microbiology and Biotechnology. 2015;**99**:7025-7034. DOI: 10.1007/s00253-015-6810-z

[27] Orozco H, Matallana E, Aranda A. Oxidative stress tolerance, adenylate cyclase, and autophagy are key players in the chronological life span of *Saccharomyces cerevisiae* during winemaking. Applied and Environmental Microbiology. 2012;**78**: 2748-2757. DOI: 10.1128/AEM.07261-11

[28] Wang C, Cui Y, Qu X. Mechanisms and improvement of acid resistance in lactic acid bacteria. Archives of Microbiology. 2018;**200**:195-201. DOI: 10.1007/s00203-017-1446-2

[29] Novo M, Gonzalez R, Beltran E, Martínez M, Yuste M, Morales P. Improved fermentation kinetics by wine yeast strains evolved under ethanol stress. LWT—Food Science and Technology. 2014;**58**:166-172. DOI: 10.1016/j.lwt.2014.03.004

[30] Pretorius I, Bauer F. Meeting the consumer challenge through genetically customized wine-yeast strains. Trends in Biotechnology. 2002; **20**:426-432

[31] Minty J, Singer M, Scholz S, Bae C, Ahn J, Foster C, et al. Design and characterization of synthetic fungal-bacterial consortia for direct production of isobutanol from cellulosic biomass. Proceedings of the National Academy of Sciences of the United States of America. 2013;**110**:14592-14597. DOI: 10.1073/pnas.1218447110

[32] Bokulich N, Ohta M, Richardson P, Mills D. Monitoring seasonal changes in winery-resident microbiota. PLoS One. 2013;**8**:e66437. DOI: 10.1371/journal.pone.0066437

[33] Jayabalan R, Malbasa RV, Loncar ES, Vitas JS, Sathishkumar M. A review on kombucha tea: Microbiology, composition, fermentation, beneficial effects, toxicity, and tea fungus. Comprehensive Reviews in Food Science and Food Safety. 2014;**13**: 538-550. DOI: 10.1111/1541-4337.12073

[34] Piao H, Hawley E, Kopf S, De Scenzo R, Sealock S, Henick-Kling T, et al. Insights into the bacterial community and its temporal succession during the fermentation of wine grapes. Frontiers in Microbiology. 2015;**6**:809. DOI: 10.3389/fmicb.2015.00809

[35] Cousin F, Le Guellec R, Schlusselhuber M, Dalmasso M, Laplace J, Cretenet M. Microorganisms in fermented apple beverages: current knowledge and future directions. Microorganisms. 2017;**5**. DOI: 10.3390/microorganisms5030039

[36] Wouters J, Ayad E, Hugenholtz J, Smit G. Microbes from raw milk for fermented dairy products. International Dairy Journal. 2002;**12**:91-109. DOI: 10.1016/S0958-6946(01)00151-0

[37] Peris D, Lopes C, Belloch C, Querol A, Barrio E. Comparative genomics among *Saccharomyces cerevisiae* × *Saccharomyces kudriavzevii* natural hybrid strains isolated from wine and beer reveals different origins. BMC Genomics. 2012;**13**:407. DOI: 10.1186/1471-2164-13-407

[38] Lv X, Huang X, Zhang W, Rao P, Ni L. Yeast diversity of traditional alcohol fermentation starters for Hong Ku glutinous rice wine brewing revealed by culture-dependent and culture-independent methods. Food Control. 2013;**34**:183-190. DOI: 10.1016/j.foodcon.2013.04.020

[39] Schwan R, Almeida E, Aparecida M, Souza-Dias G, Jespersen L. Yeast diversity in rice cassava fermentations produced by the indigenous Tapirape people of Brazil. FEMS Yeast Research. 2007;**7**:966-972. DOI: 10.1111/j.1567-1364.2007.00241.x

[40] Silva MS. Tejuino: bebida típica mexicana com potencial probiótico [Tese (doutorado)]. Lavras: Universidade Federal de Lavras (UFLA); 2016. 49 p

[41] de Melo G, Soccol V, Brar S, Neto E, Soccol C. Microbial ecology and starter culture technology in coffee processing. Critical Reviews in Food Science and Nutrition. 2015;**57**:2775-2788. DOI: 10.1080/10408398.2015.1067759

[42] Di Cagno R, Surico R, Paradiso A, De Angelis M, Salmon J, Buchin S, et al. Effect of autochthonous lactic acid bacteria starters on health-promoting and sensory properties of tomato juices. International Journal of Food Microbiology. 2009;**128**:473-483. DOI: 10.1016/j.ijfoodmicro.2008.10.017

[43] Alcántara-Hernández R, Rodríguez-Álvarez J, Valenzuela-Encinas C, Gutiérrez-Miceli F, Catañón-González H, Marsch R, et al. The bacterial community in 'taberna' a traditional

beverage of southern Mexico. Letters in Applied Microbiology. 2010;**51**:558-563. DOI: 10.1111/j.1472-765X.2010.02934.x

[44] Mousavi Z, Mousavi S, Razavi S, Emam-Djomeh Z, Kiani H. Fermentation of pomegranate juice by probiotic lactic acid bacteria. Journal of Microbiology and Biotechnology. 2011; **27**:123-128. DOI: 10.1007/s11274-010-0439-1

[45] Iranmanesh M, Ezzatpanah H, Mojgani N, Karimi M, Aminafshar M, Mohamadi M. Isolation of lactic acid bacteria from ewe milk, traditional yoghurt and sour buttermilk in Iran. European Journal of Food Research & Review. 2012;**2**:79-92

[46] Garofalo C, Osimani A, Milanović V, Aquilanti L, De Filippis F, Stellato G, et al. Bacteria and yeast microbiota in milk kefir grains from different Italian regions. Food Microbiology. 2015;**49**: 123-133. DOI: 10.1016/j.fn.2015.01.017

[47] Todorov S, Holzapfel W. Traditional cereal fermented foods as sources of functional microorganisms. In: Holzapfel W, editor. Advances in Fermented Foods and Beverages. 2015. pp. 123-152. DOI: 10.1016/B978-1-78242-015-6.00006-2

[48] Laureys D, De Vuyst L. Microbial species diversity, community dynamics, and metabolite kinetics of water kefir fermentation. Applied and Environmental Microbiology. 2014;**80**: 2564-2572. DOI: 10.1128/AEM.03978-13

[49] Rokas A. The effect of domestication on the fungal proteome. Trend Genetics. 2009;**25**:60-63. DOI: 10.1016/j.tig.2008.11.003

[50] Ivey M, Masell M, Phister T. Microbial interactions in food fermentation. Annual Review of Food Science and Technology. 2013;**4**: 141-162. DOI: 10.1146/annurev-food-022811-101219

[51] Braga R, Dourado M, Araújo W. Microbial interactions: Ecology in a molecular perspective. Brazilian Journal of Microbiology. 2016;**47**:86-98. DOI: 10.1016/j.bjm.2016.10.005

[52] Bokulich N, Ohta M, Lee M, Mills D. Indigenous bacteria and fungi drive traditional kimoto sake fermentations. Applied and Environmental Microbiology. 2014;**80**:5522-5529. DOI: 10.1128/AEM.00663-14

[53] Mas A, Padilla B, Esteve-Zarzoso B, Beltran G, Reguant C, Bordons A. Taking advantage of natural biodiversity for wine making: The WILDWINE Project. Agriculture and Agricultural Science Procedia. 2016;**8**: 4-9. DOI: 10.1016/j.aaspro.2016.02.002

[54] Liu P, Lu L, Duan C, Yan G. The contribution of indigenous non-Saccharomyces wine yeast to improved aromatic quality of Cabernet Sauvignon wines by spontaneous fermentation. LWT—Food Science and Technology. 2016;**71**:356-363. DOI: 10.1016/j.lwt.2016.04.031

[55] Ferreira-Duarte W, Ferreira de Sousa M, Ribeiro D, Freitas R. Effect of co-inoculation of *Saccharomyces cerevisiae* and *Lactobacillus fermentum* on the quality of the distilled sugar cane beverage cachaca. Journal of Food Science. 2011;**76**:307-318. DOI: 10.1111/j.1750-3841.2011.02412.x

[56] Rodríguez-Lerma G, Gutiérrez-Moreno K, Cárdenas-Manríquez M, Botello-Álvarez E, Jiménez-Islas H, Rico-Martínez R, et al. Microbial ecology studies of spontaneous fermentation: Starter culture selection for prickly pear wine production. Journal of Food Science. 2011;**76**: 346-352. DOI: 10.1111/j.1750-3841.2011.02208.x

[57] Miranda-Castilleja D, Martínez-Peniche R, Nadal M, Aldrete-Tapia A, Arvizu-Medrano S. Enological qualities

and interactions between native yeast and lactic acid bacteria from Queretaro, Mexico. Journal of Food Science. 2018; **83**:1904-1912. DOI: 10.1111/1750-3841.14197

[58] Nehme N, Mathieu F, Taillandier P. Quantitative study of interactions between *Saccharomyces cerevisiae* and *Oenococcus oeni* strains. Journal of Industrial Microbiology & Biotechnology. 2008;**35**:685-693. DOI: 10.1007/s10295-008-0328-7

[59] Nancib N, Nancib A, Boudjelal A, Benslimane C, Blanchard F, Boudrant J. The effect of supplementation by different nitrogen sources on the production of lactic acid from date juice by *Lactobacillus casei* subsp. Rhamnosus. Bioresource Technology. 2001;**78**: 149-153. DOI: 10.1016/S0960-8524(01)00009-8

[60] Steensels J, Meersman E, Snoek T, Saels V, Verstrepen K. Large-scale selection and breeding to generate industrial yeast with superior aroma production. Applied and Environmental Microbiology. 2014;**80**:6965-6975. DOI: 10.1128/AEM.02235-14

[61] Pérez-Torrado R, Querol A, Guillamón J. Genetic improvement of non-GMO wine yeasts: Strategies, advantages and safety. Trends in Food Science and Technology. 2015;**45**:1-11. DOI: 10.1016/j.tifs.2015.05.002

[62] Peterbauer C, Maishberger T, Haltrich D. Food-grade gene expression in lactic acid bacteria. Biotechnology Journal. 2011;**6**:1-15. DOI: 10.1002/biot.201100034

[63] Ostergaard S, Olsson L, Nielsen J. Metabolic engineering of *Saccharomyces cerevisiae*. Microbiology and Molecular Biology Reviews. 2000;**64**:34-50

[64] Fidalgo M, Barrales R, Ibeas J, Jimenez J. Adaptive evolution by mutations in the *FLO11* gene. PNAS. 2006;**103**:11228-11233. DOI: 10.1073/pnas.0601713103

[65] Strejc J, Siristova L, Karabin M, Almeida J, Branyik T. Production of alcohol-free beer with elevated amounts of flavouring compounds using lager yeast mutants. Journal of Institute of Brewing. 2013;**119**:149-155. DOI: 10.1002/jib.72

[66] Tilloy V, Ortiz-Julien A, Dequin S. Reduction of ethanol yield and improvement of glycerol formation by adaptive evolution of the wine yeast *Saccharomyces cerevisiae* under hyperosmotic conditions. Applied and Environmental Microbiology. 2014;**80**: 2623-2632. DOI: 10.1128/AEM.03710-13

[67] Bachmann H, Starrenburg M, Molenaar D, Kleerebezem M, van Hylckama J. Microbial domestication signatures of *Lactococcus lactis* can be reproduced by experimental evolution. Genome Research. 2012;**22**:115-124. DOI: 10.1101/gr.121285.111

[68] Cordente A, Cordero-Bueso G, Pretorius I, Curtin C. Novel wine yeast with mutations in *YAP1* that produce less acetic acid during fermentation. FEMS Yeast Research. 2013;**13**:62-73. DOI: 10.1111/1567-1364.12010

[69] Li N, Duan J, Gao D, Luo J, Zheng R, Bian Y, et al. Mutation and selection of *Oenococcus oeni* for controlling wine malolactic fermentation. European Food Research and Technology. 2015;**240**: 93-100. DOI: 10.1007/s00217-014-2310-0

[70] Sato M, Kishimoto M, Watari J, Takashio M. Breeding of brewer's yeast by hybridization between top fermenting yeast *Saccharomyces cerevisiae* and cryophilic yeast *Saccharomyces bayanus*. Journal of Bioscience and Bioengineering. 2002;**93**:509-511. DOI: 10.1016/S1389-1723(02)80101-3

[71] Garcia R, Solodovnikova N, Wendland J. Breeding of lager yeast

with *Saccharomyces cerevisiae* improves resistance and fermentation performance. Yeast. 2012;**29**:343-355. DOI: 10.1002/yea.2914

[72] Brice C, Sanchez I, Bigey F, Legras J, Blongin B. A genetic approach of wine yeast fermentation capacity in nitrogen-starvation reveals the key role of nitrogen signaling. BMC Genomics. 2014;**15**:495. DOI: 10.1186/1471-2164-15-495

[73] Mitsumasu K, Liu Z, Tang Y, Akamatsu T, Taguchi H, Kida K. Development of industrial yeast strain with improved acid- and thermo-tolerance through evolution under continuous fermentation conditions followed by haploidization and mating. Journal of Bioscience and Bioengineering. 2014;**118**:689-695. DOI: 10.1016/j.jbiosc.2014.05.012

[74] Mukai N, Nishimori C, Wilson I, Mizuno A, Takahashi T, Sato K. Beer brewing using fusant between a sake yeast and a brewer's yeast. Journal of Bioscience and Bioengineering. 2001;**91**: 482-486. DOI: 10.1016/S1389-1723(01) 80277-2

[75] Hou L. Improved production of ethanol by novel genome shuffling in *Saccharomyces cerevisiae*. Applied Biochemistry and Biotechnology. 2010; **160**:1084-1093. DOI: 10.1007/ s12010-009-8552-9

[76] Wang H, Hou L. Genome shuffling to improve fermentation properties of top-fermenting yeast by the improvement of stress tolerance. Food Science and Biotechnology. 2010;**19**: 145-150. DOI: 10.1007/s10068-010-0020-3

[77] Wei P, Li Z, He P, Lin Y, Jiang N. Genome shuffling in the ethanologenic yeast *Candida krusei* to improve acetic acid tolerance. Biotechnology and Applied Biochemistry. 2010;**49**:113-120. DOI: 10.1042/BA20070072

[78] Wei K, Cao X, Li X, Wang C, Hou L. Genome shuffling to improve fermentation properties of acetic acid bacterium by the improvement of ethanol tolerance. International Journal of Food Science and Technology. 2012; **47**:2184-2189. DOI: 10.1111/j.1365-2621. 2012.03086.x

[79] Dai Z, Nielsen J. Advancing metabolic engineering through systems biology of industrial microorganisms. Current Opinion in Biotechnology. 2015;**36**:8-15. DOI: 10.1016/j. copbio.2015.08.006

[80] Sybesma W, Hugenholt J, de-Vos W, Smid E. Safe use of genetically modified lactic acid bacteria in food: Bringing the gap between consumers, green groups, and industry. Electronic Journal of Biotechnology. 2006;**9**: 424-448. DOI: 10.2225/vol9-issue4-fulltext-12

[81] Husnik J, Volschenk H, Bauer J, Colavizza D, Luo Z, van Vuuren H. Metabolic engineering of malolactic wine yeast. Metabolic Engineering. 2006;**8**:315-323. DOI: 10.1016/j. ymben.2006.02.003

[82] Dragosits M, Mattanovich D. Adaptive laboratory evolution—Principles and applications for biotechnology. Microbial Cell Factories. 2013;**12**:64. DOI: 10.1186/1475-2859-12-64

[83] Derkx P, Janzen T, Sorensen K, Christensen J, Stuer-Lauridsen B, Johansen E. The art of strain improvement of industrial lactic acid bacteria without the use of recombinant DNA technology. Microbial Cell Factories. 2014;**13**:S5. DOI: 10.1186/ 1475-2859-13-S1-S5

[84] Cebollero E, Gonzalez-Ramos D, Tabera L, Gonzalez R. Transgenic wine yeast technology comes to age: Is it time for trangenic wine? Biotechnology

Letters. 2007;**29**:191-200. DOI: 10.1007/s10529-006-9236-y

[85] Haber J. Mating-type genes and MAT switching in *Saccharomyces cerevisiae*. Genetics. 2012;**191**:33-64. DOI: 10.1534/genetics.111.134577

[86] Bellon J, Schmid F, Capone D, Dunn B, Chambers P. Introducing a new breed of wine yeast: Interspecific hybridization between a commercial *Saccharomyces cerevisiae* wine yeast and *Saccharomyces mikatae*. PLoS One. 2013;**8**:e62053. DOI: 10.1371/journal.pone.0062053

[87] González S, Gallo L, Climent M, Barrio E, Querol A. Ecological characterization of natural hybrids from *Saccharomyces cerevisiae* and *S. kudriavzevii*. International Journal of Food Microbiology. 2007;**116**:11-18. DOI: 10.1016/j.ijfoodmicro.2006.10.047

[88] Bellon J, Eglington J, Siebert T, Pollnitz A, Rose L, de Barros M, et al. Newly generated interspecific wine yeast hybrids introduce flavour and aroma diversity to wines. Applied Microbiology and Biotechnology. 2011;**91**:603-612. DOI: 10.1007/s00253-011-3294-3

[89] Zhao D, Wu B, Zhang Y, Jia H, Zhang X, Cheng S. Identification of protoplast fusion strain Fhhh by randomly amplified polymorphic DNA. Journal of Microbiology and Biotechnology. 2009;**25**:1181-1188. DOI: 10.1007/s-11274-009-9999-0

[90] Rossi F, Rizzotti L, Felis G, Torriani S. Horizontal gene transfer among microorganisms in food: Current knowledge and future perspectives. Food Microbiology. 2014;**42**:232-243. DOI: 10.1016/j.fm.2014.04.004

[91] Frost L, Koraimann G. Regulation of bacterial conjugation: Balancing opportunity with adversity. Future Microbiology. 2010;**5**:1057-1071

[92] Shea E, Cotter P, Ross R, Hill C. Strategies to improve the bacteriocin protection provided by lactic acid bacteria. Current Opinion in Biotechnology. 2013;**24**:130-134

[93] Verraes C, Van Boxsael S, Van Meervenee E, Van Coillie, Butaye P, Catry B, et al. Antimicrobial resistance in the food chain: A review. International Journal of Environmental Research and Public Health. 2013;**10**:2643-2669. DOI: 10.3390/ijerph10072643

[94] Brenner K, Joe L, Arnold F. Engineering microbial consortia: a new frontier in synthetic biology. Journal of Trends in Biotechnology. 2008;**26**:483-489. DOI: 10.1016/j.tibtech.2018.05.004

[95] Hays S, Patrick W, Ziesack M, Oxman N, Silver P. Better together: engineering and application of microbial symbioses. Current Opinion in Biotechnology. 2015;**36**:40-49. DOI: 10.1016/j.copbio.2015.08.008

[96] Jia X, Liu C, Song H, Ding M, Du J, Ma Q, Yuan Y. Design, analysis and application of synthetic microbial consortia. Synthetic and Systems Biotechnology. 2016;**1**:109-117. DOI: 10.1016/j.synbio. 2016.02.001

Chapter 7

Perspectives and Uses of Non-*Saccharomyces* Yeasts in Fermented Beverages

Waldir Desiderio Estela Escalante

Abstract

Fermented beverages such as wine, cider and beer are normally fermented with *Saccharomyces* yeasts due to their well-known fermentative behavior. These yeasts have been extensively investigated and are used in commercial processes. On the other hand, non-*Saccharomyces* yeasts were always considered contaminants in winemaking and brewing. Most researchers in the past argued that these yeasts produce several compounds that may alter the sensory quality of wine and beers. However, recent studies have demonstrated that their fermentative metabolism can be regulated and addressed to the production of compounds of sensory importance. Currently, some non-*Saccharomyces* yeasts belonging to the genera *Kloeckera, Candida, Hanseniaspora* are getting importance due to their high potentiality to be used in the production of fermented beverages such as special wines and craft beers. The emergence of new consumption patterns and market niches demanding products with new sensory characteristics has catapulted the exploitation of these yeasts.

Keywords: non-*Saccharomyces* yeasts, fermented beverages, wine, craft beers

1. Introduction

Fermentation of wines, beers and ciders is traditionally carried out with *Saccharomyces cerevisiae* strains, the most common and commercially available yeast. They are well known for their fermentative behavior and technological characteristics which allow obtaining products of uniform and standard quality. *Saccharomyces cerevisiae* is the most used yeast in fermentative processes. In wine fermentation, strains with specific characteristics are needed, for instance, highly producers of ethanol to reach values of 11–13% v/v, typically found in this beverage. On the other hand, beers and ciders contain less amounts of ethanol with a balanced and distinctive sensory profile characteristic of each one. In recent years, new consuming trends and requirements for new and innovative products have emerged. This situation led to rethink about the existing fermented beverages and to meet the demands of consumers. Yeasts are largely responsible for the complexity and sensory quality of fermented beverages. Based on this, current studies are mainly focused on the search of new type of yeasts with technological application. Non-*Saccharomyces* yeasts have always been considered contaminants in the manufacture of wine and beer. Therefore, procedures for eliminating them are routinely utilized such as must pasteurization, addition of sulfite and sanitization of equipment and processing halls. In recent years, the negative perception about non-*Saccharomyces* yeasts has been changing due to the fact that several studies have shown that during spontaneous fermentations of wine, these yeasts play an important role in the definition of the sensory quality of the final product. Based on this evidence, the fermentative behavior of some non-*Saccharomyces* yeasts is being studied in deep with the purpose of finding the most adequate conditions and the most suitable strain to be utilized in the production of fermented beverages.

2. Yeasts

Yeasts are eukaryotic microorganisms that inhabit a variety of ecological niches such as water, soil, air and the surface of plants and fruits. Commonly, they are present during the decomposition of ripen fruits and participate in the fermentation process. In this natural environment, the yeasts find nutrients and substrates necessary for their metabolism and fermentative activity [1, 2]. Yeasts are not nutritionally demanding compared to other microorganisms such as lactic acid bacteria. For supporting their growth, they need common compounds such as fermentable sugars, amino acids, vitamins, minerals and also oxygen. Morphologically the yeasts are very diverse, being the round, ellipsoidal and oval shapes mostly predominant. During the identification, the microscopic evaluation is the first resource followed by microbiological and biochemical tests; subsequently, assays of sugar fermentation and assimilation of amino acids are necessary [3]. The production and tolerance to ethanol, organic acids and SO_2 are also important tools to differentiate among species. The reproduction of yeasts is mainly by budding, which results in a new and genetically identical cell. Budding is the most common type of asexual reproduction, although cell fission is a characteristic of yeasts belonging to the genus *Schizosaccharomyces* (**Figure 1**). Cultivation conditions leading to the starvation of nutrients such as the lack of amino acids induce sporulation, which is a mechanism used by yeasts to survive under unfavorable conditions. As a consequence of the sporulation, yeast cells undergo genetic variability. In industrial

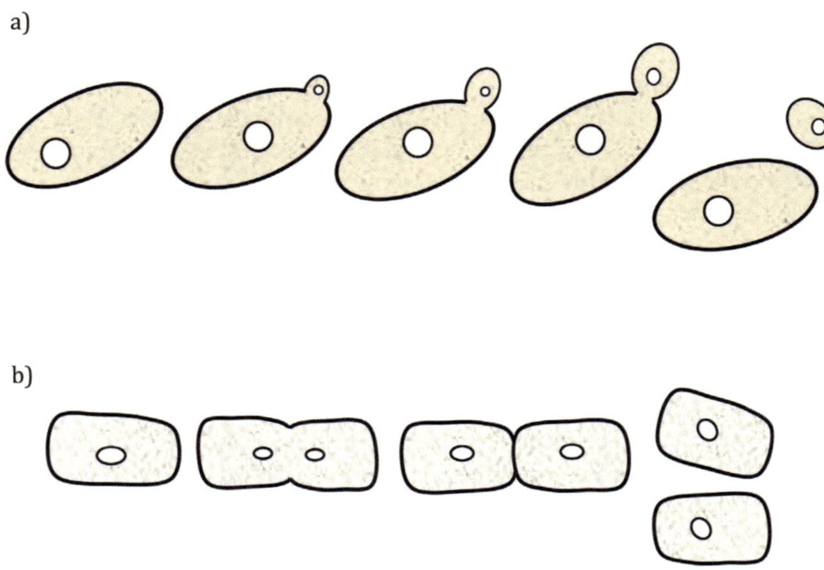

Figure 1.
Asexual reproduction of yeasts. (a) Budding, typically observed in Saccharomyces cerevisiae, Candida, Kloeckera, Brettanomyces *and (b) fission, typically observed in* Schizosaccharomyces pombe.

fermentation processes, asexual reproduction of yeasts is preferable to ensure the conservation of the genotype and to maintain their fermentative behavior over time. Regarding their metabolism, yeasts are usually characterized by fermenting a broad spectrum of sugars, among them, glucose, fructose, sucrose, maltose and maltotriose, which are found in ripen fruits and processed cereals. In addition, yeasts tolerate acidic environments with pH values around 3.5 or even less. According to technological convenience, yeasts are divided into two large groups namely *Saccharomyces* and non-*Saccharomyces*. Morphologically, *Saccharomyces* yeasts can be round or ellipsoidal in shape depending on the growth phase and cultivation conditions. *S. cerevisiae* is the most studied species and the most utilized in the fermentation of wines and beers due to its excellent fermentative capacity, rapid growth and easy adaptation. They tolerate concentrations of SO_2 that normally most non-*Saccharomyces* yeasts do not survive. However, despite these advantages, it is possible to find in the nature representatives of *S. cerevisiae* that do not necessarily present these features.

3. Non-*Saccharomyces* yeasts

Non-*Saccharomyces* yeasts are a group of microorganisms genetically diverse with specific metabolic characteristics and high potential for using in fermentation processes. In the past, many of them have been considered contaminants due to the production of compounds that alters the sensory quality of wines [4, 5]. With the purpose of eliminating them and avoiding their fermentative activity, for instance, in wine processing, disinfection of fermentation tanks and containers with sulfite is commonly performed. However, over time, the importance of non-*Saccharomyces* yeasts in spontaneous fermentation has been demonstrated since they contribute positively to the definition of the sensory quality of wines. These yeasts predominate at the initial stage of the spontaneous fermentation [6–8] until certain concentration of ethanol is reached (usually between 4 and 5% v/v), which are then inhibited due to the effect of the ethanol and the depletion of dissolved oxygen [9, 10]. At the end of the process, *Saccharomyces* yeasts, the most resistant to ethanol, predominate and complete the fermentation. It has been reported that some non-*Saccharomyces* yeasts are able to survive toward the end of the spontaneous fermentation and exert their metabolic activity, thus contributing positively to the sensory quality of wines. Based on this evidence, in recent years, many researchers have focused their studies in understanding the nature and fermentative activity of the non-*Saccharomyces* yeasts [8, 11–21]. The findings demonstrated the enormous potential of these yeasts for use in the fermentation of traditional and nontraditional beverages. Despite the fact that most non-*Saccharomyces* yeasts show some technological disadvantages compared to *Saccharomyces cerevisiae* such as lower fermentative power and production of ethanol, non-*Saccharomyces* yeasts possess characteristics that in *S. cerevisiae* are absent, for instance, production of high levels of aromatic compounds such as esters, higher alcohols and fatty acids [22, 23]. In addition, it has been reported that the fermentative activity of these yeasts is manifested in the presence of small amounts of oxygen which leads to an increase in cell biomass and the decrease in ethanol yield, a strategy that can be used to reduce the ethanol content of wines produced in coculture with *S cerevisiae* [24–26]. With the aim of exploiting the positive characteristics of non-*Saccharomyces* yeasts and reducing their negative impact, fermentations with mixed and sequential cultures with *S. cerevisiae* can be performed to produce fermented beverages with different sensory profiles [27–29]. The most important fact is related to the potential for producing a broad variety of compounds of sensory importance necessary to improve the organoleptic quality of wines and beers. The findings reported so far in literature have led to rethink the role of these yeasts in fermentative processes and to evaluate their use in the development of new products. Among the most studied non-*Saccharomyces* yeasts that reached special importance for researchers include *Candida*, *Kloeckera*, *Hanseniaspora, Brettanomyces, Pichia*, *Lanchacea* and *Kluyveromyces*, among others.

3.1 Fermentative metabolism of sugars

Either non-*Saccharomyces* or *Saccharomyces* yeasts share common pathways for the central metabolism of carbon; thus, both groups metabolize glucose through glycolysis. However, the mechanisms involved in the regulation of respire-fermentative metabolism can differ significantly among them [30]. The glycolysis operates indistinctly under aerobic and anaerobic conditions, and through it, the glucose is metabolized to pyruvate by means of a series of biochemical reactions (**Figure 2**). Under anaerobic or oxygen-limited conditions, pyruvate is converted to acetaldehyde and then to ethanol, and as a result, two net moles of ATP are generated. Under fully aerobic conditions and in the absence of any repression effect, the

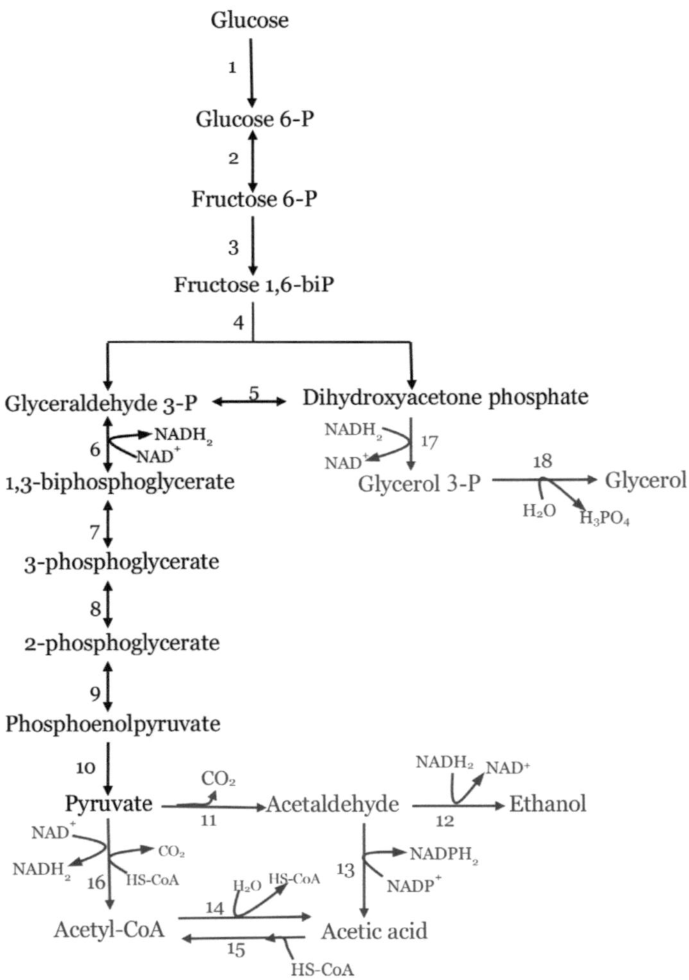

Figure 2.
Fermentative metabolism of glucose by yeasts: Glycolysis (black lines) and ethanol and glycerol production (blue lines). Enzymes: 1, hexokinase; 2, phosphoglucose isomerase; 3, phosphofructokinase; 4, fructose 1,6-bisphosphate aldolase; 5, triosephosphate isomerase; 6, glyceraldehyde 3-phosphate dehydrogenase; 7, phosphoglycerate kinase; 8, phosphoglycerate mutase; 9, enolase; 10, pyruvate kinase; 11, pyruvate decarboxylase; 12, alcohol dehydrogenase; 13, aldehyde dehydrogenase; 14, acetyl-CoA hydrolase; 15, acetyl-CoA synthetase; 16, pyruvate dehydrogenase; 17, glycerol 3-P dehydrogenase; 18, glycerol 3-phosphatase.

generation of energy is greater since glucose undergoes a complete oxidation, and as a result 36 net moles of ATP per mole of glucose are generated. The low-energy yield obtained by yeasts under anaerobic conditions forces the cell to increase the flow of glucose consumption in order to obtain a higher amount of energy in the form of ATP. As consequence, the ethanol accumulates in the fermentation medium and exerts its inhibitory effect, thus stopping the fermentative activity of the yeasts [31]. The low amount of energy generated under anaerobic conditions is used by the yeast cells in requirements for maintenance and growth. Glucose is easily transported and metabolized inside the cell; however, disaccharides such as sucrose, maltose or lactose must be first hydrolyzed to their simple forms (hexoses) which are then catabolized in the glycolysis pathway. Sucrose is hydrolyzed to fructose and glucose, maltose to two glucose units and lactose to glucose and galactose. The disaccharides are preferably hydrolyzed in the periplasmic space before entering the cytosol. Under anaerobic conditions besides ethanol, glycerol is also produced, thus contributing to restore the redox balance inside the cell. The production of glycerol increases in fermentations with musts of high specific gravity as a response to the osmotic stress [32]. It has been found that yeasts unable of metabolizing dihydroxyacetone (**Figure 2**) are not capable of producing glycerol, and as a consequence dihydroxyacetone accumulates and inhibits the fermentation. Moreover, glucose apart of being metabolized via glycolysis, it is also broken by complementary pathways that are not necessarily related to the generation of energy. The hexose monophosphate pathway (HMP) also known as the pentose phosphate cycle usually accompanies the glycolytic pathway [33]. In addition, yeasts during fermentation produce small amounts of acetic acid either from acetaldehyde or acetyl-CoA (**Figure 2**). Acetic acid is the main organic acid produced by yeasts during the fermentation of glucose, and it is responsible for the acidification and the decrease of pH of the medium. Ethanol is the most important fermentation by-product, and from the technological point of view, the production capacity of yeasts is an important parameter that determines their usability in fermentative processes. Gay Lussac defined a stoichiometric theoretical relationship to explain the production of ethanol by *Saccharomyces cerevisiae* yeasts which is:

$$\underset{\text{glucose}}{1\,C_6H_{12}O_6} \rightarrow \underset{\text{ethanol}}{2\,C_2H_5OH} + \underset{\text{carbon dioxide}}{2\,CO_2} \tag{1}$$

According to this relationship, from 180.0 grams of glucose, 92.0 grams of ethanol and 88.0 grams of carbon dioxide are produced, which results in a theoretical yield of 0.511 g ethanol/g glucose. However, in practice, besides ethanol and CO_2, the production of biomass, glycerol and other minority compounds also happens, that is:

$$C_6H_{12}O_6 + \text{nitrogen} \rightarrow C_2H_5OH + CO_2 + \text{glycerol} + \text{biomass} + \text{minority compounds} \tag{2}$$

At industrial scale, a yield of 0.45 g ethanol/g glucose is acceptable [34]. In the case of fermentations with non-*Saccharomyces* yeasts, lower yields are commonly observed. Regarding to glycerol, in the case of *S. cerevisiae,* its production represents approximately 3% of the utilized sugar. Minor compounds are represented by higher alcohols, esters, aldehydes and organic acids, among others.

3.1.1 Importance of oxygen

Oxygen is an important element during the complete oxidation of glucose since it serves as final acceptor of electrons under aerobic conditions. It is also essential for other metabolic processes such as the synthesis of structural components of the cytoplasmic membrane of yeasts. During alcoholic fermentation, as ethanol accumulates, it exerts a detrimental effect on the integrity and stability of the cytoplasmic membrane [31]. Under this condition, the supply of small amounts of oxygen to the medium through aeration promotes the synthesis of unsaturated fatty acids and sterols (mainly ergosterol) which are important components of the yeast cell membrane. Thus, the produced compounds can be used to replace the damaged fraction caused by the effect of ethanol that acts as a solvent [35, 36]. The replacement of unsaturated fatty acids and sterols is important to maintain the cell viability and allow the yeasts to complete successfully the fermentation. From the technological point of view, the supply of small amounts of oxygen is recommended in fermentations with musts of high specific gravity in order to avoid some drawbacks such as sluggish fermentation. It is also necessary for promoting the fermentative metabolism of non-*Saccharomyces* yeasts which are unable to ferment under fully anaerobic conditions [37]. The optimization of the aeration rate is very important to ensure the predominance of the fermentative metabolism and to reach the highest ethanol yield. In Crabtree-negative yeasts, as the concentration of oxygen in the medium increases above a certain value, the metabolism may become predominantly oxidative; thus, the ethanol yield decreases and the production of biomass increases. The highest ethanol yield is possible to achieve, adjusting properly the aeration rate of the fermentation medium. Aeration also affects the production of glycerol by yeasts; thus, as the concentration of oxygen increases, the production of glycerol decreases. From the technological point of view, aeration of the fermentation medium is an interesting tool to control the metabolic activity of non-*Saccharomyces* yeasts during fermentation, for instance, wines and beers [38, 39]. In addition, aeration can be also used in winemaking to improve the quality of wines since it provokes the transformation of phenols, which reduces the astringency.

3.2 Production of higher alcohols

During alcoholic fermentation, either non-*Saccharomyces* or *Saccharomyces* yeasts produce diverse volatile compounds of sensory importance such as higher alcohols, aldehydes, fatty acids and esters in different concentrations depending on the species of yeasts and the fermentation conditions. The harmonic balance of the compounds determines the sensory quality of the fermented beverage. Higher alcohols are a group of compounds that mostly confer unpleasant organoleptic character when present at high concentrations [40, 41]. In adequate concentrations, they contribute positively in defining the organoleptic quality of alcoholic beverage such as wines, beers and ciders. They are produced in the cytosol and then exported outside the yeast cell where it accumulates. Higher alcohols result from the decarboxylation of ketoacids that leads to the formation of the respective aldehydes, which are then reduced to form the corresponding higher alcohols (**Figure 3**). Ketoacids can be originated either from the metabolism of glucose or the catabolism of amino acids [42, 43], which are taken by the yeast cell from the fermentation medium. The synthesis of higher alcohols involves the participation of at least three enzymes: a transaminase, a carboxylase and an alcohol dehydrogenase. Factors that increase the metabolism of sugar and amino acids promote the synthesis of higher alcohols. The factors include temperature of fermentation, amino acid concentration and composition of the fermentation medium.

3.3 Production of esters

Esters are a group of compounds that mostly impart positive sensory characteristics to fermented beverages such as wines, beer and ciders. They are formed by the

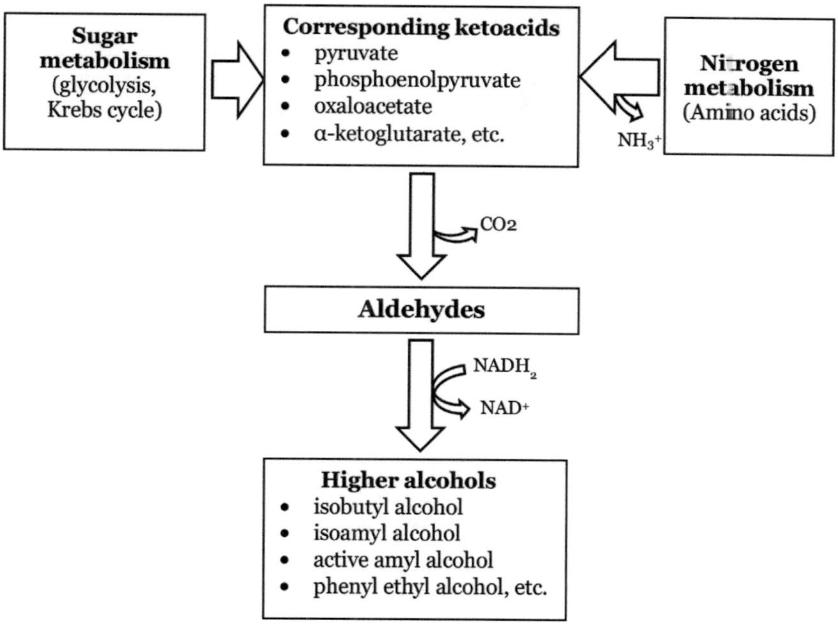

Figure 3.
Production of higher alcohols by yeast. Ehrlich's pathway and glucose catabolism.

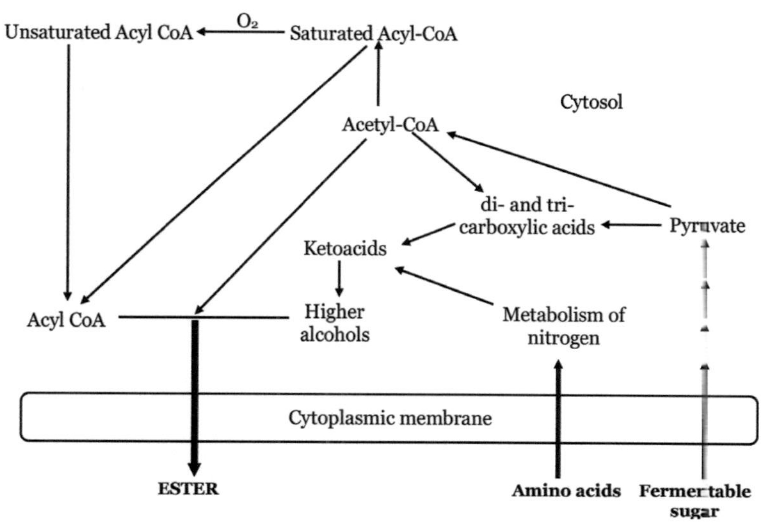

Figure 4.
Mechanisms for the production of esters by yeasts.

action of specific enzymes that catalyze the reaction between an alcohol and a volatile fatty acid (**Figure 4**). The synthesis of esters by yeast initially involves the activation of fatty acids to acyl coenzyme A mediated by energy and the subsequent condensation of the active compound with an alcohol present in the medium to form the corresponding ester [44]. From the sensory point of view, acetate esters are the most important compounds present in fermented beverages, which include ethyl acetate, butyl acetate, propyl acetate, phenyl ethyl acetate and amyl acetate, among others. The esters produced by *S. cerevisiae* involve the activity of at least three acetyltransferases (AAT, EC 2.3.1.84): an alcohol acetyltransferase, an ethanol acetyltransferase and an isoamyl alcohol acetyltransferase [45, 46]. Other enzymes such as ester synthase were also reported to participate in the synthesis of esters.

However, the relevance attributed to the activity of this enzyme is quite limited. Ethyl acetate is the most abundant ester present in wines and largely responsible for the sensory character. Studies carried out with non-*Saccharomyces* yeasts related to the ability of producing esters allowed to select species of *Hanseniaspora* and *Pichia* able to promote esterification of various alcohols such as ethanol, isoamyl alcohol and 2-phenyl ethanol to produce the corresponding esters [47].

4. Most important non-*Saccharomyces* yeasts

4.1 *Candida* yeasts

In the last years, the fermentative behavior of some *Candida* yeasts has been studied with respect to the production of wines and beers. The most studied species include *Candida stellata*, *C. zemplinina* and *C. pulcherrima*, among others [16, 20, 21, 48–50]. Representatives of *Candida* yeasts have been isolated from the early stages of spontaneous fermentation of different types of wines [8, 19, 51, 52]. The isolated species were characterized by being round in shape and smaller than *S. cerevisiae*. These yeasts are able to sediment toward the end of fermentation in a similar manner as *S. cerevisiae* [20]. Currently, the most important characteristics reported include the production of considerable amounts of ethanol and glycerol and a balanced production of volatile compounds of sensory importance, for instance, esters, fatty acids, aldehydes and higher alcohols. The production of ethanol is an important feature to define the use of yeasts in the production of fermented beverages with high ethanol contents such as wines. It has been reported that *C. zemplinina* strains are capable of producing ethanol up to 11.0% v/v [53], amount normally reached during the fermentation of sweet and semidry wines with *S. cerevisiae*. In addition, it has been demonstrated that *Candida* yeasts are capable of producing high amounts (up to 25.0 g/L) of glycerol [53–56], compound that contributes positively to the sensory quality of wines, beers and other beverages. The fermentative behavior of these yeasts was also evaluated as mixed cultures with *S. cerevisiae* [57]. The results were promising and interesting for being scaled-up to pilot fermentations. For instance, fermentation experiments of mixed cultures of *C. stellata* with *S. cerevisiae* produced higher levels of esters and fatty acids than monocultures of *S. cerevisiae* [19, 57]. Fermentations with mixed and even sequential cultures of yeasts are an interesting field of research to evaluate the potential use of non-*Saccharomyces* yeasts to produce sensory differentiated beverages. In addition, individual fermentations with *C. stellata* and *C. zemplinina* strains using immobilized systems have been also performed [53, 58]. The results showed the improvement of some technological properties such as the fermentation rate, ethanol production and the reusability of the strains in successive fermentations. Currently, studies to evaluate the usability of *C. zemplinina* strains in beer fermentation have been carried out using malt wort of 14 and 20°P, typically used in beer fermentation processes [21, 22]. The yeast strains showed a suitable fermentative behavior for the production of lager and ale beers. One interesting feature is that *Candida zemplinina* is unable to ferment maltose, the main fermentable sugar of the malt wort. This characteristic is of special importance since it would enable the production of beers with low ethanol content and particular sensory profiles.

4.2 *Kloeckera* yeasts

Yeasts species belonging to this genus have recently become of interest for the production of fermented beverages. Species such as *Kloeckera apiculata, K. javanica* and *K. corticis* were isolated from a variety of niches including the spontaneous fermentation of grape must and ciders [6, 8, 49, 59]. Most representatives present a lemon shape (apiculate yeasts) and asexual reproduction with bipolar budding. It was reported that these yeasts participate positively in the early stage of the spontaneous fermentation of wine [59, 60], strains of *Kloeckera apiculata* being the most dominant [19, 49, 51, 52]. During spontaneous fermentation, as the ethanol concentration increases, the fermentative activity of these yeasts slows down and stops toward the end of fermentation by the effect of the ethanol [61]. These yeasts are characterized by producing amounts of ethanol around 4–5% v/v, values typically found in commercial beers. It was reported that the control of aeration during fermentation has effect on the production of ethanol and compounds of sensory importance such as esters, higher alcohols and organic acids [14]. Based on the information available in literature, these yeasts are promissory for being used in brewing; however, before defining a strategy of exploitation, it is necessary to carry out more in-depth studies on the effect of temperature, wort composition and inoculation rate in the fermentative activity of these yeasts. In addition, it is also necessary to carry out studies on the behavior of these yeasts in fermentations with mixed and sequential cultures with *Saccharomyces cerevisiae* and the production of compounds of sensory importance. Studies carried out with pure cultures of *Kloeckera corticis* showed that these yeasts are capable of producing acetic acid, acetaldehyde, ethyl acetate and acetoin at high concentrations [62]. In addition, it has been reported that strains of *Kloeckera apiculata* are capable of producing higher concentrations of ethyl and isoamyl acetate than other non-*Saccharomyces* yeasts [14, 63]. From the technological point of view, techniques of cell immobilization can be an additional strategy to improve the fermentative behavior and the production of compounds of sensory importance. The ability of these yeasts to produce a variety of aromatic compounds with positive impact on the sensory quality makes them attractive and potentially exploitable in fermentation processes.

4.3 *Hanseniaspora* yeasts

Few studies have been conducted regarding the potential use of yeasts belonging to the genus *Hanseniaspora* (apiculate yeasts) in the production of fermented beverages. The studied yeasts were isolated from the spontaneous fermentation of grape musts [6, 8, 59] and include species of *Hanseniaspora uvarum*, *H. osmophila* and *H. guilliermondii*, among others. It has been shown that these yeasts play an important role during the early stage of spontaneous fermentation of wine and strains of *Hanseniaspora uvarum* (also called *Kloeckera apiculata*) are dominant [19, 51, 52]. They are characterized by tolerating and producing low amounts of ethanol that do not exceed the values of 5.0% v/v [61]. This limitation explains why these yeasts do not participate actively toward the end of spontaneous fermentation of wines where the ethanol content reaches values even higher than 10%v/v. However, the fermentative capability of these yeasts is enough to produce beers of standard ethanol content similarly to those found in the market (4.5–5%v/v). In addition, they are able to ferment a wide range of sugars including maltose, which is an important feature needed for the production of beers. Regarding the production of compounds of sensory importance, studies have reported that strains of *Hanseniaspora osmophila* are characterized by producing high concentrations of acetic acid, acetaldehyde and ethyl acetate [62]. Additionally, it was also found that strains of *Hanseniaspora uvarum* are able to produce a variety of esters that confer fruitiness to fermented beverages [11, 62, 64]. However, other studies reported that mixed cultures of *H. uvarum* with *S. cerevisiae* produce higher amounts of higher alcohols than monocultures with *S. cerevisiae*

[4, 19]. Regarding fermentation parameters, the control of aeration and temperature exerts an important effect on the dynamics and activity of *Hanseniaspora* yeasts. Both parameters are important to control the production of compounds of sensory importance, which influence the quality of fermented beverages [11, 65]. However, in view of the scarce information on the fermentative behavior of *Hanseniaspora* yeasts, particularly referring to the production of fermented beverages, additional studies are needed to perform in order to find the adequate conditions for their usage, for instance, in the production of beers with new sensory profiles.

4.4 *Brettanomyces* yeasts

Yeasts of this genus do not have a good reputation in fermentation processes such as in winemaking. For instance, representatives of *Brettanomyces bruxellensis* are considered detrimental due to the production of compounds such as 4-ethylguaiacol, 4-ethylphenol and 4-ethylcatechol which impart unpleasant sensory character to wines known as "Bretty" [5, 66]. These compounds result from the activity of a decarboxylase that acts on hydroxycinnamic acids followed by a reduction reaction [67]. The hydroxycinnamic acids are phenolic compounds naturally present in the skin and seeds of grapes. The common representatives of this genus were isolated from the spontaneous fermentation of wine, beer, cider and even kombucha [68–70]. It was also isolated from equipment and utensils utilized in fermentation processes, which are difficult to sanitize. The commonly isolated species include *Brettanomyces bruxellensis*, *B. lambicus*, *B. intermedius* and *B. anomalus*, among others [68, 69]. Particularly, strains of *B. bruxellensis* are able to ferment only in the presence of oxygen (positive Crabtree effect), a broad spectrum of sugars and even maltooligosaccharides which are not fermentable by *S. cerevisiae* [71]. Under anaerobic conditions, these yeasts are unable to ferment and produce ethanol; thus, at low concentration of sugar in the medium, the fermentation of glucose to ethanol is blocked. On the contrary, the fermentation is stimulated in the presence of oxygen, an effect known as Custer or negative Pasteur [72]. Apart from producing ethanol in the presence of oxygen, *Brettanomyces bruxellensis* also produces high concentrations of acetic acid, which acidifies and lowers the pH of the medium. However, yeasts of this genus are not entirely undesirable; some representatives participate, for instance, during the fermentation of certain beers known as "Lambic" and "Gueuze" consumed commonly in Belgium and "Coolship Ales" in North America. The fermentation of "Lambic" beer is a spontaneous process which goes through a complex succession of microorganisms where *Brettanomyces bruxellensis* participates during the final stage acidifying the product [73]. The participation of these yeasts gives the beer its characteristic acidity and dryness and additionally is responsible for the production of compounds such as ethyl phenol, ethyl acetate, ethyl caprylate, ethyl decanoate and ethyl lactate, which synergistically confer their typical aroma character [18, 74]. It has been shown that esters soften the sour taste and add fruity notes to this kind of beers [75]. Based on these findings, it was demonstrated that these yeasts and particularly *B. bruxellensis* contribute positively to defining the floral and fruity character of "Lambic" beers [18]. Beyond the contribution of *Brettanomyces* yeasts in spontaneous fermentation processes, in recent years, their use in controlled fermentations has been investigated, both in pure and in coculture with *S. cerevisiae* [15, 17]. Interesting findings were reported, indicating that the control of aeration during fermentation is a critical point to guide the fermentative metabolism toward the production of important volatile compounds that may contribute to the organoleptic character of fermented beverages.

5. Production of special wines

It is of common agreement that non-*Saccharomyces* yeasts contribute beneficially to the sensory quality of spontaneously fermented wines, an evidence that served as a starting point to pay attention to particular yeast species that could be exploited in fermentations of commercial and noncommercial fermented beverages. Non-*Saccharomyces* species are characterized by producing a greater diversity of compounds of sensory importance than *S. cerevisiae* yeasts. Although these yeasts show a low fermentation power, some species possess important fermentative features, for instance, representatives of *Kloeckera* and *Hanseniaspora* yeasts produce a variety of compounds of sensory impact, particularly esters at concentrations even higher than *S. cerevisiae*. On the other hand, *Candida zemplinina*, a fructofilic yeast, has been shown to produce glycerol in higher concentrations than *S. cerevisiae*. It is also capable of producing ethanol in concentrations high enough to produce different types of wines. In view of the complementary characteristics of both groups of yeasts (*Saccharomyces* and non-*Saccharomyces*), the use of non-*Saccharomyces* yeasts can be proposed in fermentations with mixed or sequential cultures with *S. cerevisiae* as an important strategy to improve sensory complexity and mouthfeel of wines [19, 73]. The fermentative versatility of non-*Saccharomyces* yeasts would enable the production of special wines with different and innovative sensory characteristics. In addition, among the techniques that can be implemented for enabling their practical exploitation include the selection of new strains, the development of fermentation strategies (mixed or sequential cultures with two or more yeast strains), the ratio of both strains in the inoculum (non-*Saccharomyces*/*Saccharomyces cerevisiae*) and the inoculation rate at the beginning of fermentation [57, 76]. Finally, some technological characteristics of non-*Saccharomyces* yeasts can be also modified by using cultivation techniques in bioreactors with the aim of improving, for instance, the fermentation rate. The possibility of commercializing as starter cultures is an attractive opportunity for the production of different types of wines with special sensory qualities.

6. Production of craft beers

In the last 10 years, the market of craft beers has increased in the USA, Latin America and some countries of Europe [77, 78]. This phenomenon is related to the expectation of consumers for discovering in these beers sensory characteristics different from those routinely found in commercial beers [74]. Current consumers are curious and interested in sensing new flavors and aromas that can satisfy their preferences. As consequence, new market segments have emerged in response to the broad possibility of offering new types of beers produced using different methods and techniques of fermentation. The production of craft beer is generally carried out in small-scale breweries and involves the use of non-technified processing methods. Craft beers are not usually filtered; due to this, their shelf life is relatively short, and therefore, their consumption must be within few days after bottling. There are a variety of innovative alternatives to produce different types of craft beers which include the use of new types of adjuncts either amylaceous (cereal grains) or non-amylaceous (fruit pulps or juices) and selected strains of non-*Saccharomyces* yeasts which have an enormous exploitation potential. Although most non-*Saccharomyces* yeasts produce low concentrations of ethanol, the fermentative capacity of some representatives of *Kloeckera* and *Hanseniaspora* yeasts is adequate to produce beers with an ethanol content typically found in the market

(4.5–5%v/v). Among non-*Saccharomyces* yeasts considered important in beer fermentation, *Brettanomyces lambicus* is the most representative which is involved in the production of "Lambic" and "Gueuze" beers. Currently, some studies with *Candida zemplinina* strains were performed in fermentations with pure malt wort and with different adjuncts (grape or apple juice) at different temperatures and specific gravities. The findings were promissory and showed the capability of these yeasts to ferment at low temperatures (14°C) and in medium with high specific gravity (16°P), which demonstrates the possibility for being exploited in the production of craft beers. In addition, it was also proposed that these yeasts can be used for the production of beers with low ethanol content since they are not able to ferment maltose, the main and most abundant sugar present in the wort [20, 21]. Additionally, other non-*Saccharomyces* yeasts such as *Dekkera anomala, Naumovozyma dairenensis* and *Debaryomyces* spp. have been also reported with a high potential for being used in the fermentation of beers. In view of the different fermentative behavior of non-*Saccharomyces* yeasts and the variety of compounds of sensory importance that they can produce during fermentation, their use in controlled fermentations has aroused the interest of brewers for producing beers with distinctive sensory features [23, 79].

7. Conclusion

Non-*Saccharomyces* yeasts show a great potential to be used in the production of fermented beverages mainly wines and beers. These yeasts show a variety of fermentative patterns, and depending on the fermentation conditions, they produce a wide range of volatile compounds of sensory importance. For their practical application in a particular fermentative process, it is necessary knowing the parameters that directly influence on the fermentative activity and the production of desirable volatile compounds. Among the non-*Saccharomyces* yeasts that have attracted interest of researchers due to their fermentative qualities include strains of *Candida stellata, C. zemplinina, Kloeckera apiculata* and *Hanseniaspora uvarum*. Particularly, strains of *Candida stellata* and *C. zemplinina* have become very attractive for using in fermentations of different types of wines and beers. These yeasts are capable of producing significant concentrations of glycerol, an important compound that imparts a positive impact on the sensory quality of wines and beers. *Candida* yeasts, especially *C. zemplinina*, also produce high concentrations of ethanol, high enough to drive fermentation processes of wines. On the other hand, species of *Kloeckera* and *Hanseniaspora* yeasts are characterized by producing considerable amounts of acetate esters, valuable compounds that contribute positively to the sensory character of beers. Based on this, if a fermentation process that involves the use of non-*Saccharomyces* yeasts is going to be implemented, it is necessary to select the best representatives and then define the appropriate fermentation conditions for the production of fermented beverages with the desired sensory qualities.

Conflict of interest

The author certifies that he has *no* affiliation with or involvement in any organization or entity with any financial interest or non-financial interest in the subject matter or materials discussed in this manuscript.

Author details

Waldir Desiderio Estela Escalante
Laboratory of Bioprocessing and Technology of Fermentation, Faculty of Chemistry and Chemical Engineering, Universidad Nacional Mayor de San Marcos, Lima, Peru

*Address all correspondence to: waldir.estela@unmsm.edu.pe

References

[1] Mercado L, Dalcero A, Masuelli R, Combina M. Diversity of *Saccharomyces* strains on grapes and winery surfaces: Analysis of their contribution of fermentative flora of Malbec wine from Mendoza (Argentina) during two consecutive years. Food Microbiology. 2007;**24**:403-412

[2] Clavijo A, Calderón IL, Paneque P. Diversity of *Saccharomyces* and non-*Saccharomyces* yeasts in three red grape varieties cultured in the Serranía de Ronda (Spain) vine-growing region. International Journal of Food Microbiology. 2010;**143**:241-245

[3] Barnett JA, Payne RW, Yarrow D. Yeasts: Characteristics and Identification. 2nd ed. Cambridge, UK: Cambridge University Press; 1990

[4] Ciani M, Maccarelli F. Oenological properties of non-*Saccharomyces* yeasts associated with wine-making. World Journal of Microbiology and Biotechnology. 1998;**14**:199-203

[5] Loureiro V, Malfeito-Ferreira M. Spoilage activities of *Dekkera/ Brettanomyces* spp. In: Blackburn C, editor. Food Spoilage Microorganisms. Cambridge: Woodhead Publishers; 2006. pp. 354-398

[6] Heard GM, Fleet GH. Growth of natural yeast flora during the fermentation of inoculated wines. Applied and Environmental Microbiology. 1985;**50**:727-728

[7] Fleet GH. Yeast interaction and wine flavour. International Journal of Food Microbiology. 2003;**86**:11-22

[8] Grangeteau C, Gerhards D, Terrat S, Dequiedt S, Alexandre H, Guilloux-Benatier M, et al. FT-IR spectroscopy: A powerful tool for studying the inter- and intraspecific biodiversity of cultivable non-*Saccharomyces* yeasts isolated from grape must. Journal of Microbiological Methods. 2016;**121**:50-58

[9] Pardo I, Garcia MJ, Zuñiga M, Uruburu E. Dynamics of microbial populations during fermentation of wines from the Utiel-Requena region of Spain. Applied and Environmental Microbiology. 1989;**55**:539-541

[10] Tamang JP, Fleet GH. Yeasts diversity in fermented foods and beverages. In: Satyanarayana T, Kunze G, editors. Yeast Biotechnology. Netherlands: Diversity and Applications. Springer; 2009. pp. 169-198

[11] Estela Escalante W, Rychtera M, Melzoch K, Hatta-Sakoda B, et al. Actividad fermentativa de *Hanseniaspora uvarum* y su importancia en la producción de bebidas fermentadas. Revista de la Sociedad Venezolana de Microbiología. 2011;**31**:57-63

[12] Estela Escalante W, Rychtera M, Melzoch K, Quillama Polo E, Hatta Sakoda B. Study of the fermentative activity of *Hansenula anomala* and production of chemical compounds of sensory importance. Revista Peruana de Biología. 2011;**18**(3):325-334

[13] Estela-Escalante W, Rychtera M, Melzoch K, Hatta-Sakoda B, et al. Actividad fermentativa de *Saccharomycodes ludwigii* y evaluación de la síntesis de compuestos de importancia sensorial durante la fermentación de jugo de manzana. TIP Revista Especializada en Ciencias Químico-Biológicas. 2011;**14**(1):12-23

[14] Estela-Escalante WD, Rychtera M, Melzoch K, Guerrero-Ochoa MR. Influence of aeration in the fermentative activity of *Kloeckera apiculata* during fermentation of apple juice. Acta Biológica Colombiana. 2012; **17**(2):309-321

[15] Estela-Escalante WD, Rychtera M, Melzoch K, et al. Efecto de la aireación en la producción de compuestos volátiles por cultivo mixto de *Brettanomyces intermedius* y *Saccharomyces cerevisiae* durante la fermentación de sidra. TIP Revista Especializada en Ciencias Químico-Biológicas. 2014;**17**(1):5-14

[16] Pfliegler WP, Horvath E, Kallai Z, Sipiczki M. Diversity of *Candida zemplinina* isolates inferred from RAPD, micro/minisatellite and physiological analysis. Microbiological Research. 2014;**169**:402-410

[17] Steensels J, Verstrepen KJ. Taming wild yeast: Potential of conventional and nonconventional yeasts in industrial fermentations. Annual Review of Microbiology. 2014;**68**(1):61-80. DOI: 10.1146/annurev-micro-091213-113025

[18] Crauwels S, Steensels J, Aerts G, Willems KA, Verstrepen KJ, Lievens B. *Brettanomyces bruxellensis*, essential contributor in spontaneous beer fermentations providing novel opportunities for the brewing industry. Brewing Science. 2015;**68**:110-121

[19] Liu PT, Lu L, Duan CQ, Yan GL. The contribution of indigenous non-*Saccharomyces* wine yeast to improved aromatic quality of cabernet sauvignon wines by spontaneous fermentation. LWT- Food Science and Technology. 2016;**71**:356-363

[20] Estela-Escalante WD, Rosales-Mendoza S, Moscosa-Santillán M, González-Ramírez JE. Evaluation of the fermentative potential of *Candida zemplinina* yeasts for craft beer fermentation. Journal of the Institute of Brewing. 2016;**122**:530-535

[21] Estela-Escalante WD, Moscosa-Santillán M, González-Ramírez JE, Rosales-Mendoza S. Evaluation of the potential production of ethanol by *Candida zemplinina* yeast with regard to beer fermentation. Journal of the American Society of Brewing Chemists. 2017;**75**(2):130-135

[22] Fernandez M, Úbeda JF, Briones AI. Typing of non-*Saccchromyces* yeasts with enzymatic activities of interest in wine-making. International Journal of Food Microbiology. 2000;**59**(1–20):29-36

[23] Cordero-Bueso G, Esteve-Zarzoso B, Cabellos J, Gil-Díaz M, Arroyo T. Biotechnological potential of non-*Saccharomyces* yeasts isolated during spontaneous fermentations of Malvar (*Vitis vinifera* cv. L.). European Food Research and Technology. 2013;**236**(1): 193-207. DOI: 10.1007/s00217-012-1874-9

[24] Quiros M, Rojas V, Gonzalez R, Morales P. Selection of non-*Saccharomyces* yeast strains for reducing alcohol levels in wine by sugar respiration. International Journal of Food Microbiology. 2014;**181**:85-91

[25] Contreras AC, Hidalgo PA, Henschke PJ, Chambers C, Curtin C, Varela C. Evaluation of non-*Saccharomyces* yeasts for the reduction of alcohol content in wine. Applied and Environmental Microbiology. 2015;**80**: 1670-1678

[26] Ciani M, Capece A, Comitini F, Canonico L, Siesto G, Romano P. Yeast interactions in inoculated wine fermentation. Frontiers in Microbiology. 2016;**7**(555)

[27] Gobbi M, Comitini F, Domizio P, Romani C, Lencioni L, Mannazzu I, et al. *Lachancea thermotolerans* and *Saccharomyces cerevisiae* in simultaneous and sequential co-fermentation: A strategy to enhance acidity and improve the overall quality of wine. Food Microbiology. 2013;**33**:271-281. DOI: 10.1016/j.fm.2012.10.004

[28] Loira I, Vejarano R, Banuelos MA, Morata A, Tesfaye W, Uthurry C, et al.

Influence of sequential fermentation with *Torulaspora delbrueckii* and *Saccharomyces cerevisiae* on wine quality. LWT- Food Science and Technology. 2014;**59**:915-922

[29] Canonico L, Agarbati A, Comitini F, Ciani M. *Torulaspora delbrueckii* in the brewing process: A new approach to enhance bioflavour and to reduce ethanol content. Food Microbiology. 2016;**56**:45-51. DOI: 10.1016/j.fm.2015.12.005

[30] Flores CL, Rodríguez C, Petit T, Gancedo C. Carbohydrate and energy-yielding metabolism in non-conventional yeasts. FEMS Microbiology Reviews. 2000;**24**:507-529

[31] Puligundla P, Smogrovicova D, Obulam VSR, Ko S. Very high gravity (VHG) ethanolic brewing and fermentation: A research update. Journal of Industrial Microbiology & Biotechnology. 2011;**38**:1133-1144. DOI: 10.1007/s10295-011-0999-3

[32] Prior BA, Hohmann S. Glycerol production and osmoregulation. In: Zimmermann FK, Entian KD, editors. Yeast sugar metabolism. Lancaster: Technomic Publishing; 1997. pp. 313-337

[33] Steel CC, Grbin PR, Nichol AW. The pentose phosphate pathway in the yeasts *Saccharomyces cerevisiae* and *Kloeckera apiculata*, an exercise in comparative metabolism for food and wine science students. Biochemistry and Molecular Biology Education. 2001;**29**:245-249

[34] Boudarel MJ. Contribution ál étude de la fermentation alcoolique á partir de jus de Betteraves avec. *Saccharomyces cerevisiae* [Thèse de Doctorat]. Université de Dijon, Francia; 1984

[35] Buttke TM, Jones SD, Bloch K. Effect of sterol side chains on growth and membrane fatty acid composition of *Saccharomyces cerevisiae*. Journal of Bacteriology. 1980;**144**(1):124-130

[36] Gibson BR. 125th anniversary review: Improvement of higher gravity brewery fermentation via wort enrichment and supplementation. Journal of the Institute of Brewing. 2011;**117**(3):268-284. DOI: 10.1002/j.2050-0416.2011.tb00472.x

[37] Visser W, Scheffers WA, Batenburg-Van Der Vegte WH, Van Dijken JP. Oxygen requirements of yeasts. Applied and Environmental Microbiology. 1990;**56**(12):3785-3792

[38] González R, Quiros M, Morales P. Yeast respiration of sugars by non-*Saccharomyces* yeast species: A promising and barely explored approach to lowering alcohol content of wines. Trends in Food Science and Technology. 2013;**29**(1):55-61. DOI: 10.1016/j.tifs.2012.06.015

[39] Rodrigues AJ, Raimbourg T, Gonzalez R, Morales P. Environmental factors influencing the efficacy of different yeast strains for alcohol level reduction in wine by respiration. LWT-Food Science and Technology. 2016;**65**:1038-1043

[40] Romano P, Suzzi G, Comi G, Zironi R. Higher alcohol and acetic acid production by apiculate wine yeasts. The Journal of Applied Bacteriology. 1992;**73**:126-130

[41] Vidrih R, Hribar J. Synthesis of higher alcohols during cider processing. Food Chemistry. 1999;**67**:287-294

[42] Ehrlich F. Uber eine Methode zur spaltung racemischer aminosauren mittels Hefe. Biochemische Zeitschrift. 1906;**1**:8

[43] Webb AD, Ingraha JL. Fusel oil. Advances in Applied Microbiology. 1963;**5**:317-353

[44] Nordstrom K. Possible control of volatile ester formation in brewing. In: Proc. Eur. Brew. Conv. 10th, Stockholm. 1965. pp. 195-208

[45] Yoshioka K, Hashimoto N. Ester formation by alcohol acetyltransferase from brewers' yeast. Agricultural and Biological Chemistry. 1981;**45**(10): 2183-2190

[46] Lilly M, Lambrechts MG, Pretorius IS. Effect of increased yeast alcohol acetyltransferase activity on flavor profiles of wine and distillates. Applied and Environmental Microbiology. 2000; **66**(2):744-753

[47] Rojas V, Gil JV, Manzanares P, Gavara R, Piñaga F, Flors A. Measurement of alcohol acetyltransferase and ester hydrolase activities in yeast extracts. Enzyme and Microbial Technology. 2002;**30**(2):224-230. DOI: 10.1016/S0141-0229(01)00483-5

[48] Soden A, Francis IL, Oakey H, Henschke PA. Effects of co-fermentation with *Candida stellata* and *Saccharomyces cerevisiae* on the aroma and composition of chardonnay wine. Australian Journal of Grape and Wine Research. 2000;**6**:21-30

[49] Zohre DE, Erten H. The influence of *Kloeckera apiculata* and *Candida pulcherrima* yeasts on wine fermentation. Process Biochemistry. 2002;**38**:319-324

[50] Tofalo R, Schirone M, Torriani S, Rantsiou K, Cocolin L, Perpetuini G, et al. Diversity of *Candida zemplinina* strains from grapes and Italian wines. Food Microbiology. 2012;**29**:18-26

[51] Torija MJ, Rozes N, Poblet M, Guillamon JM, Mas A. Yeast population dynamics in spontaneous fermentations comparison between two different wine-producing areas over a period of three years. Antonie Van Leeuwenhoek. 2001;**79**(3):345-352

[52] Beltran G, Torija MJ, Novo M, Ferrer N, Poblet M, Guillamon JM, et al. Analysis of yeast populations during alcoholic fermentation: A six year follow-up study. Systematic and Applied Microbiology. 2002;**25**(2): 287-293

[53] Englezos V, Rantsiou K, Torchio F, Rolle L, Gerbi V, Cocolin L. Exploitation of the non-*Saccharomyces* yeast *Starmerella bacillaris* (synonym *Candida zemplinina*) in wine fermentation: Physiological and molecular characterizations. International Journal of Food Microbiology. 2015;**199**:33-40

[54] Zara G, Mannazzu I, Del Caro A, Budroni M, Pinna MB, Murru M, et al. Wine quality improvement through the combined utilisation of yeast hulls and *Candida zemplinina/Saccharomyces cerevisiae* mixed starter cultures. Australian Journal of Grape and Wine Research. 2014;**20**:199-207

[55] Mestre MV, Maturano YP, Combina M, Mercado LA, Toro ME, Vazquez F. Selection of non-*Saccharomyces* yeasts to be used in grape musts with high alcoholic potential: A strategy to obtain wines with reduced ethanol content. FEMS Yeast Research. 2017;**17**(2):1-10. DOI: 10.1093/femsyr/fox010

[56] Rantsiou K, Englezos V, Torchio F, Risse PA, Cravero F, Gerbi F, et al. Modeling of the fermentation behavior of *Starmerella bacillaris*. American Journal of Enology and Viticulture. 2017;**68**:378-385

[57] Englezos V, Torchio F, Cravero F, Marengo F, Giacosa S, Gerbi V, et al. Aroma profile and composition of Barbera wines obtained by mixed fermentations of *Starmerella bacillaris* (synonym *Candida zemplinina*) and *Saccharomyces cerevisiae*. LWT- Food Science and Technology. 2016;**73**:567-575

[58] Balli D, Flari V, Sakellaraki E, Schoina V, Iconomopoulou M,

Bekatorou A, et al. Effect of yeast cell immobilization and temperature on glycerol content in alcoholic fermentation with respect to wine making. Process Biochemistry. 2003;**39**: 499-506

[59] Suarez-Valles B, Pando Bedrinana R, Ferandez Tasco N, Querol Simon A, Rodriguez Madrera R. Yeast species associated with the spontaneous fermentation of cider. Food Microbiology. 2007;**24**:25-31

[60] Zott K, Miot-Sertier C, Claisse O, Lonvaud-Funel A, Masneufpomarede I. Dynamics and diversity of non-*Saccharomyces* yeasts during the early stages in winemaking. International Journal of Food Microbiology. 2008;**125**: 197-203

[61] Di Maro E, Ercolini D, Coppola S. Yeast dynamics during spontaneous wine fermentation of the Catalanesca grape. International Journal of Food Microbiology. 2007;**117**(2):201-210. DOI: 10.1016/j.ijfoodmicro.2007.04.007

[62] Granchi L, Ganucci D, Messini A, Vincenzini M. Oenological properties of *Hanseniaspora osmophila* and *Kloeckera corticis* from wines produced by spontaneous fermentations of normal and dried grapes. FEMS Yeast Research. 2002;(2):403-407

[63] Plata C, Millan C, Mauricio JC, Ortega JM. Formation of ethyl acetate and isoamyl acetate by various species of wine yeasts. Food Microbiology. 2003;**20**:217-224. DOI: 10.1016/S0740-0020(02)00101-6

[64] Caridi A, Tini V. Caratteristiche enologiche di *Hanseniaspora guilliermondii*. Vini d'Italia. 1991;**23**: 51-57

[65] Maturano YP, Mestre MV, Esteve-Zarzoso B, Nally MC, Lerena MC, Toro ME, et al. Yeast population dynamics during prefermentative cold soak of cabernet sauvignon and Malbec wines. International Journal of Food Microbiology. 2015;**199**:23-32. DOI: 10.1016/j.ijfoodmicro.2015.01.005

[66] Romano A, Perello MC, Lonvaud-Funel A, Sicard G, de Revel G. Sensory and analytical re-evaluation of "Brett character". Food Chemistry. 2009;**114**: 15-19

[67] Suarez R, Suárez-Lepe JA, Morata A, Calderón F. The production of ethylphenols in wine by yeasts of the genera *Brettanomyces* and *Dekkera*: A review. Food Chemistry. 2007;**102**:10-21

[68] Martens H, Iserentant D, Verachtert H. Microbiological aspects of a mixed yeast-bacterial fermentation in the production of a special Belgian acidic ale. Journal of the Institute of Brewing. 1997;**103**:85-91

[69] Morrissey WF, Davenport B, Querol A, Dobson ADW. The role of indigenous yeasts in traditional Irish cider fermentations. Journal of Applied Microbiology. 2004;**97**:647-655

[70] Teoh AL, Heard G, Cox J. Yeast ecology of Kombucha fermentation. International Journal of Food Microbiology. 2004;**95**:119-126

[71] Verachtert H, Derdelinckx G. Belgian acidic beers: Daily reminiscences of the past. Cerevisia. 2014;**38**(4):121-128. DOI: 10.1016/j.cervis.2014.04.002

[72] Wijsman MR, van Dijken JP, van Kleeff BH, Scheffers WA. Inhibition of fermentation and growth in batch cultures of the yeast *Brettanomyces intermedius* upon a shift from aerobic to anaerobic conditions (Custers effect). Antonie Van Leeuwenhoek. 1984;**50**: 183-192

[73] Spitaels F, Wieme AD, Janssens M, Aerts M, Daniel HM, Van Landschoot A, et al. The microbial diversity of

traditional spontaneously fermented lambic beer. PLoS One. 2014;**9**(4):1-13. DOI: 10.1371/journal.pone.0095384

[74] Vanderhaegen B, Neven H, Coghe S, Verstrepen KJ, Derdelinckx G, Verachtert H. Bioflavoring and beer refermentation. Applied Microbiology and Biotechnology. 2003;**62**:140-150

[75] Verstrepen KJ, Derdelinckx G, Dufour JP, Winderickx J, Thevelein JM, Pretorius IS, et al. Flavor-active esters: Adding fruitiness to beer. Journal of Bioscience and Bioengineering. 2003;**96**: 110-118. DOI: 10.1263/jbb.96.110

[76] Comitini F, Gobbi M, Domizio P, Romani C, Lencioni L, Mannazzu I, et al. Selected non-*Saccharomyces* wine yeasts in controlled multistarter fermentations with *Saccharomyces cerevisiae*. Food Microbiology. 2011;**28**: 873-882

[77] Kell J. What You Didn't Know About The Boom In Craft Beer. 2016. Available from: http://fortune.com/2016/03/22/craft-beer-sales-rise-2015/. [Accessed: 2018-07-20]

[78] Brewers-Association. National beer sales and production data. The New Brewer. 2017. Available from: https://www.brewersassociation.org/statistics/national-beer-sales production data/. [Accessed: 2018-07-18]

[79] Johnson E. Biotechnology of non-*Saccharomyces* yeasts-the ascomycetes. Applied Microbiology and Biotechnology. 2013;**97**(2):503-517. DOI: 10.1007/s00253-012-4497-y

Chapter 8

Torulaspora delbrueckii: Towards Innovating in the Legendary Baking and Brewing Industries

Ángel De La Cruz Pech-Canul, David Ortega, Antonio Garcia-Triana and Rosa Lidia Solís-Oviedo

Abstract

Baking and brewing are among the oldest bioprocesses refined by human societies. Both fermentative processes have successfully used domesticated strains of *Saccharomyces cerevisiae* in their process as the biocatalyst throughout their evolution. However, the dominance of *S. cerevisiae* has limited the capability for diversification of many organoleptic properties of the final product, such as aroma and flavours. The use of non-*Saccharomyces* yeasts can be an enormous source of opportunities for innovation in both fermentative processes. *Torulaspora delbrueckii* is a ubiquitous yeast species, and numerous strains have been isolated from many different bioprocesses. The strains of *T. delbrueckii*, once considered microbial contamination, have recently shown several advantages over *S. cerevisiae* strains, including higher ethanol tolerance; better capabilities to consume wort sugars; higher resistance to hop/pH/osmotic stress; and freeze-thaw resistance, among others. This chapter aims to present a comprehensive review of frontier research on *T. delbrueckii* regarding its potential and prospects for the baking and brewing industries.

Keywords: alcoholic beverages, beer production, baking industry, brewing industry, *Torulaspora delbrueckii*

1. Introduction

Bread and beer are among the oldest foods in the human history. The consumption of both of these fermented products has been rooted as a basic human food, and at the present time, these are still among the most consumed foods around the world. The ubiquity of their production allowed a diversification and development of refined, artisan techniques, which currently comprises innumerable recipes [1, 2]. All the recipes include essentially the same basic ingredients such as cereals, yeast, and water. However, the organoleptic properties (aroma, flavours, etc.) of the final product differ greatly between recipes.

Since early times, both cereals and water were identified as fundamental ingredients for the preparation of beer or bread. Despite the fact that these ingredients have been recognised as essentials for centuries, the experimental approaches developed by Pasteur during the mid-nineteenth century revealed the existence of a third element much more essential to the fermentation process: yeast. The fermentation performed by yeast is undoubtedly the oldest and the largest biotechnology

IntechOpen

application. There are many types of yeast strains used for fermented foods commonly known as commercial strains: baker's yeast in bread production and brewer's yeast in beer fermentation. After centuries of selection, due to the refinement of the fermentation processes, today it is easy to find a wide variety of dedicated yeast strains that are suitable for different types or styles for either beer or bread.

The yeast strains responsible of these fermented foods are able to ferment sugars present in the flour or in the wort (starch, glucose, fructose, sucrose, and maltose, among others), which is concomitant with the production of other molecules such as CO_2, the main causes of dough leavening and the natural carbonation of beer. The type of yeast strain used in the fermentation process also greatly influences the properties displayed in the final product such as the texture of the dough and the flavour, and ideally, certain yeasts can also add some nutritional values to the final product [3].

The capabilities of the yeast strains to grow fast (fast propagation) and to produce a valuable product are still currently exploited by the industrial field. Depending on the final product, the yeast strains also possess other advantages, such as high tolerance to stresses caused by high sugar concentration or the drying/freezing of dough present in baker's yeast [2]. On the other hand, brewer's yeast which is similar to wine's yeast offers particular characteristics to the fermentation process such as an optimal flocculation, high ethanol tolerance, and rapid growth at high osmolarity [4].

Since the beginning, the food industry has mainly used *Saccharomyces* or closely related strains, which could be a result of the ubiquity of this genus. As consequence, scientific research efforts have been focused mainly on *Saccharomyces cerevisiae*, a yeast that nowadays is still the most commonly used microorganism in baking, brewing, and other fermented foods [5, 6]. Furthermore, *S. cerevisiae* has also been historically used as a model organism for the research on fundamental aspects of eukaryotic cell biology. The popularity of *S. cerevisiae* in the food industry has led to the standardisation of the organoleptic properties of the final product, which limits the capability to improve or to create new properties for the final product.

The use of non-*Saccharomyces cerevisiae* yeasts, also known as "nonconventional" or "non-commercial" yeast, offers new alternatives for the development of products with improved properties, such as biomass yield, distinct flavour complexity, aroma profile, and other advantages. Among nonconventional yeasts, *Torulaspora delbrueckii* (formerly *Saccharomyces rosei* or *S. rosei*) has been considered of oenological interest for decades.

At the present time, *T. delbrueckii* is starting to be recognised as a model organism of study because most of its biological features, like its sugar metabolism, differ greatly from the more prevalent *S. cerevisiae* [7]. These differences provide many advantages of biotechnological importance in several fermentative processes; for example, it is quite interesting how *T. delbrueckii* can adapt its physiological state in order to endure the harsh conditions present during the frozen dough preservation [8]. On the other hand, the use of *T. delbrueckii* in the brewing industry has had a positive effect on the aroma and taste of the final alcoholic beverage [9–11]. The industrial brewing process has appreciated several features of this yeast strain that also complement its suitability for the fermented food preparation processes, such as its higher ability to retain cell viability under stress conditions, high ethanol tolerance, an increased osmotic resistance, and the advantageous capability to yield a final product with lower levels of unpleasant acetaldehyde, acetoin, acetate, and ethyl acetate [12]. Fermentation with *T. delbrueckii* also provides an excellent example of improvement in the industrial process with the consequent creation of new value-added products. In the present chapter, we review the current and potential applications of *T. delbrueckii* strains in the bread and brewing industries discussing their physiological perspective.

2. The genetics of *Torulaspora delbrueckii*: an overview

Torulaspora delbrueckii has unique abilities when compared to other yeasts; the use of this microorganism has many advantages yet to be potentially exploited in the biotech industry. The progress in understanding its physicochemical and physiological mechanisms of action has been hampered by the lack of genetic and molecular tools specific for this yeast. The development of tools for metabolic engineering of a specific microorganism is essential for the improvement of industrial processes. Once the microorganism of interest has been isolated and identified, one of the first steps for the development of the genetic tools is to determine its exact genome sequence. With the advent of modern, state-of-the-art equipment and facilities dedicated to unravel the DNA sequence from diverse biological samples; nowadays, the sequencing of small genomes (<50 MB) has become even cheaper and more reliable than just a decade ago.

A pioneering work presented in 2002 described the isolation of genes from *T. delbrueckii* and their subsequent heterotrophic expression using *Saccharomyces cerevisiae* as a host [13, 14]. From this work, the first yeast genomic library of *T. delbrueckii* PYCC532 was derived. In 2011, a draft genome sequence of *T. delbrueckii* CBS 1146 was published as part of a molecular evolution study [15]. The CBS 1146 strain has been preserved since 1970 under laboratory conditions and thus raises the question regarding the potential differences when compared to a fresh strain isolated from an active alcoholic fermentation. A complementary study that addressed this question was published recently in 2015 [16], where a set of differential genes were identified. The most recent sequencing projects have had much better coverage than preliminary studies. Most recently, other *T. delbrueckii* genomes have been published (**Table 1**). For example, the first complete genome map of *T. delbrueckii* COFT1 has

Strain	Source	GenBank accession	Genome assembly level	Reference
CBS 1146 (NRRL Y-866)	Unknown. Isolated by the Wallenstein Lab., No. 129, 119,077. Deposited by the NRRL	GCA_000243375.1	Chromosome	[15]
COFT1	Isolated from the spontaneous wine fermentation at the Yalumba Wine Company (Angaston, Australia)	CP027647.1 to CP027655.1	Whole-genome map	[17]
NRRL Y-50541	Isolated from the mezcal-fermenting process at Oaxaca, Mexico	CP011778 to CP011785	Chromosome	[16, 18]
SRCM101298	Isolated from fermented food by Sung Ho Cho, Microbial Institute for Fermentation Industry, South Korea	GCA_002214845.1	Contig	[19]

Table 1.
Genomes sequencing projects developed for Torulaspora delbrueckii.

been recently assembled, having been isolated from a spontaneous wine fermentation from Australia. Its genome consists of eight chromosomes and one mitochondrial chromosome. Altogether, these published data sets are proving to be useful as they guide the design of experimental approaches to study enzymes involved in the biosynthesis and/or the catabolism of biotechnological molecules of interest.

The discovery of the circular plasmid pTD1 from *T. delbrueckii* CBS 1090 provided an excellent platform for the development of modern genetic tools. The circular pTD1 (4.8 kbp) is an unusual finding in the diverse yeast genera that normally possess linear plasmids [20]. The plasmid pTD1 belongs to the 2-μm family, and it has been shown that the members of this plasmid family keep a high-copy number with minimal impact on the host. Recently, a model was suggested for the 2-μm protein complexes required for plasmid partitioning and transcriptional regulation [21]. pTD1 also contains an AT-hook motifs (residues 222–234) which are small DNA-binding modules with a preference for binding AT-rich DNA [22] and have been frequently identified in a large number of proteins, such as transcription and chromatin remodelling factors, such as the yeast centromere-binding protein and Mif2 DNA replication origin recognition factor Orc2, respectively [21, 23]. Two decades after the discovery of pTD1, its importance has been recently brought to light when a modified version for the TD recombinase (variant TD1–40) was employed to the development and analysis of two Flp-like site-specific recombination systems. The evolved variants of the TD recombinase, unlike the wild-type enzyme, were suitable for genome engineering in *Escherichia coli* and mammalian cells [24]. The authors also suggest that its application could be potentially extended to plant and insect cells.

The allele-coupled exchange (ACE) and the allelic exchange (AE) technologies are becoming more common for the manipulation of microorganisms for biotech purposes. For example, researchers lead by Professor Nigel Minton at the Synthetic Biology Research Centre (SBRC) (University of Nottingham, UK) have successfully dedicated their efforts to develop the ACE and the AE technologies in diverse *Clostridia* strains and other Gram-positive bacteria [25, 26]. The genetic manipulation of *T. delbrueckii* was initially achieved using the genetic tools developed originally for *S. cerevisiae.* The improved gene disruption method for *T. delbrueckii* was performed using the classic PCR-based disruption cassettes, one of the most commonly used strategies for gene targeting in *S. cerevisiae* and other organisms [12]. Eventually, ACE was adapted for baker's yeast *T. delbrueckii* IGC5323 and was one of the goals for the development of genetic tools towards the metabolic engineering of *T. delbrueckii* [27].

At the present time, many attempts have been made to expand the number of selection markers available for the construction of new molecular tools for *T. delbrueckii*; however, the pursuit of selection markers remains unsuccessful [12]. A successful auxotrophic selection marker was the creation of a screening system under glucose as sole carbon source. The deletion of LGT1 gene, identified as coding for a hexose transporter, was successfully conducted, despite the fact that the deletion did not impaired glucose uptake ability [28]. According to previous works, it is likely that the genome of *T. delbrueckii* contains other hexose transporters [29]. Other approaches are still being developed towards genome editing, and trends indicate that eventually the modern CRISPR-CAS9 technique could be adapted for *T. delbrueckii*, just as it was recently fully adapted for *S. cerevisiae* [30].

3. From the lab to the kitchen: efforts towards the incorporation of scientific research into the baking and brewing industries

Results derived from scientific research have positively influenced many aspects of human wellbeing, such as food production. Many food industries are currently interested in innovation through the usage of *T. delbrueckii* strains in their fermentative processes. Consequently, the brewing and baking industries are starting to use nonconventional yeast strains in their processes.

Effective biomass production from molasses is a crucial aspect to consider in the selection of baker's yeast for the industrial process. Baker's yeast is able to propagate and to create biomass from sugarcane molasses, which contains mainly glucose, fructose, and sucrose as well as trisaccharide raffinose [31, 32]. On the other hand, invertase activity is crucial for the hydrolysis of disaccharide into free glucose and fructose monomers, required for yeast growing on molasses.

Yeast strains with high invertase activity exhibit a low production of CO_2 in the sweet dough. This last observation can be explained by the rapid entry of free sugars into the cells causing a massive increase in the osmotic pressure that affects the cellular homeostasis which eventually slows glycolysis [33–35].

Moreover, both trehalose and glycogen are known as the major store of glucose into *Saccharomyces cerevisiae* cells. A rapid increase of the levels of these sugars is an early metabolic response during conditions of oxidative, heat, or salt/osmotic stresses. It has been proposed that these sugars have several physiological functions. For example, the accumulation of these sugars has a function as glycolytic safety valves to escape "substrate-accelerated death": a phenomenon that follows when the starved yeast is exposed to the substrate, which limits their growth [36–39].

Oppositely, *Torulaspora delbrueckii* strains under hyperosmotic/frozen stresses into sweet dough have shown the ability to adapt promptly to high-osmotic-pressure environments which correlates in part with a low-invertase activity, as well as a slow rate of trehalose mobilisation, displaying a higher accumulation of trehalose than *S. cerevisiae* [8, 27]. Moreover, the intracellular trehalose accumulation, induced by desiccation of *T. delbrueckii*, protects the yeast cell and presents a lower oxidative stress, which correlates with a higher fermentative capacity, when compared to other nonconventional yeasts [40]. The trehalose content may possibly be correlated to their types of trehalase. Strain D2–4 was found to harbour two types of trehalase activities, which have different optimum reaction pH at 4.3 and 6.7. On the other hand, the freeze-sensitive mutant strain 60B3 bears additional activity at pH 5.7, which adds a third type of trehalase activity in that sensitive mutant. The change of trehalose content during the growth of the freeze-sensitive 60B3 strain was directly correlated with the change of the trehalase activity at pH 5.7. Despite the fact that higher trehalose levels are always correlated with higher stress resistance, experimental results suggest that other factors are involved in the maintenance of stress resistance [41–43].

As mentioned above, the metabolism of *T. delbrueckii* and *S. cerevisiae* differs greatly, such as their regulatory mechanisms in the adaptive response to salt stress [44]. The gene ENA1, encoding a Na^+-ATPase, is a key determinant in the *Saccharomyces cerevisiae* tolerance when it is exposed to salt stress as high concentrations of extracellular toxic monovalent cations (i.e. Na^+ and Li^+) [45]. The regulation of ENA1 required for cell survival is mainly under the control of three diverse signalling pathways, (1) high-osmolarity glycerol (HOG), (2) cell wall integrity (CWI), and (3) calcineurin/Crz1p pathways [46–48]. Glycerol production is essential for *S. cerevisiae* to deal with osmotic stresses. Hog1 phosphorylation occurs as a response to osmotic stress, and the phosphorylated Hog1 interacts with transcription factors to modulate its gene expression patterns during stress responses [49, 50].

In order to understand the high-osmolarity glycerol (HOG) pathway in *T. delbrueckii*, the Hog1 homologue in *T. delbrueckii* (*TdHog1*) was characterised as well as its mutant versions. The expression of GPD1 was not strongly affected in the *TdHog1*-deleted mutant. Also, *S. cerevisiae* and *T. delbrueckii* have divergent regulatory mechanisms that control glycerol accumulation under a moderate osmotic stress condition [51]. As a consequence of glycerol accumulation, in anaerobiosis, glycerol production of *T. delbrueckii* represents around 6% of the total carbon flux, a value that is comparable to *S. cerevisiae* under the same conditions. However, acetic acid levels are increased which allows for reduction of NAD+ generated during glycerol formation in *S. cerevisiae* as a side-effect of the overexpression of GPD1 and/or GPD2 in the presence of high-glycerol concentration. A significant relationship between glycerol and acetic acid production was not found in *Torulaspora delbrueckii* [52, 53]. When an excess of acetic acid is produced in alcoholic beverages such as a beer or wine, it provides a characteristic vinegar-like flavour or sour taste [54, 55]. A higher percentage of acetic acid also results in decreased CO2 production [9, 56–58].

Saccharomyces cerevisiae exhibits an adaptive response to cell wall stress mediated by cell wall integrity MAPK signalling factor Slt2, which once activated triggers Rlm1 phosphorylation [59]. Additionally, the *slt2*Δ mutant allowed for the discovery of a novel regulatory mechanism associated with PKA inhibition [60, 61]. During the study of *hog1* mutant from *S. cerevisiae*, it has been reported that Slt2p is rapidly dephosphorylated (1 min). On the other hand, a Tdhog1 mutant from *T. delbrueckii* showed a significant reduction of the phospho-Slt2p signal, and it was delayed around 30–60 min [51].

The induction of the ENA1 gene is mediated by calcineurin which plays a role in the dephosphorylation of Crz1. Two Crz1-binding regions have been identified into the ENA1 promoter; the antagonistic regulation of ENA1 is via protein kinase A (PKA) that is involved in the Crz1 phosphorylation [62]. Additionally, phosphatases Ppz1 and Ppz2, individually or both, influenced the expression of ENA1. For example, a higher increase of the ENA1 expression in Ppz1 mutants was observed which was correlated to an increase halotolerance. Interestingly, Ppz1 showed to be dependent of an intact calcineurin/Crz1-signalling pathway to keep its ENA1 promoter activity [63]. During the analysis of TdCRZ1, the homologue to *CRZ1* in *Torulaspora delbrueckii*, the authors tried to enhance the salt tolerance of *S. cerevisiae* HS13. So, the TdCrz1p was linked to the freeze tolerance capability, a very important feature with great potential for industrial applications [44].

4. Yeast cocultures: *Torulaspora delbrueckii*—combining to enhance the product quality

At the present time, commercial strains of *Torulaspora delbrueckii* are used in the bread and brewing industries and are summarised in **Table 2**. The success of *T. delbrueckii* relies mainly on the superior flavour that its fermentation can provide to the final product and also in its incredible ability to withstand stress conditions described previously. These properties will lead to improve the product quality and enhance the flavour complexity. However, there are still some challenges to overcome to employ a pure culture of *T. delbrueckii* in industrial fermentations.

Name	Supplier	Industry		Reference
		Bakery	Brewery	
Biodiva™TD291	Lallemand		✓	[64]
ZYMAFLORE® ALPHA$^{TD\ n.\ sacch}$	Laffort		✓	[10]
H299–18	Nikka Uisukii KK	✓		[65]
NS8422 (FERM P-12709)	Nikka Whiskey KK	✓		[66]

Table 2.
A brief list of Torulaspora delbrueckii commercially available.

For this reason, these yeast strains are usually employed in co-fermentations with *Saccharomyces cerevisiae* and/or other yeast strains [9, 10]. For example, in mixed fermentations, it plays an important role to enhance its organoleptic properties such as flavour, aroma, and a final product with low-alcohol content [9].

The current key market players for global yeast market are listed below:

- AB Mauri
- Biospringer
- Chr. Hansen Holding A/S
- Lesaffre
- AB Vista
- Alltech
- Angel Yeast Co., Ltd.
- Biorigin—Art in Natural Ingredients
- DSM N.V.
- ICC
- Kerry Group
- Lallemand Inc.
- Leiber GmbH
- Minn-Dak Yeast Company
- Ohly
- Oriental Yeast Co., Ltd.
- Pacific Ethanol, Inc.
- Pakmaya
- Suboneyo Chem. Pharmaceuticals Pvt. Lim.
- Synergy Flavours

The flavour profiles of co-fermentations in brewing showed significant differences, revealing a species-dependent relationship. Analysis of the main volatile compounds on the beers produced by *T. delbrueckii* and *S. cerevisiae* in the pure cultures and their simultaneous co-fermentation at different ratios was performed. *T. delbrueckii* was able to increase the levels of higher alcohols, where β-phenyl ethanol was excluded. These results are opposite to the data obtained in winemaking, where lower levels of higher alcohols are detected. β-phenyl ethanol and ethyl butyrate levels were lowered when a major presence of *T. delbrueckii* was present in the inoculum ratio [9–11]. A yeast population change has been correlated with the inoculum size ratio and the type of cell-to-cell interactions that occur during mixed culture fermentation. The faster decay of *T. delbrueckii* during cocultures with *S. cerevisiae* is notable below a 2:1 ratio. The last observation could be related to multiple factors, for example, due to the *T. delbrueckii*'s killer activity: a kind of immune system that secretes protein toxins, which become lethal to other yeast species [67, 68].

Sequential inoculation of *T. delbrueckii* with *S. cerevisiae* has shown higher levels of desired aroma compounds compared to simultaneous inoculation, exemplified by the enhanced production of 4-vinyl guaiacol (clove-like aroma) [69].

Unlike the production of beer and wine, co-fermentation with *T. delbrueckii* during dough preparation has been barely explored; only simultaneous co-fermentations have been performed. *T. delbrueckii* JK08 and *P. anomala* JK04 exhibited a superior flavour and mouthfeel, respectively, as well as an improvement in the colour, when compared to *S. cerevisiae*. Even when these strains did not fulfil the exact criteria of commercial baker's yeasts [70], the use of these three yeasts together has been proven to enhance the bread quality [70].

5. Conclusion

The history of fermented foods has long accompanied the evolution of the human civilisation. While the ingredients may have changed, their selection has also been shaped to meet new consumer demands. In fact, over centuries, man has refined the art of fermented food by pure empirical observation, for example, through the selection of the best cereals with better performing characteristics or through the domestication of yeast strains. Despite the fact that the fermented food industry has mastered the domestication of *Saccharomyces cerevisiae*, the use of nonconventional yeast strains has proved to be advantageous for the fermented food industry.

Once considered a microbial contamination, *Torulaspora delbrueckii* has been shown to have a positive influence on several organoleptic properties for the final products of the brewing and bread industries. For example, when this nonconventional yeast is used in the brewing industry, the aromatic profiles and flavours of the beer are enhanced; and some strains have the peculiarity to produce naturally less-ethanol content while retaining all its improved properties. Additionally, many of its other biological features were conveniently suitable for the industrial processes, such as its robustness potential to resist frozen/thaw stress. These advantages will be useful for biotechnological exploitation that will lead to innovation of new products or even to process improvement for the food industry. As usual in new trends in science, to date, the information regarding *T. delbrueckii* genetics and its metabolic pathways remain scarce. Fortunately, the scientific community is starting to focus their efforts to deeply understand the nature of this splendid genus. Continued scientific research will gradually lead to the accumulation of more data that will impact positively the fermented food industry.

Acknowledgements

The authors acknowledge to the National Council of Science and Technology from Mexico (CONACyT) and to the Autonomous University of Chihuahua.

Angel de la Cruz Pech-Canul was supported by CONACyT through the "Cátedras CONACyT para Jóvenes Investigadores" programme (Project No. 609).

Conflict of interest

The authors declare that they no conflicts of interest.

Author details

Ángel De La Cruz Pech-Canul[1]*, David Ortega[2], Antonio Garcia-Triana[3] and Rosa Lidia Solís-Oviedo[3]

1 CONACyT—Faculty of Chemical Sciences, Autonomous University of Chihuahua, Circuito Universitario s/n, Chihuahua, México

2 Centre for Biomolecular Sciences, The University of Nottingham, Nottingham, United Kingdom

3 Faculty of Chemical Sciences, Autonomous University of Chihuahua, Circuito Universitario s/n, Chihuahua, México

*Address all correspondence to: angelpechcanul@gmail.com; apech@conacyt.mx

References

[1] Chavan RS, Chavan SR. Sourdough technology—A traditional way for wholesome foods: A review. Comprehensive Reviews in Food Science and Food Safety. 2011;**10**(3):169-182

[2] Donalies UE, Nguyen HT, Stahl U, Nevoigt E. Improvement of *Saccharomyces* yeast strains used in brewing, wine making and baking. Advances in Biochemical Engineering/Biotechnology. 2008;**111**:67-98

[3] Burrow S. Baker's yeast. In: Rose AH, Harrison JS, editors. The Yeasts: Biology of yeasts. 3. 2nd ed. London and New York: Academic Press; 1969. pp. 349-420

[4] Stratford M. Lectin-mediated aggregation of yeasts—Yeast flocculation. Biotechnology and Genetic Engineering Reviews. 1992;**10**(1):283-342

[5] Lodolo EJ, Kock JLF, Axcell BC, Brooks M. The yeast *Saccharomyces cerevisiae*—The main character in beer brewing. FEMS Yeast Research. 2008;**8**(7):1018-1036

[6] Heitmann M, Zannini E, Arendt E. Impact of *Saccharomyces cerevisiae* metabolites produced during fermentation on bread quality parameters: A review. Critical Reviews in Food Science and Nutrition. 2018;**58**(7):1152-1164

[7] Alves-Araújo C, Pacheco A, Almeida MJ, Spencer-Martins I, Leão C, Sousa MJ. Sugar utilisation patterns and respiro-fermentative metabolism in the baker's yeast *Torulaspora delbrueckii*. Microbiology. 2007;**153**(3):898-904

[8] Hernandez-Lopez MJ, Prieto JA, Randez-Gil F. Osmotolerance and leavening ability in sweet and frozen sweet dough. Comparative analysis between *Torulaspora delbrueckii* and *Saccharomyces cerevisiae* baker's yeast strains. Antonie van Leeuwenhoek. 2003;**84**(2):125-134

[9] Canonico L, Agarbati A, Comitini F, Ciani M. *Torulaspora delbrueckii* in the brewing process: A new approach to enhance bioflavour and to reduce ethanol content. Food Microbiology. 2016;**56**:45-51

[10] Tataridis P, Kanellis A, Logothetis S, Nerantzis E. Use of non-saccharomyces *Torulaspora delbrueckii* yeast strains in winemaking and brewing. Zbornik Matice srpske za prirodne nauke. 2013;**124**:415-426

[11] Canonico L, Comitini F, Ciani M. *Torulaspora delbrueckii* contribution in mixed brewing fermentations with different *Saccharomyces cerevisiae* strains. International Journal of Food Microbiology. 2017;**259**:7-13

[12] Pacheco A, Santos J, Chaves S, Almeida J, Leão C, Sousa MJ. The emerging role of the *Torulaspora delbrueckii* in bread and wine production: Using genetic manipulation to study molecular basis of physiological responses. In: Eissa AA, editor. Structure and Function of Food Engineering. London: IntechOpen; 2012

[13] Hernandez-Lopez MJ, Prieto JA, Randez-Gil F. Isolation and characterisation of the gene URA3 encoding the orotidine-5-phosphate decarboxylase from *Torulaspora delbrueckii*. Yeast. 2002;**19**(16):1431-1435

[14] Alves-Araujo C, Hernandez-Lopez MJ, Sousa MJ, Prieto JA, Randez-Gil F. Cloning and characterisation of the MAL11 gene encoding a high-affinity maltose transporter from *Torulaspora delbrueckii*. FEMS Yeast Research. 2004;**4**(4-5):467-476

[15] Gordon JL, Armisen D, Proux-Wera E, OhEigeartaigh SS, Byrne KP,

Wolfe KH. Evolutionary erosion of yeast sex chromosomes by mating-type switching accidents. Proceedings of the National Academy of Sciences of the United States of America. 2011;**108**(50):20024-20029

[16] Gomez-Angulo J, Vega-Alvarado L, Escalante-García Z, Grande R, Gschaedler-Mathis A, Amaya-Delgado L, et al. Genome sequence of *Torulaspora delbrueckii* NRRL Y-50541, isolated from Mezcal fermentation. Genome Announcements. 2015;**3**(4):e00438-e00415

[17] Tondini F, Jiranek V, Grbin PR, Onetto CA. Genome sequence of australian indigenous wine yeast *Torulaspora delbrueckii* COFT1 using nanopore sequencing. Genome Announcements. 2018;**6**(17):e00321-18

[18] Segura LE. Identificación y caracterización por métodos moleculares de levaduras aisladas del proceso de elaboración del mezcal en el estado de Oaxaca. Guadalajara, Mexico: CIATEJ-CONACYT; 2010

[19] Benson DA, Karsch-Mizrachi I, Lipman DJ, Ostell J, Wheeler DL. GenBank: Update. Nucleic Acids Research. 2004;**32**(Database issue):D23-DD6

[20] Blaisonneau J, Sor F, Cheret G, Yarrow D, Fukuhara H. A circular plasmid from the yeast *Torulaspora delbrueckii*. Plasmid. 1997;**38**(3):202-209

[21] McQuaid ME, Pinder JB, Arumuggam N, Lacoste Jessica SC, Chew Joyce SK, Dobson MJ. The yeast 2-μm plasmid Raf protein contributes to plasmid inheritance by stabilising the Rep1 and Rep2 partitioning proteins. Nucleic Acids Research. 2017;**45**(18):10518-10533

[22] Reeves R, Nissen M. The A.T-DNA-binding domain of mammalian high mobility group I chromosomal proteins. A novel peptide motif for recognising DNA structure. The Journal of Biological Chemistry. 1990;**265**(15):8573-8582

[23] Aravind L, Landsman D. AT-hook motifs identified in a wide variety of DNA-binding proteins. Nucleic Acids Research. 1998;**26**(19):4413-4421

[24] Voziyanova E, Anderson RP, Shah R, Li F, Voziyanov Y. Efficient genome manipulation by variants of site-specific recombinases R and TD. Journal of Molecular Biology. 2016;**428**(5 Pt B): 990-1003

[25] Minton NP, Ehsaan M, Humphreys CM, Little GT, Baker J, Henstra AM, et al. A roadmap for gene system development in *Clostridium*. Anaerobe. 2016;**41**:104-112

[26] Sheng L, Kovacs K, Winzer K, Zhang Y, Minton NP. Development and implementation of rapid metabolic engineering tools for chemical and fuel production in *Geobacillus thermoglucosidasius* NCIMB 11955. Biotechnology for Biofuels. 2017;**10**:5

[27] Hernandez-Lopez MJ, Blasco A, Prieto JA, Randez-Gil F. Ura^- host strains for genetic manipulation and heterologous expression of *Torulaspora delbrueckii*. International Journal of Food Microbiology. 2003;**86**(1):79-86

[28] Pacheco A, Almeida MJ, Sousa MJ. Improved gene disruption method for *Torulaspora delbrueckii*. FEMS Yeast Research. 2009;**9**(1):153-160

[29] Alves-Araujo C, Hernandez-Lopez MJ, Prieto JA, Randez-Gil F, Sousa MJ. Isolation and characterisation of the LGT1 gene encoding a low-affinity glucose transporter from *Torulaspora delbrueckii*. Yeast. 2005;**22**(3):165-175

[30] Mans R, Wijsman M, Daran-Lapujade P, Daran J-M. A protocol for introduction of multiple genetic

modifications in *Saccharomyces cerevisiae* using CRISPR/Cas9. FEMS Yeast Research. 2018;**18**(7):foy063-foyfoy

[31] Pejin D, Dosenovic I, Milic M, Razmovski R, Karadzic V, Grbic J. Molasses quality for baker's yeast production as influenced by its microbiological contamination and chemical composition. Zuckerindustrie (Germany). 1996;**121**:424-427

[32] Rosen K. Production of baker's yeast. In: Berry DR, Russell I, Stewart GG, editors. Yeast Biotechnology. Dordrecht: Springer Netherlands; 1987. pp. 471-500

[33] Thevelein JM, Hohmann S. Trehalose synthase: Guard to the gate of glycolysis in yeast? Trends in Biochemical Sciences. 1995;**20**(1):3-10

[34] Myers DK, Lawlor DT, Attfield PV. Influence of invertase activity and glycerol synthesis and retention on fermentation of media with a high sugar concentration by *Saccharomyces cerevisiae*. Applied Environmental Microbiology. 1997;**63**(1):145-150

[35] Somsen OJ, Hoeben MA, Esgalhado E, Snoep JL, Visser D, van der Heijden RT, et al. Glucose and the ATP paradox in yeast. Biochemical Journal. 2000;**352**(Pt 2):593-599

[36] Blomberg A. Metabolic surprises in *Saccharomyces cerevisiae* during adaptation to saline conditions: Questions, some answers and a model. FEMS Microbiology Letters. 2000;**182**(1):1-8

[37] François J, Parrou JL. Reserve carbohydrates metabolism in the yeast *Saccharomyces cerevisiae*. FEMS Microbiology Reviews. 2001;**25**(1):125-145

[38] Teusink B, Walsh MC, van Dam K, Westerhoff HV. The danger of metabolic pathways with turbo design. Trends in Biochemical Sciences. 1998;**23**(5):162-169

[39] Postgate JR, Hunter JR. Acceleration of bacterial death by grown substrates. Nature. 1963;**198**:273

[40] Gamero-Sandemetrio E, Payá-Tormo L, Gómez-Pastor R, Aranda A, Matallana E. Non-canonical regulation of glutathione and trehalose biosynthesis characterises non-*Saccharomyces* wine yeasts with poor performance in active dry yeast production. Microbial Cell. 2018;**5**(4):184-197

[41] Van Dijck P, Colavizza D, Smet P, Thevelein JM. Differential importance of trehalose in stress resistance in fermenting and nonfermenting *Saccharomyces cerevisiae* cells. Applied and Environmental Microbiology. 1995;**61**(1):109-115

[42] Yokoigawa K, Murakami Y, Kawai H. Trehalase activity and trehalose content in a freeze-tolerant yeast, *Torulaspora delbrueckii*, and its freeze-sensitive mutant. Bioscience, Biotechnology, and Biochemistry. 1995;**59**(11):2143-2145

[43] Alves-Araujo C, Almeida MJ, Sousa MJ, Leao C. Freeze tolerance of the yeast *Torulaspora delbrueckii*: Cellular and biochemical basis. FEMS Microbiology Letters. 2004;**240**(1):7-14

[44] Hernandez-Lopez MJ, Panadero J, Prieto JA, Randez-Gil F. Regulation of salt tolerance by *Torulaspora delbrueckii* calcineurin target Crz1p. Eukaryotic Cell. 2006;**5**(3):469-479

[45] Märquez J, Serrano R. Multiple transduction pathways regulate the sodium-extrusion gene PMR2/ENA1 during salt stress in yeast. FEBS Letters. 1996;**382**(1):89-92

[46] Panadero J, Hernández-López MJ, Prieto JA, Randez-Gil F. Overexpression of the calcineurin target CRZ1 provides freeze tolerance and enhances the fermentative capacity of baker's yeast. Applied and Environmental Microbiology. 2007;**73**(15):4824-4831

[47] Cyert MS. Calcineurin signalling in *Saccharomyces cerevisiae*: How yeast go crazy in response to stress. Biochemical and Biophysical Research Communications. 2003;**311**(4):1143-1150

[48] Rodríguez-Peña JM, García R, Nombela C, Arroyo J. The high-osmolarity glycerol (HOG) and cell wall integrity (CWI) signalling pathways interplay: A yeast dialogue between MAPK routes. Yeast. 2010;**27**(8):495-502

[49] Westfall PJ, Patterson JC, Chen RE, Thorner J. Stress resistance and signal fidelity independent of nuclear MAPK function. Proceedings of the National Academy of Sciences. 2008;**105**(34):12212-12217

[50] García-Marqués S, Randez-Gil F, Prieto J. Nuclear versus cytosolic activity of the yeast Hog1 MAP kinase in response to osmotic and tunicamycin-induced ER stress. FEBS Letters. 2015;**589**(16):2163-2168

[51] Hernandez-Lopez MJ, Randez-Gil F, Prieto JA. Hog1 mitogen-activated protein kinase plays conserved and distinct roles in the osmotolerant yeast *Torulaspora delbrueckii*. Eukaryotic Cell. 2006;**5**(8):1410-1419

[52] Brandam C, Lai QP, Julien-Ortiz A, Taillandier P. Influence of oxygen on alcoholic fermentation by a wine strain of *Torulaspora delbrueckii*: Kinetics and carbon mass balance. Bioscience, Biotechnology, and Biochemistry. 2013;**77**(9):1848-1853

[53] Renault P, Miot-Sertier C, Marullo P, Hernández-Orte P, Lagarrigue L, Lonvaud-Funel A, et al. Genetic characterisation and phenotypic variability in *Torulaspora delbrueckii* species: Potential applications in the wine industry. International Journal of Food Microbiology. 2009;**134**(3):201-210

[54] Mas A, Torija MJ, MDC G-P, Troncoso AM. Acetic acid bacteria and the production and quality of wine vinegar. The Scientific World Journal. 2014;**2014**:6

[55] Ingledew WM. Effect of bacterial contaminants on beer. A review. Journal of the American Society of Brewing Chemists. 1979;**37**(3):145-150

[56] Kaur K, Singh N. Effect of acetic acid and cmc on rheological and baking properties of flour. Journal of Food Quality. 1999;**22**(3):317-327

[57] Semić A, Oručević S, Bauman I, Muminović Š, Spaho N, Klepo B. Effects of increasing sourness of bread dough on bread quality. In: Proceedings of the 5th International Congress Flour Bread, 7th Croatian Congress of Cereal Technologists. Osijek, Croatia: Josip Juraj Strossmayer University, Agriculture Faculty in Osijek; 21-23 October 2009

[58] Goold HD, Kroukamp H, Williams TC, Paulsen IT, Varela C, Pretorius IS. Yeast's balancing act between ethanol and glycerol production in low-alcohol wines. Microbial Biotechnology. 2017;**10**(2):264-278

[59] Sanz AB, García R, Rodríguez-Peña JM, Arroyo J. The CWI pathway: Regulation of the transcriptional adaptive response to cell wall stress in yeast. Journal of Fungi. 2018;**4**(1):1

[60] García R, Bravo E, Diez-Muñiz S, Nombela C, Rodríguez-Peña JM, Arroyo J. A novel connection between the cell wall integrity and the PKA pathways regulates cell wall stress response in yeast. Scientific Reports. 2017;7:5703

[61] Martín H, Rodríguez-Pachón JM, Ruiz C, Nombela C, Molina Ma. Regulatory mechanisms for modulation of signalling through the cell integrity Slt2-mediated pathway in *Saccharomyces cerevisiae*. Journal of Biological Chemistry 2000;**275**(2):1511-1519

[62] Ruiz A, Ariño J. Function and regulation of the *Saccharomyces cerevisiae* ENA sodium ATPase system. Eukaryotic Cell. 2007;**6**(12):2175-2183

[63] Ruiz A, Yenush L, Ariño J. Regulation of ENA1 Na(+)-ATPase gene expression by the Ppz1 protein phosphatase is mediated by the calcineurin pathway. Eukaryotic Cell. 2003;**2**(5):937-948

[64] Petruzzi L, Capozzi V, Berbegal C, Corbo MR, Bevilacqua A, Spano G, et al. Microbial resources and enological significance: Opportunities and benefits. Frontiers in Microbiology. 2017;**8**:995

[65] Hideaki H, Sato Y. inventors. *Torulaspora delbrueckii* h299-18 and production of frozen dough for bread using the same. Japan patent JP2579723B2; 1994

[66] Lino S, Takeuchi T, Yoshida O, inventors. Baker's yeast and frozen bread dough prepared by using the yeast. Japan patent JP3142941B2; 1992

[67] Toh DWK, Chua JY, Liu SQ. Impact of simultaneous fermentation with *Saccharomyces cerevisiae* and *Torulaspora delbrueckii* on volatile and non-volatile constituents in beer. LWT. 2018;**91**:26-33

[68] Kun-Farkas G, Rezessy-Szabó J, Zákány F, Hoschke A. Interaction of Saccharomyces and non Saccharomyces yeast strains in an alcoholic fermentation process. Acta Alimentaria-ACTA ALIMENT. 2005;**34**:81-90

[69] Holt S, Mukherjee V, Lievens B, Verstrepen KJ, Thevelein JM. Bioflavoring by non-conventional yeasts in sequential beer fermentations. Food Microbiology. 2018;**72**:55-66

[70] Wahyono A, Kang WW, Park HD. Characterisation and application of *Torulaspora delbrueckii* JK08 and *Pichia anomala* JKO4 as baker's yeasts. Journal of Food and Nutrition Research. 2015;**54**(3):205-217